# Adult Nursing
# at a Glance

This title is also available as an e-book.
For more details, please see
**www.wiley.com/buy/9781118474556**
or scan this QR code:

# Adult Nursing at a Glance

**Andrée le May**
Professor of Nursing
School of Health Sciences
University of Southampton

**Series Editor: Ian Peate**

WILEY Blackwell

This edition first published 2015 © 2015 by John Wiley & Sons, Ltd.

*Registered Office*
John Wiley & Sons, Ltd, The Atrium, Southern Gate, Chichester, West Sussex, PO19 8SQ, UK

*Editorial Offices*
9600 Garsington Road, Oxford, OX4 2DQ, UK
The Atrium, Southern Gate, Chichester, West Sussex, PO19 8SQ, UK
350 Main Street, Malden, MA 02148-5020, USA

For details of our global editorial offices, for customer services and for information about how to apply for permission to reuse the copyright material in this book please see our website at www.wiley.com/wiley-blackwell

*Library of Congress Cataloging-in-Publication Data*

Le May, Andrée, author.
  Adult nursing at a glance / Andrée le May.
    1 online resource.
  Includes bibliographical references and index.
  Description based on print version record and CIP data provided by publisher; resource not viewed.
  ISBN 978-1-118-47453-2 (Adobe PDF) – ISBN 978-1-118-47454-9 (ePub) –
ISBN 978-1-118-47455-6 (pbk.)
I. Title.
[DNLM:   1. Nursing Process.   2. Nursing.   WY 100.1]
  RT41
  610.73–dc23
                                        2014021564
A catalogue record for this book is available from the British Library.

Wiley also publishes its books in a variety of electronic formats. Some content that appears in print may not be available in electronic books.

Cover image: Intravenous infusion. LIFE IN VIEW/SCIENCE PHOTO LIBRARY

Cover design by Meaden Creative

Set in 9.5/11.5pt Minion by SPi Publisher Services, Pondicherry, India
Printed and bound in Singapore by Markono Print Media Pte Ltd

1   2015

# Contents

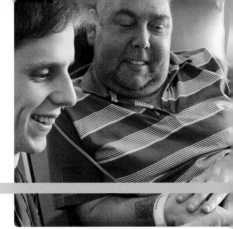

v

**Section 2**

# Nursing people with common disorders 44

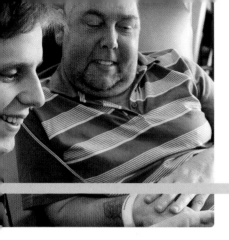

# About this book

Adult Nursing at a Glance brings together up-to-date evidence and essential knowledge from various sources (see Acknowledgements), blended with a lifetime's experience of nursing practice, research and teaching, in an easy-to-follow introductory or revision text for student nurses.

The essential components of excellent nursing are set out in Section 1, highlighting the skills that all students need to develop from the outset of their studies. Organisational and leadership skills, which are usually developed at a later stage in a student's journey, draw the book to a close in Section 3. The central section focuses on the systems of the body, applying the essential components of excellent nursing, set out in Section 1, to the care of people with the most common disorders of these systems.

## Section 1: Essentials of excellent nursing care

This section provides summaries of essential elements of nursing. It is built on the premise that excellent care is not just about what we do but also how we do it. Fundamental to excellent nursing is the merging of technically competent care with the maintenance and/or enhancement of the patient's (and their family's and carer's) dignity. Care that is technically competent but does not promote the patient's dignity is inadequate: care that promotes dignity but is not technically competent is also inadequate.

In this section you will find chapters focusing on:
- Safeguarding dignity
- Skilled appropriate communication
- Accurate assessment and monitoring
- Tailored symptom control and management
- Attentive risk assessment and management
- Tailored health education and promotion
- Thorough discharge planning
- Evaluation of the outcomes of care and care processes
- Research and service development.

These nine themes are central to excellent nursing. They are detailed in this section and each is linked to a 'symbolic character'. These characters are taken forward throughout Section 2 to draw attention to particular aspects of care that focus on, for example, health education and promotion or discharge planning related to the disorder covered. This approach is designed to appeal to those of you who are visual learners, as well as those who are non-visual learners, thereby making critical messages easy to remember. The dignity character appears as a watermark on every single right hand page in Section 2 to emphasise the crucial position of dignity within all aspects of nursing care.

## Section 2: Nursing people with common disorders

This Section's two-page summaries focus on common disorders. Illustrations of, for example, anatomy and physiology, pathology, or critical features of nursing care take up the left hand page: explanatory summarised text forms the right hand page. The symbolic characters introduced in Section 1 run throughout this section detailing the likely key elements of nursing for the disorders covered.

Each system in this section starts with a chapter presenting an overview of the system; this is followed by one focusing on signs, symptoms, assessment and emergencies. The subsequent chapters then outline only the most common disorders associated with that system. The book does not attempt to cover all the disorders that a nurse will encounter, but the principal conditions described will give a firm basis for you to consider how to manage other conditions – the details of which can be consulted elsewhere.

*You should use the checklists under 'Essentials of best practice' as prompts to explore further, using your experience and knowledge, what aspects of nursing care you might add for a person with each of the conditions concerned.*

## Section 3: Essential skills – leadership and organisational

Organisational aspects of care focus on:
- Leadership
- Management
- Managing people and difficult situations
- Research utilisation
- Time management
- Continuing professional development
- Practice development.

Nursing is not simply about providing excellent, up-to-date individualised care to people and their families and carers, but is also about creating the best environment within which to provide care. This section will enable you to understand how to help achieve that.

# Acknowledgements

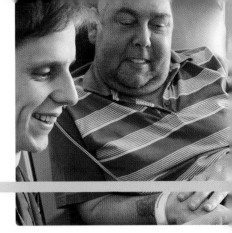

Information is synthesised from the following sources, with permission:

Aaronson PI, Ward JPT & Connolly MJ (2012) *The Cardiovascular System at a Glance*. Oxford, Wiley Blackwell.

Brooker C & Nicol M (2011) (Eds) *Alexander's Nursing Practice*. Edinburgh, Churchill Livingstone Elsevier.

Davey P (Ed) (2014) *Medicine at a Glance*, 4th edn. Oxford, Wiley Blackwell.

Dougherty L & Lister S (Eds) (2011) *The Royal Marsden Hospital Manual of Clinical Nursing Procedures. Student Edition*, 8th edn. Oxford, Wiley Blackwell.

Grace P & Borley N (Eds) (2009) *Surgery at a Glance*. Oxford, Wiley Blackwell.

Macintosh M & Moore T (Eds) (2011) *Caring for the Seriously Ill Patient*. London, Hodder Arnold.

O'Brien L (Ed) (2012) *District Nursing Manual of Clinical Procedures*. Oxford, Wiley Blackwell.

Peate I & Nair M (Eds) (2011) *Fundamentals of Anatomy and Physiology for Student Nurses*. Oxford, Wiley Blackwell.

www.patient.co.uk

Other more specific sources and websites are detailed in the text and in the References.

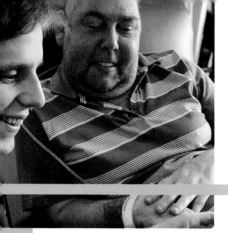

# How to use your revision guide

## Features contained within your revision guide

**The overview page** gives a summary of the topics covered in each part.

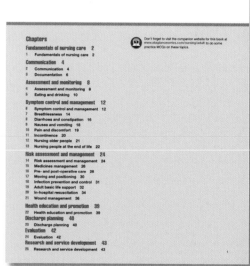

**Essentials of excellent nursing care**

**Section 1**

Don't forget to visit the companion website for this book at www.ataglanceseries.com/nursing/adult to do some practice MCQs on these topics.

**Each topic** is presented in a double-page spread with clear, easy-to-follow diagrams supported by succinct explanatory text.

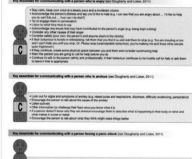

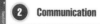

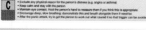

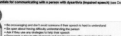

Nine central nursing themes are discussed in the book and these are represented by **symbolic characters** to highlight particular aspects of care.

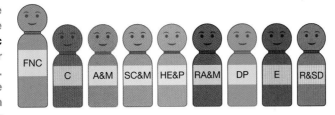

**FNC:** Fundamental nursing care
**C:** Communication with healthcare team, patient & family
**A&M:** Accurate assessments & regular monitoring
**SC&M:** Symptom control & management
**HE&P:** Health education & promotion
**RA&M:** Risk assessment & management
**DP:** Discharge planning
**E:** Evaluation
**R&SD:** Research & service development

The **dignity character (FNC)** appears as a watermark on every single right hand page in section 2 to emphasise the crucial position of dignity within all aspects of nursing care.

**Patient information** boxes list key resources that provide additional information.

**The website icon** indicates that you can find accompanying resources on the book's companion website.

---

**Patient information**

Useful information can be obtained from:
BAPEN at www.bapen.org.uk (the most up-to-date information about MUST can be downloaded from this website).

---

For consistency between paper and electronic versions of this book we use the words 'above' or 'below' in the text to direct you to illustrations.

# The anytime, anywhere textbook

## Wiley E-Text

Your book is also available to purchase as a **Wiley E-Text: Powered by VitalSource** version – a digital, interactive version of this book which you own as soon as you download it.

Your **Wiley E-Text** allows you to:

**Search:** Save time by finding terms and topics instantly in your book, your notes, even your whole library (once you've downloaded more textbooks)

**Note and Highlight:** Colour code, highlight and make digital notes right in the text so you can find them quickly and easily

**Organise:** Keep books, notes and class materials organised in folders inside the application

**Share:** Exchange notes and highlights with friends, classmates and study groups

**Upgrade:** Your textbook can be transferred when you need to change or upgrade computers

**Link:** Link directly from the page of your interactive textbook to all of the material contained on the companion website

The **Wiley E-Text** version will also allow you to copy and paste any photograph or illustration into assignments, presentations and your own notes.

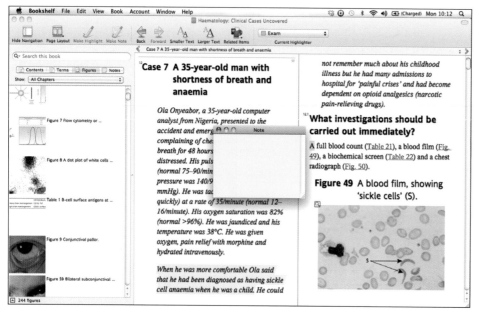

# Wiley E-Text
### Powered by VitalSource®

### *To access your Wiley E-Text:*

- Visit **www.vitalsource.com/software/bookshelf/downloads** to download the Bookshelf application to your computer, laptop, tablet or mobile device.

- Open the Bookshelf application on your computer and register for an account.

- Follow the registration process.

## CourseSmart

**CourseSmart** gives you instant access (via computer or mobile device) to this Wiley-Blackwell e-book and its extra electronic functionality, at 40% off the recommended retail print price. See all the benefits at: **www.coursesmart.com/students**

### *Instructors ... receive your own digital desk copies!*
**CourseSmart** also offers instructors an immediate, efficient, and environmentally-friendly way to review this book for your course.

For more information visit **www.coursesmart.com/instructors**.

With CourseSmart, you can create lecture notes quickly with copy and paste, and share pages and notes with your students. Access your **CourseSmart** digital book from your computer or mobile device instantly for evaluation, class preparation, and as a teaching tool in the classroom.

Simply sign in at **http://instructors.coursesmart.com/bookshelf** to download your Bookshelf and get started. To request your desk copy, hit 'Request Online Copy' on your search results or book product page.

We hope you enjoy using your new book. Good luck with your studies!

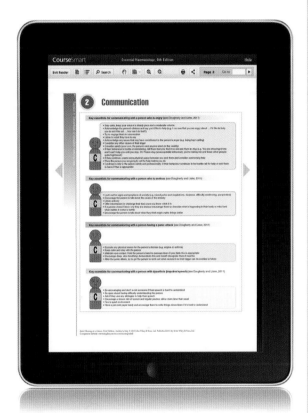

**Course**Smart
Learn Smart. Choose Smart.

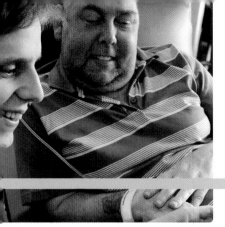

# About the companion website

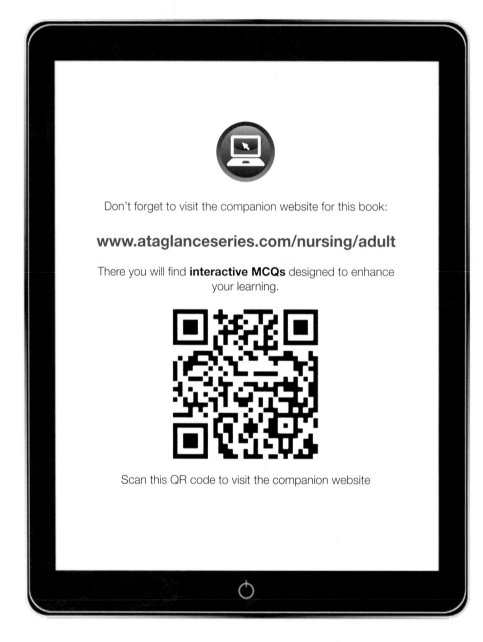

Don't forget to visit the companion website for this book:

## www.ataglanceseries.com/nursing/adult

There you will find **interactive MCQs** designed to enhance your learning.

Scan this QR code to visit the companion website

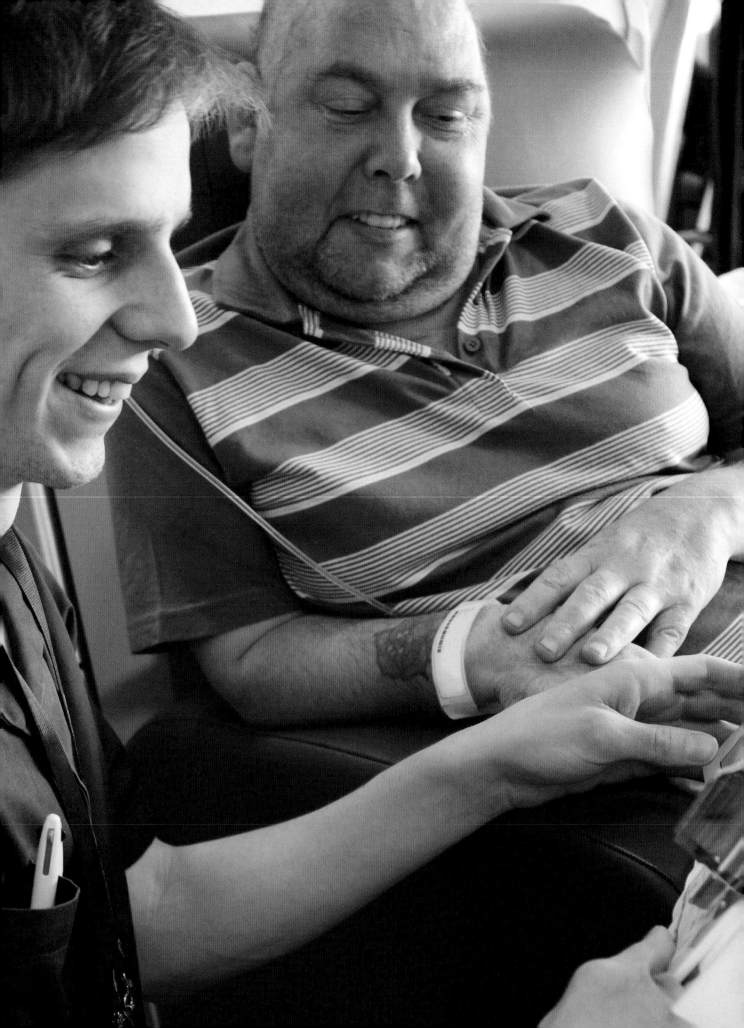

# Essentials of excellent nursing care

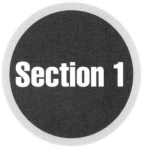

**Section 1**

## Chapters

Don't forget to visit the companion website for this book at www.ataglanceseries.com/nursing/adult to do some practice MCQs on these topics.

# 1 Fundamentals of nursing care

- Treat each person as an individual
- Listen to and respect their views
- Work with patients and their families/carers to identify their individual needs and decide, with them, what care is required to meet these needs (and ensure that it is carried out)
- Promote privacy
- Offer choice whenever possible
- Ensure patients and their families/carers know what is happening, what to expect and what their role in care entails
- Ensure people can voice satisfaction and dissatisfaction with care without fearing reprisal
- Question practice that you think is inappropriate

**FNC**

- Safeguarding dignity
- Skilled appropriate communication
- Accurate assessment and monitoring
- Tailored symptom control and management
- Attentive risk assessment and management
- Tailored health education and promotion
- Thorough discharge planning
- Evaluation of the outcomes of care and care processes
- Research and service development

*Adult Nursing at a Glance*, First Edition. Andrée le May. © 2015 John Wiley & Sons, Ltd. Published 2015 by John Wiley & Sons, Ltd.
Companion website: www.ataglanceseries.com/nursing/adult

# The fundamentals of nursing care

- Excellent care is about what we do **and** how we do it.
- Fundamental to excellent nursing is the merging of technically competent care with the maintenance and/or enhancement of the patient's (and their family's and carer's) dignity.
- Care that is technically competent but does not promote the patient's dignity is inadequate: care that promotes dignity but is not technically competent is also inadequate.
- Excellent nursing is therefore underpinned by the following:
  - safeguarding dignity;
  - skilled appropriate communication;
  - accurate assessment and monitoring;
  - tailored symptom control and management;
  - attentive risk assessment and management;
  - tailored health education and promotion;
  - thorough discharge planning;
  - evaluation of the outcomes of care and care processes;
  - research and service development.

# Maintaining the patient's dignity

- Dignity is often said to be hard to define. The available definitions tend to focus on either the professional view of dignity or the public's view. The challenge is to integrate them.
- Professional definitions of dignity are often abstract and are inclined to focus on the behaviours, values and attitudes that professionals need to have, for example 'Dignity is concerned with how people feel, think and behave in relation to the worth or value of themselves and others. To treat someone with dignity is to treat them as being of worth, in a way that is respectful of them as valued individuals' (RCN, 2008: www.rcn.org.uk).
- Public reports (e.g. Francis, 2013), however, suggest that patients and the public see dignity in more pragmatic terms focusing on whether or not certain important aspects of daily living can be completed whilst relying on others for assistance, for example being able to go to the toilet when needed, having privacy, being able to wash after using the toilet; having food and drink that can be consumed when needed and when wanted, being helped with eating and drinking if necessary; being listened to and having opinions respected.
- Integrating the professional and the public views of dignity is important to the provision of excellent care so that the patient and his/her family feel that they have experienced competent individualised care that allowed them to maintain their dignity.
- Dignity is maintained by:
  - What nurses do. (e.g.)
  Work with patients and their families/carers to identify their individual needs and decide, with them, what care is required to meet these needs.
  - How nurses do it. (e.g.)
  Treat each patient as an individual.
  Listen to and respect their views.
  Work in partnership with each patient and their family/carers.
  Offer choice wherever possible.
  Promote privacy.
  Ensure people can voice satisfaction *and* dissatisfaction with care without fearing reprisal.
  - When nurses do it. (e.g.)
  Identify with patients (and their family/carers) mutually convenient times for care whenever possible.
  Ensure that medications, designed to fit the patient's needs rather than the treatment plan are given on time (particularly night sedation).

The following pages detail the essentials of technically competent care which need to accompany the maintenance of the patient's (and their family's and carer's) dignity to ensure best practice.

# 2 Communication

## Key essentials for communicating with a person who is angry (see Dougherty and Lister, 2011)

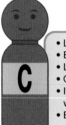

- Stay calm, keep your voice at a steady pace and a moderate volume
- Acknowledge the person's distress and say you'd like to help (e.g. I can see that you are angry about … I'd like to help you to sort this out … how can I do that?)
- Try to engage them in conversation
- Listen to what they have to say
- Acknowledge any issues that may have contributed to the person's anger (e.g. being kept waiting)
- Consider any other causes of their anger
- Consider safety (your own, the person's and anyone else's in the vicinity)
- If their behaviour is hostile or intimidating, tell them that you find it so and ask them to stop (e.g. You are shouting at me and I can't help you until you stop. Or: Please stop (unacceptable behaviour), you're making me and these other people quite frightened.)
- If they continue, create some physical space between you and them and consider summoning help
- Warn the person you are going to call for help before you do
- Continue to talk to the person calmly and professionally: if their behaviour continues to be hostile call for help or ask them to leave if that is appropriate

## Key essentials for communicating with a person who is anxious (see Dougherty and Lister, 2011)

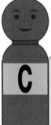

- Look out for signs and symptoms of anxiety (e.g. raised pulse and respirations, dizziness, difficulty swallowing, perspiration)
- Encourage the person to talk about the cause of the anxiety
- Listen actively
- Offer information (or challenge their fear) once you know what it is
- If a person doesn't know why they are anxious encourage them to describe what is happening in their body or mind and what makes it worse or better
- Encourage the person to talk about what they think might make things better

## Key essentials for communicating with a person having a panic attack (see Dougherty and Lister, 2011)

- Exclude any physical reason for the person's distress (e.g. angina or asthma)
- Keep calm and stay with the person
- Maintain eye contact. Hold the person's hand to reassure them if you think this is appropriate
- Encourage deep, slow breathing: demonstrate this and breath alongside them if need be
- After the panic attack, try to get the person to work out what caused it so that trigger can be avoided in future

## Key essentials for communicating with a person with dysarthria (impaired speech) (see Dougherty and Lister, 2011)

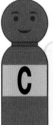

- Be encouraging and don't avoid someone if their speech is hard to understand
- Be open about having difficulty understanding the person
- Ask if they use any strategies to help their speech
- Encourage a slower rate of speech and regular pauses: allow more time than usual
- Find a quiet environment
- Have a pen and paper ready and encourage them to write things down/draw if it's hard to understand

# Communication

- Communication permeates everything that nurses do.
- Communication is the transfer of information between one person and another, and their reaction to it.
- Being able to communicate effectively with patients, their families/carers and colleagues is an essential feature of skilled nursing practice.
- Nurses can use skilled communication to enhance care.
- Communication includes a variety of different verbal and non-verbal cues and skills.
- Verbal communication comprises speech and language. This includes the way we use words, tones and inflections; the way we phrase what we say and the questions that we ask in order to communicate what we are thinking and feeling.
- Non-verbal communication comprises many things: touch, facial expressions, eye contact and the way we look at each other, gestures, body movements, posture and body positions, our use of space, the clothes we wear and our appearance and even the timing of communication.
- Non-verbal communication often supports verbal communication but it is a powerful way of communicating information on its own.
- Silence is also a powerful means of communication.
- Written communications are also important to
  - convey information between members of the multi-disciplinary team and other colleagues;
  - to help patients and their families/carers retain information about their illness and treatment.
- Communication is influenced by many things, for example culture, age, mood, emotion, uncertainty, stress, anxiety, knowledge and skills.
- The effectiveness of communication can be affected by age-related or disease-linked problems such as hearing loss, sight loss or alterations, speech alterations, emotions, mood, memory changes and cognitive impairment.
- Nurses should minimise age/disease related barriers to effective communication and also reduce organisational barriers such as lack of privacy, having insufficient time to clarify uncertainties or misunderstandings and communicating complicated information in noisy environments that make talking and hearing difficult.
- Altered mental capacity may mean that a patient is unable to communicate their wishes, understand information given to them or use it in decision making. Where altered mental capacity is suspected the person's capacity for decision making should be reviewed by the multi-disciplinary team.
- Effective communication is about using the right verbal and non-verbal skills for the person (or people) involved in each interaction (see above for tips on how to interact in difficult situations).

## Useful communication skills

- Establishing rapport.
- Active and empathic listening.
- Responding appropriately.

- Not being afraid to keep quiet (or to speak out).
- Using questions to find out more (particularly open questions).
- Using reinforcement (e.g. 'go on', nodding) to encourage communication.
- Using story-telling to find out more or engage people in conversation.
- Using touch appropriately, particularly expressive touch.
- Observing people's reactions and changing your communication style in response to them.
- Being non-judgemental and open.
- Showing respect and maintaining dignity through both actions and words.
- Remembering that the 'little things' (e.g. smiling and eye contact) are important.
- Evaluating how well your interactions with people go is important for either reinforcing effective skills or improving things for next time.

## Communicating with older people

Older people use healthcare more than others. Many have difficulties communicating which you will have to overcome. Here are some tips to help you:

- Make sure that spectacles, hearing aids and dentures are appropriate, clean, working and worn.
- Ensure lighting is glare free and shows your face.
- Make sure the patient knows you're there – stand or sit in the person's visual field, at the same level as they are, get their attention by saying their name and identifying yourself clearly at the start of the conversation; always say something when you are leaving.
- Make sure you have the person's attention before you speak – touch may be useful here or eye contact, but saying their name and that you are there may work just as well.
- Check that your mouth, gestures and facial expressions can be seen so that anyone who lip reads can do this easily.
- Don't shout; reduce background noise. Sometimes you might have to speak slightly more slowly and a little louder than usual.
- Pause between sentences and check that you've been understood.
- Leave enough time for communication – it's just as important as any other aspect of care.
- Keep calm and patient and allow enough time for responses. Don't be afraid of silence.
- Reinforce communication – use nods or say something so that the person knows you've listened to and understood them.
- Avoid child-like or patronising language.
- If you're writing information, make sure you use a large black felt pen and check that the size and style of your writing can be read.
- If any interaction becomes too heated leave and say that you'll come back later – and come back later!
- Check that any call bells or alarm systems can be reached before you leave.
- Encourage regular eye, hearing and dental checks.
- Refer if necessary to a speech and language therapist.

# **3** Documentation

## Principles of good record keeping (NMC, 2009: 5)

1. 'Handwriting should be legible.
2. All entries to records should be signed. In the case of written records, the person's name and job title should be printed alongside the first entry.
3. In line with local policy, you should put the date and time on all records. This should be in real time and chronological order, and be as close to the actual time as possible.
4. Your records should be accurate and recorded in such a way that the meaning is clear.
5. Records should be factual and not include unnecessary abbreviations, jargon, meaningless phrases or irrelevant speculation.
6. You should use your professional judgement to decide what is relevant and what should be recorded.
7. You should record details of any assessments and reviews undertaken, and provide clear evidence of the arrangements you have made for future and ongoing care. This should also include details of information given about care and treatment.
8. Records should identify any risks or problems that have arisen and show the action taken to deal with them.
9. You have a duty to communicate fully and effectively with your colleagues, ensuring that they have all the information they need about the people in your care.
10. You must not alter or destroy any records without being authorised to do so.
11. In the unlikely event that you need to alter your own or another healthcare professional's records, you must give your name and job title, and sign and date the original documentation. You should make sure that the alterations you make, and the original record, are clear and auditable.
12. Where appropriate, the person in your care, or their carer, should be involved in the record keeping process.
13. The language that you use should be easily understood by the people in your care.
14. Records should be readable when photocopied or scanned.
15. You should not use coded expressions of sarcasm or humorous abbreviations to describe the people in your care.
16. You should not falsify records.'

## Box 3   NMC Guidance on Record Keeping (2009: 3) states that good record keeping can:

- 'help to improve accountability
- show how decisions related to patient care were made
- support the delivery of services
- support effective clinical judgements and decisions
- support patient care and communications
- make continuity of care easier
- provide documentary evidence of services delivered
- promote better communication and sharing of information between members of the multi-professional healthcare team
- help to identify risks, and enable early detection of complications
- support clinical audit, research, allocation of resources and performance planning
- help to address complaints or legal processes.'

Source: www.nmc-uk.org/Documents/NMC-Publications/NMC-Record-Keeping-Guidance.pdf

*Adult Nursing at a Glance*, First Edition. Andrée le May. © 2015 John Wiley & Sons, Ltd. Published 2015 by John Wiley & Sons, Ltd.
Companion website: www.ataglanceseries.com/nursing/adult

# Documentation

- Accurate documentation promotes continuity of care.
- Clearly, succinctly and accurately recording care given, or to be given, is a vital part of communication within the health care team and between services.
- Care and observations of a patient's condition are recorded through a variety of paper and/or electronic means including:
  - patient records (e.g. including nursing assessments);
  - care plans;
  - medication charts;
  - observational charts (e.g. vital signs, fluid balance, Glasgow Coma Scale, pain scales);
  - printouts from monitors (e.g. ECGs);
  - risk assessment charts (e.g. early warning scores, pressure ulcer risk assessment);
  - letters/emails/text messages;
  - photographs (e.g. of wounds).
- Written information is an indispensable way of recording care.
- Written information should be presented so that it can be understood by the intended reader. Handwriting should be clear and information should be presented without using ambiguous terms or abbreviations.
- Professional and statutory bodies lay down guidance for record keeping ensuring consistency across the branches/specialties of nursing (above).
- Whilst record keeping is an essential part of care, all necessary steps should be taken not to allow it to drive patient care or to intrude excessively into the time devoted to patient contact.

# 4 Assessment and monitoring

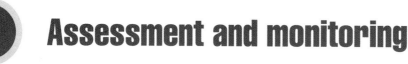

More detail about system assessment is provided in Section 2

## Temperature – key features (see Dougherty and Lister, 2011)

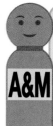

- **Balance** between heat production and heat loss
- **Core body temperature** is normally between 36–37.5°C. Temperature above or below this range affects body function
- **Temperature varies** with time of day – diurnal variation (higher in evening than morning) and location (cooler further from core)
- **Temperature can be taken** with a glass thermometer orally, rectally, axillary or in the ear using a tympanic membrane thermometer

## Cardiovascular system – key features to assess (see Dougherty and Lister, 2011)

- **Pulse** – count rate (normal range 55–90/min); feel rhythm (normally regular sequence) and amplitude (strength) for 60 seconds
- **Apical beat** – listen with stethoscope: compare rate with radial pulse in patients with atrial fibrillation
- **Blood pressure (BP)** – normal range 110–140 mmHg systolic/ 70—90 mmHg diastolic. Taken electronically or manually
- **Electrocardiogram (ECG)** – shows electrical activity of heart: 12 lead usually in hospital: ambulatory in community
- **Pulse oximetry** – electronic probe positioned on end of finger – gives pulse rate and oxygen saturation (normal 95–100%)
- **Skin colour and condition** (e.g. flushed, pallor, cyanosis: dry, cold, warm, sweaty, clammy)

## Respiratory system – key features to assess (see Dougherty and Lister, 2011)

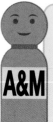

- **Breathing** – measure rate (normal range 12–18 breaths/min: <8 + >27 emergency: >24 regular monitoring), rhythm (steady – expiration usually lasts twice as long as inspiration) and depth (shallow, gasping, deep). Chest expansion – normally each side equal
- **Skin colour** – cyanosis (blue tone to skin and mucous membranes – usually seen if oxygen saturation 85–90%)
- **Oxygen saturation** using pulse oximetry (normal 95–100%: lower but still normal in patients with chronic respiratory conditions)
- **Accessory muscle use** in respiratory distress (abdominal, sternomastoid and scalene) to increase respiration
- **Respiratory distress** considered if sentence cannot be completed in one breath. Level of consciousness may be compromised
- **Lung function assessments** can be made through measurement of, for example, peak expiratory flow (PEF), forced vital capacity (FVC)
- **Sputum production** – colour, frothiness, amount, ease of expectoration, blood

## Neurological system – key features to assess (see Dougherty and Lister, 2011)

- **Level of consciousness** – arousability and awareness. Alterations can be slight to severe. Measure using Glasgow Coma Scale
- **Pupillary activity** – examine size (pinpoint, small, mid-sized), reactiveness to light ((un)reactive), equal/unequal size and reactions
- **Motor function** – muscle strength, tone, coordination, reflexes (e.g. blink, gag and swallow), abnormal movements (e.g. seizures)
- **Sensory function** – vision (central and peripheral), hearing and understanding, sensations (superficial light touch and deep pain)
- **Vital signs** – temperature, respiration, pulse and blood pressure

## Fluid intake and output – key features

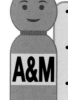

- **Intake and output** are normally balanced (fluid balance). Monitor for signs of fluid overload or dehydration
- **Intake includes** oral intake from food and drinks (~2 litres), all parenteral/intravenous fluids and any enteral intake
- **Output includes** urine, faeces (~100 ml/day), perspiration (~200 ml/day), gastric secretions and drains

## Box 4 Useful examples of measurement scales to help with assessment and monitoring

Nutrition: Malnutrition Universal Screening Tool (MUST)
Pressure ulcer risk: Waterlow Scale
Pain: Visual/Verbal/Numeric Analogue Scales: Pain Strategies Questionnaire (PSQ): body maps
Anxiety: Hospital Anxiety and Depression (HAD) Scale
Depression: HAD Scale
Memory loss: Mini Mental State Examination (MMSE)
Deteriorating condition: Modified Early Warning System (MEWS)

*Adult Nursing at a Glance*, First Edition. Andrée le May. © 2015 John Wiley & Sons, Ltd. Published 2015 by John Wiley & Sons, Ltd.
Companion website: www.ataglanceseries.com/nursing/adult

## Assessment and monitoring

- Assessment is the systematic collection of key information to inform care. Monitoring is the regular updating of this information.
- Assessment and monitoring are iterative processes.
- Accurate assessment and ongoing monitoring of a patient's physical and mental health is critical to the provision of effective, safe and timely care and the plotting of progress/deterioration.
- Assessment and monitoring of the patient's relatives' responses to the illness/condition and its consequences also needs to be made.
- All nurses, regardless of the healthcare setting they work in, undertake various types of assessment and monitoring.
- Skilled assessment is linked to the ability to prioritise care that needs to be done urgently and care that can wait.
- Successful assessment and monitoring involves nurses merging hard data (e.g. from measurement equipment and assessment scales) with soft data (e.g. from talking, watching and listening to patients, their families and their healthcare team members) to form a complete picture of the patient's condition and their response(s) to it and to nursing care and treatments.
- Assessments can range from the comprehensive (e.g. covering physical, psychological, social, emotional, spiritual and cultural dimensions) to the specific (e.g. taking a temperature or monitoring wound healing).
- Making a comprehensive nursing assessment should be done in partnership with the patient and their family/carers and underpins the delivery of the fundamentals of nursing care (Chapter 1).
- Comprehensive assessments may not always be possible or appropriate, for example in the emergency department where a patient's needs are prioritised through triage or in the GP practice where a patient is attending for one particular activity (e.g. suture removal).
- All nursing assessments should inform and be informed by those made by other healthcare workers.
- The specific assessment and monitoring of elements of a patient's health can help in the early detection of general health problems (e.g. hypertension), in establishing the effectiveness of treatments (e.g. in type 1 diabetes), in determining the progression of an acute illness (e.g. an infection) or a long-term condition (e.g. multiple sclerosis), the impact of a one type of illness on another (e.g. acute respiratory infection on asthma) and the generation of an illness because of another (e.g. depression resulting from COPD).
- Accurate baseline assessments are essential if improvement or deterioration of a patient's health is to be swiftly identified and managed appropriately through ongoing monitoring.
- The results of assessment and monitoring need to be accurately recorded in a patient's care plan or notes.
- Initial assessments and deviations from the expected course of a patient's condition need to be effectively communicated to relevant healthcare team members.
- Following an initial nursing assessment the majority of ongoing monitoring is likely to focus on four key areas:
  - the patient's physical health and present condition set against the treatment plan;
  - the patient's mental health and present condition set against the treatment plan;
  - any special requirements the patient has;
  - the patient's and the carer's requirements for social support.

## Physical health

The most frequent assessments made by nurses are associated with assessing a patient's physical health through recording how various body systems function. Recording 'vital signs' includes assessments of temperature control, the cardiovascular system and the respiratory system. Other common assessments focus on the neurological system, nutritional status, fluid intake and output, urinalysis, deteriorating physical condition, pain, pressure ulcer risk, faecal elimination and functional independence. Some assessments of physical health are guided by measurement scales (above) and nursing models. Others will rely on observation, auscultation, touch/feeling combined with recordings made by appropriate equipment.

## Mental health

People with acute physical illnesses and long-term conditions may also have mental health needs. It is important that nurses can recognise *both* physical and mental health conditions. Most commonly nurses need to be able to recognise when a patient (or their carer) is anxious, depressed, confused or disorientated and know how to seek specialist advice. There are a variety of pre-determined questions and scales (above) that can be used to help make initial assessments but it's important to remember that much can be learnt from talking with someone and observing their general demeanour.

People with mental health problems also have physical illnesses requiring care from non-mental health specialists: in these instances planning and providing individualised, appropriate care will require close liaison between the mental health and acute/community/ primary care teams.

## Special requirements

Sometimes assessments are undertaken to determine a patient's requirements for particular equipment (e.g. pressure relieving equipment) or aides for daily living (e.g. special cutlery/crockery). These assessments are frequently made with a specialist nurse or allied healthcare professional and closely linked to the patient's carers' abilities too. The use and suitability of any equipment should be regularly monitored and adjusted to suit changing needs.

## Requirements for social support

Social support is a term which can mean different things – here it is used to focus attention on two interlinked aspects of care:
1 the patient's needs for and opportunities for company and interaction in order to minimise social isolation;
2 the practical support a patient needs to live at home.
Assessing someone's level of social support and resultant needs may seem intrusive and will need to be sensitively handled. In hospital this assessment may begin close to admission and continue throughout a patient's stay in preparation for timely discharge. In the community, for a patient requiring nursing longer, these requirements may change over time. Ensuring the best fit between a patient's requirements and what is provided is reliant on the multi-disciplinary team working together in partnership with the patient and family. Providing appropriate social support may necessitate liaison across health, social and third sector organisations.

# 5 Eating and drinking

**Nutritional assessment includes:**
- **Asking patients/families/carers about nutritional needs** (identify allergies or intolerances and dislikes and preferences)
- **Routinely recording (and dating) patient's weight and height** on admission to hospital if possible
- **Assessing patients using validated scales if signs of malnourishment** (e.g. MUST): refer to dietician
- **Observing the patient's appearance** (e.g. pallor, skin tone, oedema)
- **Assessing a patient's requirements for help with eating and drinking** – discuss with appropriate therapist
- **Regularly monitoring food and fluid intake and discussing this with the patient, their family/carers and your colleagues**
  - **Checking food intake** (and also output – constipations/diarrhoea)
  - **Checking fluid intake and output**
    - **Intake and output** are normally balanced (fluid balance). Monitor for signs of fluid overload or dehydration
    - **Intake includes** oral intake from food and drinks (~2 l), all parenteral/intravenous fluids and any enteral intake
    - **Output includes** urine, faeces (~100 ml/day), perspiration (~200 ml/day), gastric secretions and drains

## Box 5   Useful ways to assess and monitor nutritional status

**Malnutrition Universal Screening Tool** (MUST) (BAPEN, 2003)
This scale is a five step screening tool. It identifies adults who are malnourished, at risk of malnutrition or are obese. MUST combines the results of BMI measurement, unplanned weight loss and acute disease scores to obtain an overall malnutrition risk score (0 – 2+). This score can then be used, with its integral management guidelines, to develop the best plan of care with the patient and/or their carers.

**Body Mass Index** (BMI)
Tables showing BMI shade in weights which are indicative of obesity, being overweight or underweight as well as a healthy weight.

**Food diary**
Useful way to track what is eaten and drunk over a period of time (e.g. 5 days). Templates available on the internet. Food diaries are the most used in primary care.

**To evaluate how much importance you and your colleagues put on nutritional needs ask yourself these questions**
(based on Bond, 1997: 11-12)

1. What do you do to ensure that patients are well fed?
2. How much time do you spend on nutrition related activities?
3. Do you really know what happens at meal times?

*Adult Nursing at a Glance*, First Edition. Andrée le May. © 2015 John Wiley & Sons, Ltd. Published 2015 by John Wiley & Sons, Ltd.
Companion website: www.ataglanceseries.com/nursing/adult

# Eating and drinking

- The body requires particular nutrients to stay healthy (proteins, fats, carbohydrates, vitamins, minerals and fluid).
- Eating and drinking the right things are important in maintaining health and aiding recovery from illnesses, surgery or accidents.
- In ill health or following surgery the body may require extra nutrients for repair.
- Imbalances of nutrients can alter the body's homeostasis.
- Malnutrition is any imbalance between the person's nutritional needs and their diet.
- Malnutrition can be assessed using the Malnutrition Universal Screening Tool (MUST) (above).
- Eating and drinking difficulties can occur because of:
  - nausea and/or vomiting;
  - a sore mouth or ill-fitting dentures;
  - difficulty swallowing;
  - difficulty using equipment, for example cutlery following paralysis, or severe dementia;
  - anorexia;
  - early satiety;
  - allergies or intolerances;
  - particular diseases (e.g. diabetes).
- Nurses, alongside dieticians, catering staff, occupational therapists, physiotherapists, speech and language therapists and healthcare assistants have an important role to play in making sure that patients consume an appropriate diet whilst in hospital.
- Consuming an appropriate diet is not just about eating and drinking the right things, it is also about the functional ability to eat and drink (e.g. having sufficient dexterity to open food packaging, having dentures that fit and are in place, being able to reach drinks or meals that are left at the bedside, having the right adapted cutlery/plates/mats or being able to swallow).
- Nurses need to assess if a patient has consumed an appropriate amount of food and drink each day. This will involve finding out if food is left uneaten, why this happened and making appropriate changes (e.g. see above).
- Practice nurses, health visitors, GPs and dieticians also have a valuable role to play in advising people about lifestyle changes that affect their eating and drinking habits.
- Nutrition screening will include:
  - asking about usual diet (food **and** drink);
  - asking about food preferences/allergies;
  - asking about normal food habits (e.g. does the patient usually eat breakfast? Which meal is the largest during the day? Are sandwiches eaten for supper?);
  - discussing feeding difficulties (e.g. using special cutlery, ill-fitting dentures, sore mouth);
  - checking weight, height and Body Mass Index (BMI) on admission and weight at specified intervals during hospital stay if appropriate;
  - checking BMI in primary care to determine the need for life style changes in relation to weight gain or loss;
  - observing the patient (e.g. pallor, skin tone, under/overweight, oedema, mood);
  - noting results from blood tests (e.g. for anaemia);
  - evaluating nutritional intake (e.g. are meals left unfinished? Is there a mismatch between fluid intake and output? Does the person feel hungry after eating?).
- Some people will require nutritional support e.g. oral supplements/ sip feeds (high calories, high protein or high vitamin) or feeding using special preparations put directly into the gastro-intestinal tract via a naso-gastric (NG) tube or a percutaneous endoscopic gastrostomy (PEG) or intravenously using total parenteral nutrition (TPN).
- Some people will have special dietary requirements, for example people with coeliac disease require a gluten free diet, people with constipation may require a high fibre diet, people with heart failure or cirrhosis of the liver may have a low salt diet to help, alongside diuretics, control oedema.
- Poor wound healing may be linked to malnutrition, for example vitamin C deficiency.
- Eating and drinking are social activities and being isolated in doing these may increase feelings of social isolation in some groups of people (e.g. older people eating by themselves in their rooms in residential or nursing homes).

## Patient information

Useful information can be obtained from:
BAPEN at www.bapen.org.uk (the most up-to-date information about MUST can be downloaded from this website).

# 6 Symptom control and management

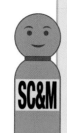

Common symptoms requiring consideration are:
- Pain and discomfort
- Anxiety, fear and uncertainty
- Nausea
- Vomiting
- Breathlessness
- Constipation
- Diarrhoea
- Incontinence of either urine or faeces (or both)
- Pyrexia
- Tiredness
- Dizziness

# Symptom control and management

- Symptoms are aspects of an illness that are noticed by a patient (e.g. pain, nausea, vomiting, breathlessness, diarrhoea, constipation, incontinence, tiredness, anxiety, fear and discomfort): signs are aspects that are noticed by other people (e.g. pallor, cyanosis, clamminess, wakefulness and rapid breathing).
- Patients may require help to control and manage both symptoms and signs.
- Working with each patient, their family/carer and the multi-disciplinary team to alleviate a person's symptoms and signs is a central component of nursing care.
- Patients may have several signs and symptoms that cause them discomfort and concern. Nurses need to be able to identify these and work out, with others, the best way(s) to alleviate them.
- Patients most commonly need help with:
  - alleviating or controlling pain;
  - reducing discomfort related to specific procedures;
  - managing fear, uncertainty and anxiety;
  - alleviating nausea (and vomiting);
  - minimising breathlessness;
  - improving diarrhoea and constipation;
  - managing continence;
  - minimising tiredness.
- Patients often know what will help them best, so asking them (or their family/carers) should be your first action.
- Techniques used to control signs and symptoms may be pharmacological or non-pharmacological (e.g. for pain several techniques may be used, analgesic drugs, deep breathing, guided imagery or simply talking to someone about their pain and concerns).
- The severity of some symptoms can be measured using rating or visual analogue scales, for example for pain and anxiety.
- Measuring signs and symptoms allows comparisons to be made between baseline and subsequent measurements so the effectiveness (or not) of any intervention can be judged.
- The details of how a patient's signs and symptoms are to be alleviated should be recorded in their care plan or nursing notes and regularly reviewed and updated in conjunction with others in the multi-disciplinary team.
- The following pages detail the essentials of symptom control and management for:
  - breathlessness;
  - diarrhoea;
  - constipation;
  - nausea;
  - vomiting;
  - pain and discomfort;
  - incontinence.
- Some groups of people have particular requirements related to the stage of their life that they are at, for example older people and people nearing or at the end of their lives. Particular attention is focused on these two groups of people in Chapters 12 and 13.

# 7 Breathlessness

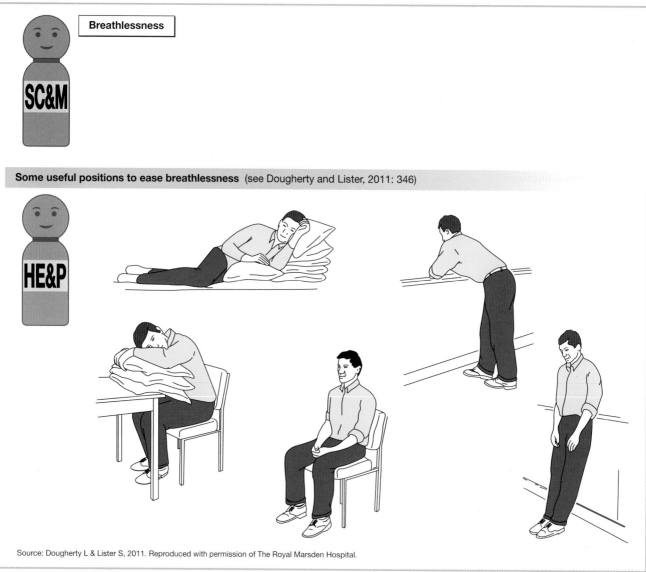

**Breathlessness**

SC&M

**Some useful positions to ease breathlessness** (see Dougherty and Lister, 2011: 346)

HE&P

Source: Dougherty L & Lister S, 2011. Reproduced with permission of The Royal Marsden Hospital.

# SC&M breathlessness

• Breathlessness (dyspnoea) is a very frightening and debilitating symptom. It can be acute or chronic.

• Acute and chronic breathlessness are largely attributed to cardiac and/or pulmonary causes.

• Acute breathlessness may also be caused by e.g. pain, diabetic ketoacidosis, drug overdoses (e.g. aspirin), trauma, altitude sickness.

• Chronic breathlessness may also be caused by severe anaemia, anxiety, thromboembolic disease, obesity and thyroid disease.

• Breathlessness can be assessed using the MRC Dyspnoea Scale (Chapter 37).

• Hyperventilation is sometimes known as behavioural breathlessness. The management of hyperventilation is different to the management of breathlessness described below and involves careful explanation of the situation, use of a calm manner to relieve anxiety, rebreathing using a paper bag or cupped hands if hyperventilation has been confirmed. Relaxation techniques can be helpful.

# Essentials of best practice

• Find out more about the current episode of breathlessness. Ask about any triggers and if anything in particular relieves breathlessness – this is particularly important in chronic breathlessness.

• Assess the general level of distress that the breathlessness is causing: colour of skin, cyanosis, pallor, clamminess, respiratory rate and quality, pulse (Chapter 37).

• Call for medical advice if a new acute episode or worsening of the patient's condition.

• Note the time when you became aware of the patient's condition.

• Reassure the patient and tell them what you are planning to do. Keep calm and explain simply and clearly what is happening and what you would like them to do. Enabling the patient and family/ carers to feel confident in you will be supportive and should reduce their feelings of anxiety.

• If the patient is prescribed oxygen or drugs to reduce breathlessness, make sure these are given immediately you become aware of the symptoms. Evaluate the success (or not) of these interventions and report this to a senior colleague or doctor.

• If appropriate loosen any restricting clothing that the patient is wearing.

• Ask the patient to sit in a more upright position (this may require your assistance and re-positioning the pillows and backrest). Sometimes leaning slightly forward is useful too (above) using a table/bed table as a support.

• Consider using controlled breathing techniques: ask the patient to focus on their breathing to make it slower and deeper. Ask them to relax their shoulders and upper chest. This should reduce fast, ineffective, shallow breathing. Sometimes patients will be able to do this more effectively if you also do the same thing, for example sitting at their level, talking them through each action and doing it so that they can concentrate on mirroring your behaviour.

• If breathlessness continues once an acute episode has subsided, adapt activities of daily living to suit the patient. Discuss this with other colleagues (e.g. occupational therapist, physiotherapist, specialist respiratory nurse) and the patient's family and carers.

• Discuss lifestyle modifications at an appropriate time (e.g. exercise, smoking cessation, weight and diet).

**8** # Diarrhoea and constipation

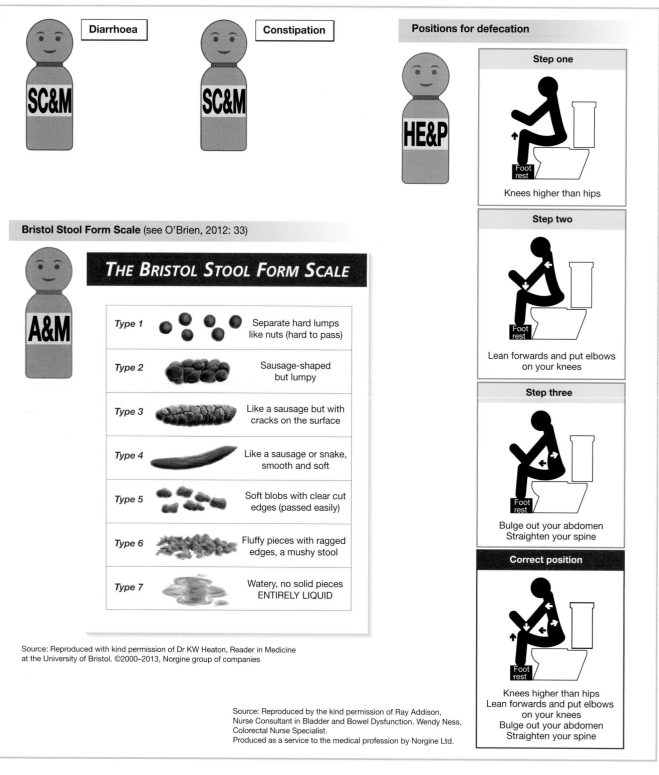

**Diarrhoea** — SC&M

**Constipation** — SC&M

**Positions for defecation** — HE&P

### Step one
Knees higher than hips

### Step two
Lean forwards and put elbows on your knees

### Step three
Bulge out your abdomen
Straighten your spine

### Correct position
Knees higher than hips
Lean forwards and put elbows on your knees
Bulge out your abdomen
Straighten your spine

**Bristol Stool Form Scale** (see O'Brien, 2012: 33) — A&M

## THE BRISTOL STOOL FORM SCALE

| Type 1 | Separate hard lumps like nuts (hard to pass) |
| Type 2 | Sausage-shaped but lumpy |
| Type 3 | Like a sausage but with cracks on the surface |
| Type 4 | Like a sausage or snake, smooth and soft |
| Type 5 | Soft blobs with clear cut edges (passed easily) |
| Type 6 | Fluffy pieces with ragged edges, a mushy stool |
| Type 7 | Watery, no solid pieces ENTIRELY LIQUID |

Source: Reproduced with kind permission of Dr KW Heaton, Reader in Medicine at the University of Bristol. ©2000–2013, Norgine group of companies

Source: Reproduced by the kind permission of Ray Addison, Nurse Consultant in Bladder and Bowel Dysfunction. Wendy Ness, Colorectal Nurse Specialist.
Produced as a service to the medical profession by Norgine Ltd.

# SC&M diarrhoea and constipation

• Diarrhoea and constipation are alterations to normal bowel patterns.
• Diarrhoea is characterised by frequently passing loose/ watery stools (above).
• Constipation is characterised by infrequently passing hard, difficult to pass stools. These stools may be small or large (above).
• Both diarrhoea and constipation can be accompanied by abdominal pain, bloating and flatulence.
• Diarrhoea is commonly caused by diet (e.g. excess ingestion of bran/fibre supplements, allergies and food intolerances), infections, medications (e.g. antibiotics, antihypertensive drugs), bowel diseases (irritable bowel syndrome, inflammatory bowel disease) and anxiety.
• Constipation is commonly caused by diet (e.g. insufficient fibre and dehydration), lack of exercise and immobility, metabolic disorders (e.g. diabetes mellitus, uraemia), obstruction (e.g. megacolon, cancer, anal fissures), neuropathies (e.g. Parkinson's disease, multiple sclerosis), bowel disease (e.g. irritable bowel syndrome) and depression.
• Diarrhoea and constipation can be acute or chronic.
• Diarrhoea can accompany constipation and often manifests as faecal incontinence. In this case more fluid stool passes around the obstruction caused by the impacted stool.

# Essentials of best practice: constipation

• Find out about the current episode of constipation and whether or not constipation is a common feature in the patient's life.
• Ask about any possible triggers and ways of relieving constipation that the patient might have used.
• Constipation can often be relieved by reviewing and altering drug regimes, diet and exercise.
• Increasing physical exercise increases peristalsis and may reduce constipation.

• Dietary alteration centres on increasing the amount of fibre in the diet and reducing refined products.
• Dehydration may be linked to constipation so increasing the amount of fluids consumed in a day may help (around ~2 l is the usual daily intake).
• Introducing more time for defecation during the day may be useful – many people simply do not allow enough time or ignore the urge to defecate.
• Thinking more about the position used for defecating might be helpful. Crouching is the best position so to mimic this sitting on the toilet with knees raised slightly by using a footstool may be helpful (opposite).
• Laxatives may be suggested, starting with the lowest dose. Once constipation resolves then laxatives should be stopped.
• Sometimes enemas/suppositories are needed to manage chronic constipation. These should be administered in line with the manufacturers' recommendations and local policy.

# Essentials of best practice: diarrhoea

• Find out more about the current episode of diarrhoea.
• Ask about any possible triggers and ways of relieving diarrhoea that the patient might have used.
• If in hospital, try to make sure the patient is close to a toilet or has a commode within the bed space. Make sure curtains are easily closable and can be securely fastened.
• Acute diarrhoea is often mild and self-limiting and care is given in the community. Advice should be given about hydration (Chapter 44), when to consult a doctor (Chapter 44) and the use of antidiarrhoeal over-the-counter drugs (e.g. loperamide) and/or rehydration medication (e.g. dioralyte).
• If infective diarrhoea is suspected, advice about infection control and hand washing should be given.
• Chronic diarrhoea needs to be managed in relation to the underlying cause. Some antidiarrhoeal drugs may be prescribed.
• Discuss lifestyle modifications if appropriate.

---

**Essentials of stoma care (colostomy and ileostomy)** (based on Dougherty and Lister, 2011)

• The patient is likely to be anxious and uncertain about what to expect: explanations should be simple and realistic without being frightening. They will need to be tailored to the patient's cognitive and emotional level. Leave enough time for questioning and reassurance. Remember that a patient may want to discuss how the stoma will affect their everyday life, for example their body image, relationship with others including sexual relationships, how to manage their stoma in public places
• A stoma specialist nurse should be consulted and visit the patient prior to (if possible) surgery. They will site the stoma
• Pre-operative information given should be consistent with the information from the stoma specialist. You should ensure the patient knows the sort of stoma to be formed (e.g. colostomy/ileostomy), whether it is permanent or temporary and its likely position. Discussing these things also allows you to talk about the likely consistency of faeces (e.g. a colostomy using the sigmoid colon will produce formed stool, looser more liquid stool will come from an ileostomy formed from the ileum because water has not yet been absorbed at this point in the intestine) and the frequency with which the stoma may work. If you are in any doubt about these things ask the stoma specialist or a senior colleague
• Patients may be worried about leakage from the stoma bag. Information about the type of appliance, the way it is held in place, its sturdiness, and whether it is a fixed or drainable appliance will help. Showing the patient pre-operatively what the appliance looks and feels like, how it is secured, emptied and changed may allay some fears. Encouraging a patient to manage their stoma as soon as possible after its formation is a good way to build confidence. Remember to talk about odour prevention since this is important but may be embarrassing for a patient to raise themselves
• The stoma and surrounding skin can be cleaned with mild soap and water: make sure it is dried thoroughly but gently before the appliance is reapplied. Techniques for appliance changing and emptying will differ between manufacturers
• Preparation for discharge from hospital involves making sure that the patient is able to care for their stoma, has enough supplies, has the contact details of community stoma specialists and an appointment to see their GP for a prescription for more supplies
• Continuity of care between the hospital and primary care teams is crucial
• Helping patients to manage colostomies and ileostomies is also an important part of a nurse's job (above)

# 9 Nausea and vomiting

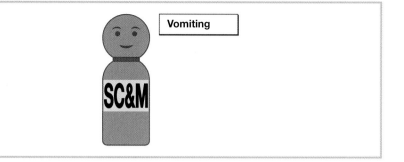

## SC&M nausea and vomiting

• Nausea and vomiting are very distressing and debilitating symptoms.
• Nausea may be experienced on its own or be accompanied by vomiting.
• The key to managing these two symptoms is to work out what is causing them. This involves communication with the multidisciplinary team, the patient and their family/carers in order to identify triggers.
• Nausea and vomiting may be caused by constipation, drugs, infection, dyspepsia, pain and anxiety. Vomiting might also be caused by raised intracranial pressure, tumours, blockages in the GI tract, uraemia.

## Essentials of best practice

• Ask about the current episode of nausea and/or vomiting and find out if anything has triggered it (or might trigger future episodes, e.g. particular smells or foods). Avoiding triggers is important although often difficult to achieve in a hospital ward.

• Treatment for vomiting may include the patient being nil by mouth to rest the gut and relieve symptoms. If this is the case an intravenous infusion will be sited and fluid balance monitoring will be essential.
• Always record vomiting and try to estimate the amount of vomit. Note also characteristics, for example the presence of bile and blood, and record. Report these immediately if present.
• If the patient is not nil by mouth make sure that something to drink is within reach and that the type of drink won't trigger feelings of nausea or vomiting.
• Make sure that a covered vomit bowl is easily reachable and so too is the call bell.
• Consider using anti-emetics and discuss this with the patient and the doctor. Review success or not of anti-emetics and give regularly as prescribed.
• If nausea is associated with pain or anxiety, ensure that these symptoms are addressed.
• If infection is suspected, use infection control procedures and advise the patient's family/carers about these.

*Adult Nursing at a Glance*, First Edition. Andrée le May. © 2015 John Wiley & Sons, Ltd. Published 2015 by John Wiley & Sons, Ltd.
Companion website: www.ataglanceseries.com/nursing/adult

# 10 Pain and discomfort

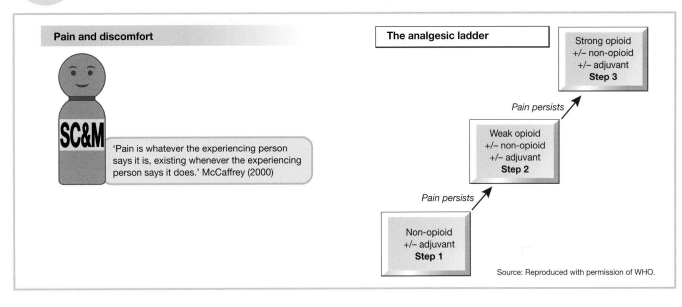

**Pain and discomfort**

SC&M

'Pain is whatever the experiencing person says it is, existing whenever the experiencing person says it does.' McCaffrey (2000)

**The analgesic ladder**

Strong opioid
+/– non-opioid
+/– adjuvant
**Step 3**

*Pain persists*

Weak opioid
+/– non-opioid
+/– adjuvant
**Step 2**

*Pain persists*

Non-opioid
+/– adjuvant
**Step 1**

Source: Reproduced with permission of WHO.

## SC&M pain and discomfort

- Pain and discomfort are distressing and debilitating symptoms.
- Pain is an individual experience (see McCaffrey's definition above).
- Pain has physical, emotional and sociocultural components.
- Pain can be influenced by the environment in which it is experienced and also the other people involved in that experience (e.g. family, carers, nurses).
- Pain can be acute or chronic (or on a continuum between the two). Acute pain usually has a limited onset and points to a clear cause. Chronic pain is prolonged, lasting beyond the course of an acute disease or healing associated with it.
- Chronic pain can impact on a person's life in many ways causing, for example, isolation, debilitation, altered lifestyle, altered personality, depression and altered functional ability.
- Pain may be experienced on its own or be accompanied by other symptoms which will also need alleviating.
- Managing pain, as with other symptoms, involves working out what is causing it and how best to alleviate it. This involves communication with the patient and their family/carers and the multi-disciplinary team.
- Effective assessment and management of pain is a key component of nursing care.

## Essentials of best practice

- Pain must be assessed thoroughly and regularly if it is to be managed well. Appropriate assessment and monitoring of pain and the effectiveness of analgesia are critical.
- Pain may be assessed using pain scales, but talking about pain is just as important.
- Anxiety exacerbates pain.

- Different types of pain require different approaches to their management.
- Surgical pain can be anticipated and a plan to manage pain should be determined prior to surgery whenever possible.
- In pre-existing pain it is important to find out more about the current episode of pain (e.g. location, intensity), what triggered it, how the patient usually manages and copes with pain and what they have tried to alleviate the pain with what effect.
- When considering chronic pain it is useful to consider other factors that might impact on the pain and contribute to a lowered pain threshold or be impacted by the pain (e.g. anxiety, depression, lifestyle, functional ability, fatigue, family/carers' reactions and tolerance).
- A variety of pain assessment tools are available (e.g. pain rulers, visual analogue scales, 'smiley faces', body maps).
- Pain assessment in vulnerable groups of people needs to be handled sensitively and innovatively (e.g. older people with dementia, people whose attitude to pain may be to put up with it, people with learning disabilities who may find it hard to express themselves, people who are confused or unconscious). Appropriate communication is a central feature of effective pain management.
- There are various approaches that can be used to achieve successful pain management (pharmacological (analgesics) or non-pharmacological management).
- Non-pharmacological management includes information giving, relaxation techniques, meditation, hypnosis, acupuncture, TENS, heat/cold therapies, therapies that result in distraction (e.g. art, music, guided imagery).
- The pharmacological management of pain can be guided by the WHO's 'analgesic ladder' (above).
- Analgesia can be administered by any route.
- Non-pharmacological and pharmacological techniques can be combined.

*Adult Nursing at a Glance*, First Edition. Andrée le May. © 2015 John Wiley & Sons, Ltd. Published 2015 by John Wiley & Sons, Ltd.
Companion website: www.ataglanceseries.com/nursing/adult

# 11 Incontinence

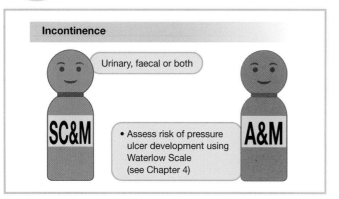

## SC&M incontinence

• From the point of view of an incontinent person, incontinence may simply be defined as passing urine or faeces in an inappropriate place. From a health professional's view, incontinence is the involuntary leakage of faeces or urine.

• Incontinence may be transient, for example after childbirth, or it may be a continuing problem associated with odour, leakage, exposure, secrecy, embarrassment and fear of not reaching the toilet in time.

• Urinary incontinence is usually categorised into different types:
  • stress urinary incontinence (SUI) which is the inability of the urethral sphincter to stay shut when pressure is exerted on the bladder by the abdomen (e.g. while sneezing, coughing or laughing, or while exercising);
  • urge incontinence which occurs when the detrusor muscle of the bladder contracts before the person wishes it to do so;
  • mixed stress and urge incontinence;
  • overflow incontinence as a result of urinary retention (e.g. prostatic hypertrophy, faecal impaction);
  • reflex incontinence due to, for example, spinal cord damage;
  • functional incontinence is when a person could be continent but can't get to the toilet/commode in time because of, for example, mobility or cognitive problems or impaired dexterity.

• Faecal incontinence may be caused by the following:
  • structural changes, for example incompetent anal sphincter, pelvic floor damage (e.g. from childbirth) or haemorrhoidectomy;
  • diminished rectal sensation, for example due to diabetic neuropathy or megacolon;
  • constipation (and associated dehydration, inadequate diet, minimal exercise etc.);
  • excessive diarrhoea;
  • neurological disorders such as Parkinson's disease, multiple sclerosis;
  • cognitive impairment, for example dementia;
  • brain damage, for example frontal lobe carcinoma, stroke;
  • specific conditions of the bowel, for example inflammatory bowel disease.

• Incontinence can lead to skin excoriation and the risk of developing pressure ulcers (Chapter 4).

• Incontinence can be managed in different ways depending on its cause and the person's ability/motivation to control it. Some possibilities require no specialist intervention although the advice of a continence nurse is always helpful (below). Others require specialist tests and intervention from continence nurses and/or urologists, these include:
  • pharmacological management (e.g. in faecal incontinence making bowel evacuation more predictable by the use of bulking agents, constipating agents, suppositories, enemas) may work well;
  • bio feedback may be successful for some people;
  • exercises, such as pelvic floor exercise, anal sphincter contracting exercises;
  • electrical stimulation of the pelvic floor;
  • anal plugs;
  • catheters urethral and supra-pubic: self-catheterisation;
  • surgery.

## Essentials of best practice

• Find out more about the person's incontinence. Take a urine specimen and test it to rule out infection. Ask about constipation and diarrhoea.

• Ask about any possible triggers and ways of relieving incontinence that the patient or their carers might have developed.

• Refer for specialist assessment.

• Discuss methods of continence management prior to the assessment, for example:
  • pads and close fitting pants (for women and men) suitable for their level of incontinence (during the day and at night) and the person's usual routines;
  • penile sheaths with leg bags and pouches (and close fitting pants) for men. Pouches enable the man to tuck his penis into them, which for some men provides a more secure fit than pads and pants and reduces urinary leakage (and increases confidence);
  • discuss bed protection at night with incontinence pads or absorbent sheets;
  • discuss access to toilets, commodes and urinary bottles for men; and mobility aids;
  • discuss skin care and the need to use a protective barrier cream and washing after changing pads and pouches.

• Make an assessment for pressure ulcer risk.

• Arrange a follow-up meeting to review the person's care and the advice/treatment given by the continence specialist.

### Patient information

Useful advice may be obtained about continence aids from:
The Bladder and Bowel Foundation (B&BF) who produce information and have a support helpline: www.bladderandbowelfoundation.org.uk.
AgeUK: www.ageuk.org.
See also the relevant specific disease focused charities and support groups.

*Adult Nursing at a Glance*, First Edition. Andrée le May. © 2015 John Wiley & Sons, Ltd. Published 2015 by John Wiley & Sons, Ltd.
Companion website: www.ataglanceseries.com/nursing/adult

# 12 Nursing older people

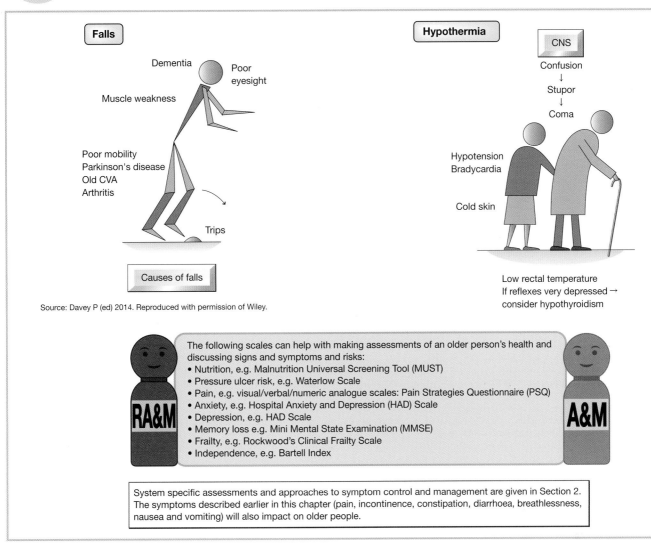

**Falls**

Dementia

Poor eyesight

Muscle weakness

Poor mobility
Parkinson's disease
Old CVA
Arthritis

Trips

Causes of falls

Source: Davey P (ed) 2014. Reproduced with permission of Wiley.

**Hypothermia**

CNS

Confusion
↓
Stupor
↓
Coma

Hypotension
Bradycardia

Cold skin

Low rectal temperature
If reflexes very depressed →
consider hypothyroidism

RA&M

The following scales can help with making assessments of an older person's health and discussing signs and symptoms and risks:
• Nutrition, e.g. Malnutrition Universal Screening Tool (MUST)
• Pressure ulcer risk, e.g. Waterlow Scale
• Pain, e.g. visual/verbal/numeric analogue scales: Pain Strategies Questionnaire (PSQ)
• Anxiety, e.g. Hospital Anxiety and Depression (HAD) Scale
• Depression, e.g. HAD Scale
• Memory loss e.g. Mini Mental State Examination (MMSE)
• Frailty, e.g. Rockwood's Clinical Frailty Scale
• Independence, e.g. Bartell Index

A&M

System specific assessments and approaches to symptom control and management are given in Section 2. The symptoms described earlier in this chapter (pain, incontinence, constipation, diarrhoea, breathlessness, nausea and vomiting) will also impact on older people.

## Nursing older people

• Growing old affects different people in different ways – some people remain healthy until their death in their 80s or 90s whilst others have multiple health problems requiring complex care by their late 60s or 70s.
• An older person's requirements of nursing care will vary as they pass through old age and will be significantly different from those of younger people. This is not an ageist statement: it simply emphasises the different needs that people have at different stages of their lives and the need for nurses to attend to older people as individuals rather than en masse.
• Some older people's needs will be multi-faceted because of their individual blend of:
  • multiple symptoms associated with natural ageing and multiple pathologies;
  • poly-pharmacy and connected drug interactions and side-effects (which may also lead e.g. to non-compliance);
  • sensory impairments (e.g. hearing and sight) and communication challenges as a consequence of aging and diseases;
  • level of frailty.

This mixture is overlaid by social and environmental features of ageing, for example available social support, levels of isolation, support with daily living and the match (or mismatch) between living environments and needs.
• Some older people will also be prone to the problems associated with growing older, for example unsteadiness resulting in falls and trips and hypothermia (above), isolation, malnutrition, cognitive impairment and depression. These problems may be overlaid on existing long-term conditions or acute illnesses.
• Integrated person-centred multi-disciplinary, multi-agency care will be required by many older people.
• Many older people will experience minimal health problems and their regular encounters with nurses will be limited to their annual flu vaccination or health check with the practice nurse.
• Whatever an older person's level of need for nursing care and symptom management and control, all nurses should provide care that is tailored to the person (and, where appropriate, their family/carers), sensitive to their needs (and preferences) and aims to promote confidence in the care given as well as feelings of safety and security.

*Adult Nursing at a Glance*, First Edition. Andrée le May. © 2015 John Wiley & Sons, Ltd. Published 2015 by John Wiley & Sons, Ltd.
Companion website: www.ataglanceseries.com/nursing/adult

# 13 Nursing people at the end of life

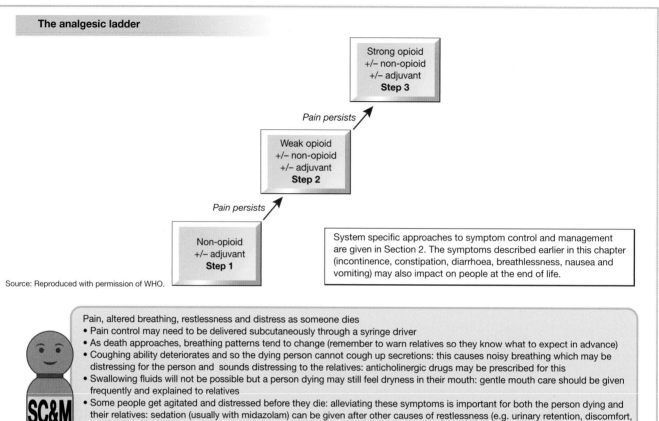

**The analgesic ladder**

> Strong opioid
> +/– non-opioid
> +/– adjuvant
> **Step 3**

*Pain persists*

> Weak opioid
> +/– non-opioid
> +/– adjuvant
> **Step 2**

*Pain persists*

> Non-opioid
> +/– adjuvant
> **Step 1**

System specific approaches to symptom control and management are given in Section 2. The symptoms described earlier in this chapter (incontinence, constipation, diarrhoea, breathlessness, nausea and vomiting) may also impact on people at the end of life.

Source: Reproduced with permission of WHO.

**SC&M**

Pain, altered breathing, restlessness and distress as someone dies
- Pain control may need to be delivered subcutaneously through a syringe driver
- As death approaches, breathing patterns tend to change (remember to warn relatives so they know what to expect in advance)
- Coughing ability deteriorates and so the dying person cannot cough up secretions: this causes noisy breathing which may be distressing for the person and sounds distressing to the relatives: anticholinergic drugs may be prescribed for this
- Swallowing fluids will not be possible but a person dying may still feel dryness in their mouth: gentle mouth care should be given frequently and explained to relatives
- Some people get agitated and distressed before they die: alleviating these symptoms is important for both the person dying and their relatives: sedation (usually with midazolam) can be given after other causes of restlessness (e.g. urinary retention, discomfort, pain) have been ruled out
- Encourage relatives to talk to the person: reassure them that hearing is the last sense to fade and show them through your example that this is an appropriate thing to do

*Adult Nursing at a Glance*, First Edition. Andrée le May. © 2015 John Wiley & Sons, Ltd. Published 2015 by John Wiley & Sons, Ltd.
Companion website: www.ataglanceseries.com/nursing/adult

# Nursing people at the end of their lives

- Palliative and end of life care are different but interlinked aspects of nursing care.
- Palliative care is fundamentally about symptom relief and control in order to increase the quality of life experienced by people with life limiting illnesses and diseases. Although palliative care will focus on any symptom the most common symptom needing palliation is likely to be pain (physical, emotional and spiritual pain) (see Chapter 10).
- As the end of life draws closer, attention will move to the palliation (easing) of symptoms associated with the process of dying. These are largely pain, alterations to breathing and restlessness and distress (above).
- In addition nurses need to focus on the person's family and friends who may be made anxious and distressed by these symptoms thereby increasing their own feelings of anxiety, uncertainty and imminent loss.
- Nursing care needs to focus also on the environment – death can occur in many places: some people will die at home, in a care home or a residential home or in a hospice, others will die in hospital – in the ward, the ED, a side room. Whichever it is, nurses should, if possible, create a private, comfortable area and stay with the patient (and their family if they wish).
- Excellent nursing care at the end of life is a balance of technical competence to ease symptoms, the promotion/facilitation of appropriate physical, emotional, cultural and spiritual comfort and skilled communication to reduce anxiety by explanations, listening and 'being there' to create (if possible) an environment within which intense and mixed emotions can be felt and expressed.

- During and after death there may be particular wishes or customs that the dying person and their family/friends would want to be performed. Nurses need to know what these are and to help to facilitate them if possible.
- After death there are several formalities that need to be undertaken (e.g. certification of death by a doctor, arranging for the person's body to be removed). Using the gap between death and the finalisation of these aspects of care to allow relatives to be alone with the patient's body may be a helpful for them – ask them if they would like this. Remember, though, if they do want this to arrange to come back in a short time to see how they are. Some people will want to be by themselves in these circumstances and a quiet comfortable room close at hand should be found. Tea and coffee will usually be appreciated at this time too.
- The family/friends may want to help lay the person out (last offices) and you should ask if they'd like to help you do this. Some people may prefer to stay and watch rather than help, others will want to leave and come back later, some people will want to stay and help or maybe do something particularly important, for instance combing the person's hair or washing their hands or helping put on a favourite or special garment. For some people being able to join you in at this final stage of care may be a comforting act of farewell.
- Nurses rarely get 'used' to death: they and their colleagues often continue to find death distressing through their careers, especially if it is unexpected or the patient has been known for a long time. Taking a little time for yourself after a patient's death, even if it is only a short break on the ward, is important. Talking about the person's death with colleagues and maybe the person's relatives is also an important part of protecting yourself from the burn-out that nurses and doctors sometimes feel.

# 14 Risk assessment and management

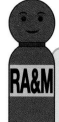

Always assess and manage risk in relation to:
- patients
- carers/family
- colleagues
- your work environment (e.g. a ward, a patient's home, a consulting room)

*Adult Nursing at a Glance*, First Edition. Andrée le May. © 2015 John Wiley & Sons, Ltd. Published 2015 by John Wiley & Sons, Ltd.
Companion website: www.ataglanceseries.com/nursing/adult

# Risk assessment and management

- Avoiding harm and keeping people safe is a vital dimension of nursing care.
- In order to do this nurses need to be able to:
  - identify, assess and report (as necessary) actual and potential threats to a person's safety and health (risk is the chance that someone might be harmed by one of these);
  - understand the cause(s) of these risks and what can be done to lessen them;
  - implement ways to avoid, reduce or control them (management);
  - evaluate the success of their actions.
- These risks could include a patient's likelihood of falling at home, of taking the wrong medication at the wrong time if self-medicating, of acquiring an infection whilst in hospital or of developing a venous thromboembolism after a period of inactivity.
- Organisational policies and procedures should guide the assessment and management of risks to patients, their families/carers, colleagues and yourself.
- Sometimes checklists (e.g. pre-operatively) or risk measurement scales (e.g. for assessing risk of developing pressure ulcers) are used to ensure that risks are assessed and minimised.
- Risk management is a term also used by organisations to describe the structures and processes they have put in place and use to identify and manage risk.
- Patient safety incidents are unintended or unforeseen events which could have harmed or did harm a patient. These should always be taken seriously and investigated to work out what went wrong and what could be done to stop the same thing happening again. Learning from this analysis is important. This process should usually be blame free.
- Knowing the part you play in maintaining patient safety is critical – a good example of this is the relationship between thorough hand washing and infection control.
- Being mindful of the safety of colleagues and yourself is also important.
- If you think that a patient or a colleague is at risk, tell someone.

# Seven steps to patient safety

The National Patient Safety Agency produced seven steps to patient safety. Using this sort of framework to improve patient safety may be useful within an organisation, unit, ward or team:

1 Build a culture which is open and fair.
2 Lead and support people by making a clear, strong focus on patient safety.
3 Develop systems and processes to manage risks and identify and assess things that could go wrong.
4 Encourage the reporting of incidents and near misses.
5 Openly communicate with and involve patients/the public.
6 Learn how and why incidents happen and share lessons.
7 Implement solutions into practice, processes and systems to prevent harm.

# Medicines management

## Medicines Management includes safe administration

The principles of this are detailed in the NMC's Standard 8: Administration.

**NB Students must never administer or supply medicinal products without direct supervision.**

'As a *registrant*, in exercising your professional accountability in the best interests of your patients:

- you must be certain of the identity of the patient to whom the medicine is to be administered
- you must check that the patient is not allergic to the medicine before administering it
- you must know the therapeutic uses of the medicine to be administered, its normal dosage, side effects, precautions and contra-indications
- you must be aware of the patient's plan of care (care plan or pathway)
- you must check that the prescription or the label on medicine dispensed is clearly written and unambiguous
- you must check the expiry date (where it exists) of the medicine to be administered
- you must have considered the dosage, weight where appropriate, method of administration, route and timing
- you must administer or withhold in the context of the patient's condition, (for example, Digoxin not usually to be given if pulse below 60) and co-existing therapies, for example, physiotherapy
- you must contact the prescriber or another authorised prescriber without delay where contra-indications to the prescribed medicine are discovered, where the patient develops a reaction to the medicine, or where assessment of the patient indicates that the medicine is no longer suitable (see Standard 25)
- you must make a clear, accurate and immediate record of all medicine administered, intentionally withheld or refused by the patient, ensuring the signature is clear and legible. It is also your responsibility to ensure that a record is made when delegating the task of administering medicine.

*In addition*:
- Where medication is not given, the reason for not doing so must be recorded.
- You may administer with a single signature any prescription only medicine (POM), general sales list (GSL) or pharmacy (P) medication.

*In respect of controlled drugs*:
- These should be administered in line with relevant legislation and local standard operating procedures.
- It is recommended that for the administration of controlled drugs a secondary signatory is required within secondary care and similar healthcare settings.
- In a patient's home, where a registrant is administering a controlled drug that has already been prescribed and dispensed to that patient, obtaining a secondary signatory should be based on local risk assessment.
- Although normally the second signatory should be another registered healthcare professional (for example doctor, pharmacist, dentist) or student nurse or midwife, in the interest of patient care, where this is not possible, a second suitable person who has been assessed as competent may sign. It is good practice that the second signatory witnesses the whole administration process. For guidance, go to www.dh.gov.uk and search for safer management of controlled drugs: guidance on standard operating procedures.
- In cases of direct patient administration of oral medication from stock in a substance misuse clinic, it must be a registered nurse who administers, signed by a second signatory (assessed as competent), who is then supervised by the registrant as the patient receives and consumes the medication.

You must clearly countersign the signature of the student when supervising a student in the administration of medicines. These standards apply to all medicinal products.'

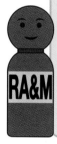

# Medicines management

- Medicines management, in the widest sense is 'the clinical, cost-effective and safe use of medicines to ensure patients get the maximum benefit from the medicines they need, while at the same time minimising potential harm' (MHRA, 2004: quoted by NMC 2013).
- In nursing, medicines management refers to prescribing, dispensing, storage, administration and disposal of medicinal products.
- NB Students must never engage in any aspect of medicines management without direct supervision.
- Medicinal products are 'any substance or combination of substances presented for treating or preventing disease in human beings or in animals. Any substance or combination of substances which may be administered to human beings or animals with a view to making a medical diagnosis or to restoring, correcting or modifying physiological functions in human beings or animals is likewise considered a medicinal product.' Council Directive 65/65/EEC.
- Avoiding harm and keeping people safe is a vital dimension of medicines management. In order to do this, nurses need to ensure that they comply with their professional and statutory body's standards.
- In the UK the NMC has issued 26 specific standards for medicines management (NMC, 2013 update) to be adhered to by registered nurses (example above).
- Standards focus on:
  - methods of supplying and/or administration;
  - checking any direction to administer a medicinal product;
  - dispensing prescription medicines and patients' own medicines;
  - storage and transportation;
  - administration of medicines (above);
  - assessment of the effectiveness of, and a patient's response to, medicines;
  - assessment of patients who are self-administering medicines or whose carers are doing this for them;
  - communication with patients about medicines;
  - titration when a range of doses is prescribed to ensure the best response by the patient (e.g. symptom control);
  - preparing medications in advance or using medications prepared by another person without observation;
  - administering medications obtained over the internet;
  - use of compliance aids;
  - disposal of medicinal products;
  - unlicensed medicines;
  - complementary and alternative therapies;
  - delegation and accountability;
  - student supervision;
  - management of adverse events;
  - reporting of adverse reactions;
  - controlled drugs.
- As you progress through your nursing course you will gain supervised experience of all aspects of medicines management so that on registration as a nurse you will be able to adhere to the standards laid down by your professional and statutory body.
- Some nurses have gained specialist qualifications enabling them to prescribe medicinal products.
- As a student, regardless of seniority, you are responsible for reporting patients' adverse reactions to medicinal products immediately to either a senior nursing colleague or a doctor. Documenting these reactions is essential.
- Any deviations from medication plans that you observe should also be reported to your seniors.

**Pre- and post-operative care**

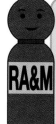

## Essentials of pre-operative care

**Ensure the patient:**
- Knows what operation is to be performed and has consented to it
- Knows what is likely to happen in the anaesthetic room and recovery suite
- Has enough time to discuss concerns (and the family has time too)
- Wears the correct identification band (and allergy bands if appropriate)
- Is assessed for risks of VTE and pressure ulcers
- Understands the regime for fasting prior to surgery
- Knows about any special feature of their surgery (e.g. equipment, hair removal from the operation site, post-operative care)
- Knows what to expect when they return to the ward (e.g. pain relief, equipment, observations)
- Has a set of baseline observations to compare post-operative observations against

## Essentials of immediate post-operative care once a patient is returned to the ward

**Ensure that:**
- You know what operation has been performed and what post-operative care has been given in the recovery suite
- You know any specific post-operative care required on the ward
- Regular observations are made of temperature, pulse, blood pressure and respiration rate and quality
- Deviations from the normal ranges for these observations are reported immediately
- Wounds are regularly inspected for oozing and bleeding: ischaemia
- Drains are patent and their contents inspected for blood
- Fluid balance is recorded: deviations from the norm are reported
- IVIs are working and fluids and drugs given as prescribed
- Pain relief is given regularly
- Nausea/vomiting are relieved appropriately (a covered vomit bowl is close by)
- The call bell is within easy reach
- You tell the patient what you are doing (they may remain drowsy post-operatively)
- You hand over all relevant information to colleagues at the end of your shift
- You document observations and care clearly in all relevant places

**In good, safe surgery, everyone – even the student or porter – should feel able to speak up if something seems not to be right.**

*Adult Nursing at a Glance*, First Edition. Andrée le May. © 2015 John Wiley & Sons, Ltd. Published 2015 by John Wiley & Sons, Ltd.
Companion website: www.ataglanceseries.com/nursing/adult

# Pre- and post-operative care

- Avoiding harm and keeping people safe before, during and after surgery is a critical component of nursing.
- Pre-operative care is the physical and psychological care provided to a patient (and their family/carers) prior to surgery.
- Intra-operative care is provided during surgery by theatre nurses, operating department technicians, anaesthetists and surgeons.
- Post-operative care is care provided following surgery in the theatre recovery area and on the ward.
- Pre-operatively assessments need to be made of the patient's physical condition and their risk of developing:
  - venous thromboembolism (VTE) (anti-embolic stockings applied appropriately and prophylaxis given as prescribed);
  - pressure ulcers (pressure relieving equipment available);
  - pulmonary aspiration (due to inhaling gastric contents during the induction of anaesthesia or during surgical manipulations) (fasting procedure instituted correctly);
  - surgical site infections or difficulties closing skin/applying dressings (removal of hair as appropriate using clippers or depilation creams rather than shaving which risks cutting the skin);
  - toxic shock syndrome in women who are menstruating and using tampons (discuss using sanitary pads rather than tampons during surgery: if tampons are left in situ for more than 6 hours infection may develop);
  - allergic reactions to products used during surgery (e.g. latex gloves, skin cleansing fluids, dressings, dressing tapes).
- Pre-operatively attention should also be paid to increasing the patient's knowledge about the surgery and its consequences and alleviating anxiety by listening to concerns and giving simple and truthful information. Family and carers will also be anxious.
- Check consent has been given for surgery (usually obtained by the surgeon), the patient is wearing an identification band with their name and hospital number clearly marked, an allergy band is worn if appropriate, the operation site has been clearly marked by the surgeon, and that the right patient is taken for surgery together with all of their relevant documentation.
- Intra-operative care starts once the patient has been handed over to the theatre staff and continues until the patient is discharged from the recovery suite.
- Specific checks are made in the anaesthetic room and the operating theatre to safeguard the patients prior to surgery. Primarily these relate to ensuring that the right patient is being operated on, the right operation is about to be performed, any risks associated with the operation have been recognised (e.g. amount of blood loss), any risks associated with the patient (e.g. previous medical history, allergies, risk of VTE) have been recognised.
- After the operation is completed and before the patient leaves the operating theatre, more checks are made. These focus on the equipment used, any tests/specimens taken, the information recorded about the procedure, any problems experienced and instructions to be carried out during the immediate post-operative recovery period.
- Following surgery, patients are cared for in the recovery suite attached to the theatre until their condition is stable and they are conscious.
- Once returned to the ward routine post-operative care commences. Initially this includes:
  - regular observations of vital signs (pulse, blood pressure and respirations);
  - checking the wound/drains for bleeding (dressings soaked with blood indicate excessive bleeding) and checking for ischaemia;
  - recording fluid intake and output;
  - ensuring that pain is managed appropriately;
  - noting and reporting any unusual behaviours (confusion, restlessness);
  - ensuring that nausea and/or vomiting are managed appropriately;
  - coaxing the patient to drink and noting their tolerance of fluids;
  - encouraging the patient to pass urine if no catheter is inserted or following its removal.
- Deviations from the norm should be reported immediately. For example. decreased blood pressure may suggest hypovolaemic shock (e.g. due to bleeding, vomiting), increased pulse may suggest low circulating blood levels (e.g. due to bleeding) (NB: increased respiratory rate coupled with shallow breathing may occur before tachycardia and hypotension are noted).
- If gastro-intestinal surgery has been performed, peristalsis usually returns to normal after about 48 hours and meals/snacks should only be introduced after confirmation with the medical team. Patients may describe cramps, wind or hunger as bowel function returns. Listening for bowel sounds with a stethoscope may be required following GI tract surgery.
- Once the immediate post-operative period is over and the patient is feeling hungry, easily digestible food (and fluid) should be gradually re-introduced. Monitoring the patient's tolerance of food is important. Small frequent meals may be better tolerated than large meals. Establishing good nutrition is essential for healing.
- Wound care is an important facet of post-operative care as is ensuring strict infection control procedures.
- Encouraging mobility and deep breathing exercises are essential in reducing the likelihood of VTE. However a person in pain is unlikely to want to move so mobilisation and pain management should be considered alongside each other.
- Remember to discuss the patient's progress with them and their family/carers. An encouraging and realistic approach is important during the recovery period and can help alleviate anxiety, encourage compliance with post-operative instructions and exercises and build the patient's (and the family's) confidence in preparation for discharge from the ward.
- Specific pre- and post-operative care may be necessary for certain operations. You should check if this is the case with senior colleagues, doctors and specialist nurses to ensure that the right specialist preparation or care is carried out.

# 17 Moving and positioning

**Essentials of safe moving and positioning**

- Undertake an initial assessment of a patient's needs and capabilities in relation to moving and positioning (day and night)
  The Health and Safety Executive (HSE) (2013) recommends focusing on:
  - o 'the extent of the individual's ability to support their own weight and any other relevant factors, for example pain, disability, spasm, fatigue, tissue viability or tendency to fall
  - o the extent to which the individual can participate in/co-operate with transfers
  - o whether the individual needs assistance to reposition themselves/sit up when in their bed/chair and how this will be achieved, e.g. provision of an electric profiling bed
  - o the specific equipment needed … and, if applicable, type of bed, bath and chair, as well as specific handling equipment, type of hoist and sling; sling size and attachments
  - o the assistance needed for different types of transfer, including the number of staff needed – although hoists can be operated by one person, hoisting tasks often require two staff to ensure safe transfer
  - o the arrangements for reducing the risk and for dealing with falls, if the individual is at risk.'
- Make a plan to meet these needs and reduce risks. Discuss this with the patient and their family, and your colleagues. Record it
- Update the assessment and plan as the patient's needs change
- Before you move someone or a piece of equipment carry out a rapid risk assessment of the situation at that time
- Report any near misses or accidents appropriately

## Moving and positioning

- Nurses undertake many activities that involve moving and positioning patients (or equipment involved in their care). These include helping a person move from one place to another, to transfer between their bed and chair, to change position in bed, to undertake activities of daily living such as transferring to the toilet, having a bath or shower and dressing.
- Inappropriate moving and positioning practice may cause:
  - discomfort and a lack of dignity for the person being moved;
  - accidents which can hurt the person being moved and the person doing the moving;
  - back pain and musculoskeletal disorders for the nurse which can lead to time off work or an inability to continue working in that job.
- When you make your initial assessment of a patient, include a risk assessment focused on their moving and positioning needs. Record this for others to use and make sure it is updated when the patient's condition or needs change.
- Use the risk assessment to plan a person's care and minimise risk to them and to you and your colleagues.

- In addition to any initial moving and positioning assessment, every time you undertake nursing care make a rapid assessment of any risk involved. Take appropriate action to manage any risk so that no harm will be caused.
- To reduce the risks of inappropriate moving and positioning, employers offer regular annual mandatory training.
- It is important to minimise the risk of undignified care, accidents and harm by adhering to your organisation's manual handling policies and following the principles of good practice above.
- Always tell others if their moving and positioning practices are deficient.

### Patient information

The Health and Safety Executive (HSE) has a web page on moving and handling in health and social care:
www.hse.gov.uk/healthservices/moving-handling.htm.

# 18 Infection prevention and control

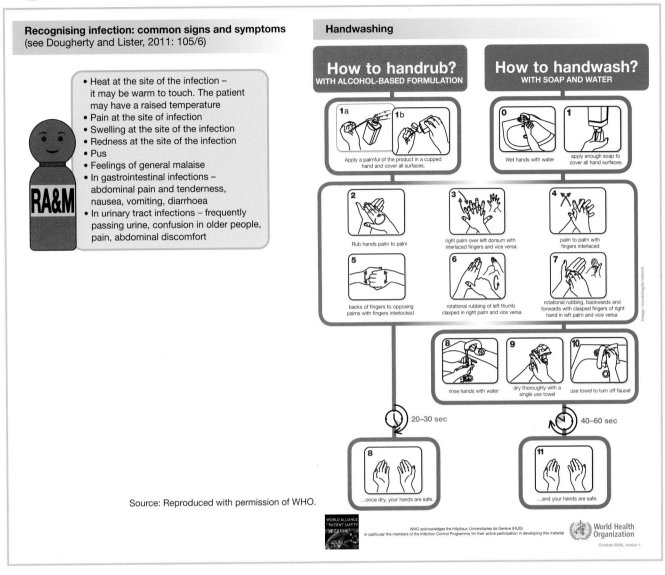

**Recognising infection: common signs and symptoms**
(see Dougherty and Lister, 2011: 105/6)

**RA&M**

- Heat at the site of the infection – it may be warm to touch. The patient may have a raised temperature
- Pain at the site of infection
- Swelling at the site of the infection
- Redness at the site of the infection
- Pus
- Feelings of general malaise
- In gastrointestinal infections – abdominal pain and tenderness, nausea, vomiting, diarrhoea
- In urinary tract infections – frequently passing urine, confusion in older people, pain, abdominal discomfort

**Handwashing**

**How to handrub?**
WITH ALCOHOL-BASED FORMULATION

**1a** **1b** Apply a palmful of the product in a cupped hand and cover all surfaces.

**2** Rub hands palm to palm

**3** right palm over left dorsum with interlaced fingers and vice versa

**4** palm to palm with fingers interlaced

**5** backs of fingers to opposing palms with fingers interlocked

**6** rotational rubbing of left thumb clasped in right palm and vice versa

**7** rotational rubbing, backwards and forwards with clasped fingers of right hand in left palm and vice versa

20–30 sec

**8** ...once dry, your hands are safe.

**How to handwash?**
WITH SOAP AND WATER

**0** Wet hands with water

**1** apply enough soap to cover all hand surfaces.

**8** rinse hands with water

**9** dry thoroughly with a single use towel

**10** use towel to turn off faucet

40–60 sec

**11** ...and your hands are safe.

Source: Reproduced with permission of WHO.

WHO acknowledges the Hôpitaux Universitaires de Genève (HUG), in particular the members of the Infection Control Programme, for their active participation in developing this material

World Health Organization

October 2006, version 1.

## Infection prevention and control

- Infection control and prevention is part of everyone's life; for example, we wash our hands after using the toilet or before we eat and we stay at home when we are ill and likely to pass on infections to other people.
- Nurses deliver care to people who may be infectious or vulnerable to cross-infection from other people, and so need to take extra precautions.
- Nurses protect people against infections in several ways. These include:
  - health education and promotion (e.g. teaching about infection control, encouraging vaccinations and immunisations);
  - preventing cross-infection between patients in hospital or in the community by vigilant handwashing (or the use of alcohol gel), the correct use of gloves, gowns and masks, the correct disposal of infected materials and sharps, and the use of isolation if appropriate (either to protect an immuno-compromised person from developing infection or to stop other patients from coming into contact with someone whose illness is contagious);
  - preventing wound infections, bladder infections or IVI-site infections by using scrupulous aseptic techniques;
  - recognising infection so treatment can be started as soon as possible (above);
  - ensuring that anti-infective medications are taken as prescribed;
  - ensuring that the rules of basic hygiene are adhered to, for example offering bed-bound patients handwashing or hand cleansing facilities after using a bedpan, bottle or commode, or before meals.

*Adult Nursing at a Glance*, First Edition. Andrée le May. © 2015 John Wiley & Sons, Ltd. Published 2015 by John Wiley & Sons, Ltd.
Companion website: www.ataglanceseries.com/nursing/adult

# 19 Adult basic life support

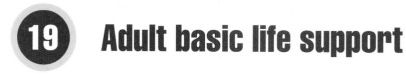

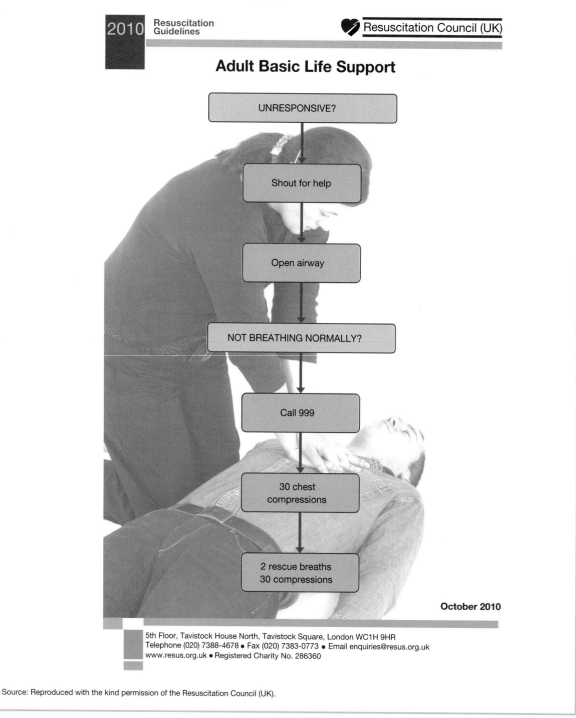

**Adult Basic Life Support**

2010 Resuscitation Guidelines

Resuscitation Council (UK)

## Adult Basic Life Support

UNRESPONSIVE?

Shout for help

Open airway

NOT BREATHING NORMALLY?

Call 999

30 chest compressions

2 rescue breaths
30 compressions

October 2010

5th Floor, Tavistock House North, Tavistock Square, London WC1H 9HR
Telephone (020) 7388-4678 ● Fax (020) 7383-0773 ● Email enquiries@resus.org.uk
www.resus.org.uk ● Registered Charity No. 286360

Source: Reproduced with the kind permission of the Resuscitation Council (UK).

*Adult Nursing at a Glance*, First Edition. Andrée le May. © 2015 John Wiley & Sons, Ltd. Published 2015 by John Wiley & Sons, Ltd.
Companion website: www.ataglanceseries.com/nursing/adult

# Basic life support

- Nurses deliver care to people who may have cardiac or respiratory arrests. Knowing what to do in these situations is critical for patients (and their families).
- All nurses are updated regularly on basic life support techniques (those above are current as this book is being written). Updates can be obtained from the Resuscitation Council (UK) www.resus.org.uk.
- You will be reading this after you have had your own training in BLS: this chapter is a reminder of the key points.
- Not all nurses work in a hospital with easily accessible equipment and skilled arrest teams. Figure 19 above shows the basic steps in providing life support in a person's home. In-hospital life support is detailed in Chapter 20.
- Always know the resuscitation wishes of patients.
- If you are nursing in the community, always have a mobile phone with you so you can quickly call for help if needed.
- Always make a mental record (then a written record) of the time you started (and stopped if this is appropriate) BLS.
- In addition to the steps opposite you need to remember that you:
  - open the airway by turning the person onto their back, tilting their head back and lifting their chin;

- compress the chest to a depth of 5–6 cm for every compression;
- compress the chest at a rate of 100/120 per minute: this should be continuous with minimal interruption for rescue breaths;
- after 30 compressions open the airway again and give 2 rescue breaths;
- rescue breaths need to be given steadily and quickly. One breath should take 1–2 seconds; watch the chest fall before giving the next. Both rescue breaths should be given within 5 seconds (if the first rescue breath of each sequence doesn't make the chest rise, check the airway for obstructions and head tilt and chin lift);
- return immediately to chest compressions;
- do not stop the 30 compressions: 2 rescue breaths routine until either:
  - help arrives,
  - the person shows signs of regaining consciousness and starts to breathe normally,
  - or you are too exhausted to continue.

Now read the most up-to-date guidelines from the Resuscitation Council.

# 20 In-hospital resuscitation

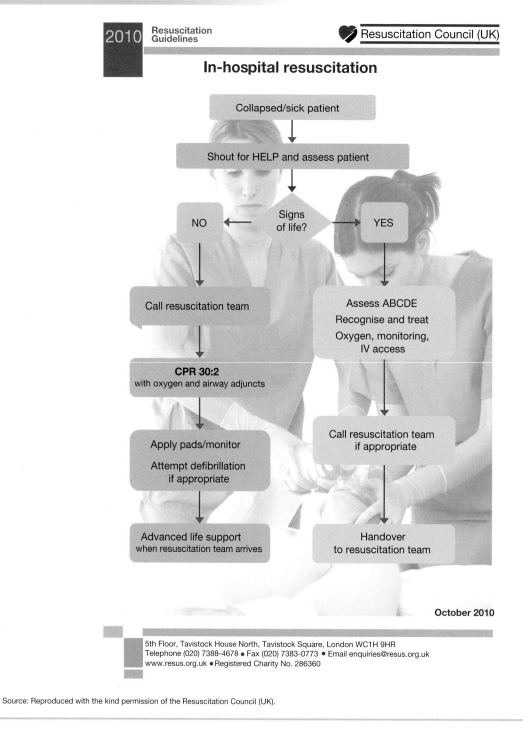

In-hospital resuscitation

**2010** Resuscitation Guidelines

Resuscitation Council (UK)

## In-hospital resuscitation

Collapsed/sick patient

↓

Shout for HELP and assess patient

↓

Signs of life?

NO ← → YES

**NO branch:**

Call resuscitation team

↓

**CPR 30:2**
with oxygen and airway adjuncts

↓

Apply pads/monitor

Attempt defibrillation
if appropriate

↓

Advanced life support
when resuscitation team arrives

**YES branch:**

Assess ABCDE

Recognise and treat

Oxygen, monitoring,
IV access

↓

Call resuscitation team
if appropriate

↓

Handover
to resuscitation team

October 2010

5th Floor, Tavistock House North, Tavistock Square, London WC1H 9HR
Telephone (020) 7388-4678 ● Fax (020) 7383-0773 ● Email enquiries@resus.org.uk
www.resus.org.uk ● Registered Charity No. 286360

Source: Reproduced with the kind permission of the Resuscitation Council (UK).

*Adult Nursing at a Glance*, First Edition. Andrée le May. © 2015 John Wiley & Sons, Ltd. Published 2015 by John Wiley & Sons, Ltd.
Companion website: www.ataglanceseries.com/nursing/adult

# In-hospital resuscitation

- Nurses deliver care to people who may have cardiac and respiratory arrests. Knowing what to do in these situations is critical for patients (and their families).
- All nurses are updated regularly on in-hospital resuscitation techniques (those in the figure are current as this book is being written). Updates can be obtained from the Resuscitation Council (UK) www.resus.org.uk.
- You will be reading this after you have had your own training in hospital resuscitation: this chapter is a reminder of the key points.
- Always know how to get help on every new ward/department you work on and that you also know the hospital telephone number to ring to get the resuscitation team.
- Always know the resuscitation wishes of patients.
- If you are the first person to find a collapsed patient, you will need to quickly decide if they have or do not have signs of life since this will determine what you do after you have called for help. Use the ABCDE assessment.

**A**irway (voice, breath sounds)
**B**reathing (rate, chest movements)
**C**irculation (pulse, skin colour, sweating, blood pressure, ECG)
**D**isability (level of consciousness, limb movements, pupillary light reflexes, blood glucose)
**E**xposure (and examine) (look at the skin, wounds, temperature).

- Always make a mental record (then a written record) of the time you started resuscitation, if this is appropriate.
- In addition to the steps above you need to remember that if you are the first person finding a person who has had an arrest (the left hand side of the figure above) that you:
  - open the airway by turning the person flat on their back, tilting their head back (unless contra-indicated, e.g. cervical spine injury) and lifting their chin;
  - compress the chest to a depth of 5–6 cm for every compression;
  - compress the chest at a rate of 100/120 per minute: this should be continuous with minimal interruption for rescue breaths;
  - after 30 compressions open the airway again and give 2 rescue breaths;
  - rescue breaths need to be given steadily and quickly. One breath should take 1–2 seconds; watch the chest fall before giving the next. Both rescue breaths should be given within 5 seconds (if the first rescue breath of each sequence doesn't make the chest rise check the airway for obstructions and head tilt and chin lift);
  - return immediately to chest compressions;
  - do not stop the 30 compressions:2 rescue breaths routine until either
    - help arrives,
    - or the person shows signs of regaining consciousness and starts to breathe normally.

- Help will arrive very quickly (although it may feel like a long time to you). Once others are there they will take over the CPR from you but you may be asked to do other specific things (record observations, draw up drugs, bring equipment, talk to other patients in the same ward) or you might not be needed anymore once the specialist resuscitation team has arrived (there will be at least five of them). There may not be enough space for you to stay.
- If you are nursing a patient who collapses but has not had a respiratory or cardiac arrest, you should call for help immediately and make a thorough assessment of their condition. Use the ABCDE to do this and take whatever action is appropriate.
- If you hear a call for help because a patient has collapsed/arrested, you should call the resuscitation team immediately then collect the resuscitation equipment returning with it as quickly as possible to the patient's bed-space.

Now read the most up-to-date guidelines from the Resuscitation Council.

## 21 Wound management

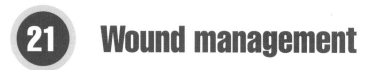

### The principles of wound management

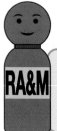

- Make sure that the patient knows when you are going to change dressings and that suitable analgesia has been given before hand
- Ensure privacy
- Pick the right dressings for the wound (e.g. alginates, occlusive, hydrocolloid, hydrogel, foams)
- Pick the right cleansing agents
- Ensure that you have all the equipment needed before starting to expose the wound
- Remember handwashing/cleansing with antibacterial substances and asepsis throughout the procedure
- Evaluate the wound every time a dressing is changed (Dougherty and Lister, 2011): record
    o size
    o wound bed (necrotic – black, slough – yellow, granulating – red, epithelialising – pink)
    o skin around the wound (e.g. intact, healthy, inflamed – allergy to dressing/tape)
    o exudate (amount)
    o odour
    o bleeding
    o pain
    o infection (take swab)
- Record observations

### Recognising infection: common signs and symptoms (see Dougherty and Lister, 2011: 105/6)

- Heat around the site of the infection. The patient may have a raised temperature
- Pain at the site of infection
- Swelling at the site of the infection
- Redness at the site of the infection
- Pus
- Feelings of general malaise

### Handwashing and cleansing: see Figure 18 for correct handwashing technique

*Adult Nursing at a Glance*, First Edition. Andrée le May. © 2015 John Wiley & Sons, Ltd. Published 2015 by John Wiley & Sons, Ltd.
Companion website: www.ataglanceseries.com/nursing/adult

# Wound management

- Wound management is a very important aspect of nursing in the hospital and the community.
- Wounds may be deliberately formed (surgical incisions) or be the result of injury (accident) or a complication of illness (e.g. diabetes) or altered circulation (leg ulcers) which may sometimes be coupled with pressure (e.g. pressure ulcers).
- Wounds can be acute (short lived) or chronic (long term).
- Wound healing can be achieved in a number of different ways:
  - joining the edges of a wound together by sutures, staples or other forms of closure (healing by primary intention);
  - if wound edges cannot be brought together the wound is left to heal through contraction and epithelialisation (healing by secondary intent);
  - the edges of some wounds cannot be joined immediately and will be left for a short time before joining (healing by tertiary intent).

- There are four broad phases to wound healing:
  - haemostasis (Chapter 59);
  - inflammation;
  - proliferation – epithelialisation;
  - maturation – the wound becomes strengthened, scar tissue is formed, thins and fades.
- Selecting the correct wound dressing is a central part of wound healing. Various options are available (above).
- Wound healing can be delayed by poor nutrition, alterations in temperature, ongoing excess exudate, poor dressing (or inappropriate) technique or use of dressings.
- During all procedures associated with wounds (e.g. dressing, drain emptying or removal, suture removal), nurses must ensure that they protect patients, through asepsis, against acquired infections.

Table 21 Dressing groups. Please refer to manufacturer's recommendations with regard to individual products.

| Dressings | Description | Advantages | Disadvantages |
|---|---|---|---|
| Activated charcoal | Contains a layer of activated charcoal that traps and reduces odour-causing molecules<br>*Example*: Carbonet, Clinisorb | Easy to apply as either primary or secondary dressing; can be combined with another dressing with absorbency<br>*Example*: Kaltocarb | Need to obtain a good seal to prevent leakage of odour; some dressings lose effectiveness when wet[a] |
| Adhesive island | Consists of a low adherent absorbent pad located centrally on an adhesive backing<br>*Example*: Mepore and Pad, Opsite Post-Op | Quick and easy to apply; protects the suture line from contamination and absorbs exudate/blood | Only suitable for light exudate; some can cause skin damage (excoriation, blistering) if applied incorrectly |
| Alginates | A textile fibre dressing made from seaweed; the soft woven fibres gel as they absorb exudate and promote autolytic debridement. Available as a sheet, ribbon or packing<br>*Example*: Kaltostat, Sorbsan, Algisorb | Are suitable for moderate to heavy exudate; can be used on infected wounds; useful for sinus and fistula drainage; have haemostatic properties; can be irrigated out of wound with warm saline | Cannot be used on dry wounds or wound with hard necrotic tissue (eschar); sometimes a mild burning or 'drawing' sensation is reported on application[a] |
| Anti-microbials | These topical dressings can be used as primary or secondary dressings and are available as a primary layer (*example*: Acticoat) and impregnated in other dressings (*examples*: Aquacel Ag, Mepilex Ag, Allevyn Ag) or as a cream (*example*: Flamazine) | Suitable for chronic wounds with heavy exudate that need protection from bacterial contamination by providing a broad range of anti-microbial activity; can reduce or prevent infection | Cannot be used during radiotherapy; sometimes sensitivity occurs with the use of silver and some skin staining can occur; instructions vary with products and dressings are expensive<br>Evidence base for use is controversial and needs monitoring[a] |
| Capillary wound dressings | Composed of 100% polyester filament outer layers and a 65% polyester and 35% cotton woven inner layer; outer layer draws exudate, interstitial fluid and necrotic tissue into the inner layer via a capillary action<br>*Example*: Vacutex | Suitable for light to heavy exudate; debride necrotic tissue; protect and insulate the wound; maintain a moist environment and prevent maceration; encourage development of granulation tissue; can be cut to any shape and are available in large rolls; can be used as a wick to drain sinus and cavity wounds | Can be hard to cut and are quite stiff to fit into wounds; cannot be used on malignant wounds or where there is the risk of bleeding due to the 'drawing' action and resultant increase in blood flow to the wound bed<br>Expensive and should be used on a named patient basis |
| Collagen | This protein is fibrous and insoluble and produced by fibroblasts. Collagen encourages collagen fibres into the granulation tissue. It is available in sheets/gels<br>*Example*: Promogran | Conforms well to wound surface, maintains a moist environment, suitable for most wounds to accelerate healing. Supports ECM | Not recommended for necrotic wounds[a] |
| Foams | Produced in a variety of forms, most being constructed of polyurethane foam and may have one or more layers; foam cavity dressings are also available<br>*Examples*: Allevyn, Mepilex, Biatain, PolyMem | Suitable for use with open, exuding wounds; highly absorbent, non-adherent and maintain a moist wound bed<br>Available for low–high exudates and/or bordered to simplify dressing choice | May be difficult to use in wounds with deep tracts and need a combined approach with an alginate or in fungating wounds |

*(Continued)*

**Table 21** (*Continued*)

| Dressings | Description | Advantages | Disadvantages |
|---|---|---|---|
| Honey – most widely used is Manuka honey | Available as tubes of liquid honey (*example*: Actibalm) or impregnated dressings (*example*: Activon Tulle; Mesitran (with hydrogel sheet)) | Suitable for acute and chronic infected, necrotic or sloughy wounds; provides a moist wound environment; non-adherent; antibacterial; assists with wound debridement; eliminates wound malodour; has an anti-inflammatory effect | Can be messy to use and causes leakage if excess exudate is present[a] May have a burning/drawing effect when first applied |
| Hydrocolloid | Usually consists of a base material containing gelatin, pectin and carboxymethylcellulose combined with adhesives and polymers; base material may be bonded to either a semi-permeable film or a film plus polyurethane foam; some have a border | Suitable for acute and chronic wounds with low to no exudate; provides a moist wound environment; promotes wound debridement; provides thermal insulation; waterproof and barrier to micro-organisms; easy to use | May release degradation products into the wound; strong odour produced as dressing interacts with exudate; some hydrocolloids cannot be used on infected wounds |
| Hydrofibre | Same consistency as hydrocolloid but in a soft woven sheet (also available with silver or combined with Duoderm in Combiderm) *Example*: Aquacel | Forms a soft, hydrophilic, gas-permeable gel on contact with the wound and manages exudate whilst preventing maceration of wound edge Easy to remove without trauma to wound bed | Does not have haemostatic property of alginates[a] |
| Hydrogels | Contain 17.5–90% water depending on the product, plus various other components to form a gel or solid sheet *Examples*: AquaForm Gel, Granugel, Geliperm (Sheet) | Suitable for light exudate wounds; absorb small amounts of exudate; donate fluid to dry necrotic tissue; reduce pain and are cooling; low trauma at dressing changes; can be used as carrier for drugs | Cool the wound surface; use with caution in infected wounds; can cause skin maceration due to leakage if too much gel is applied or the wound has moderate to heavy exudate[a] Moderate care of sheets so they do not dry out |
| Semi-permeable films | Polyurethane film with a hypoallergenic acrylic adhesive; have a variety of application methods often consisting of a plastic or cardboard carrier *Examples*: Tegaderm, Opsite | Only suitable for shallow superficial wounds; prophylactic use against friction damage; useful as retention dressing; allow passage of water vapour; allow monitoring of the wound | Possibility of adhesive trauma if removed incorrectly; do not contain exudate and can macerate, slip or leak Should not be used to cover an Allevyn dressing |
| Skin barrier film | Alcohol-free liquid polymer that forms a protective film on the skin *Example*: Cavilon (also comes as a barrier cream) | Non-cytotoxic; does not sting if applied to raw areas of skin; high wash-off resistance; protects the skin from body fluids, friction and shear and the effects of adhesive products | Requires good manual dexterity to apply; may cause skin warming on application |

Dealey (2005); Hess (2005).
[a] Requires a secondary dressing.
Dressing Data Cards are also available from World Wide Wounds (2004).
Source: Dougherty L & Lister S, 2011. Reproduced with permission of The Royal Marsden Hospital.

# 22 Health education and promotion

---

**Basic principles of educating someone about health issues**

**HE&P**

- Work out what the person needs to know
- Work out what the person does know
- Work out the best way to fill the gap (if there is one): start from where the person is
- Remember that when people are ill/uncomfortable/anxious their concentration levels may be poor
- Be clear and concise in what you say and always use simple easy-to-follow language
- Remember to give information in small chunks and check the person's understanding of what you said
- Remember to supplement oral information with written information
- Always tell a person where to get advice if they forget what you say or something unexpected or unexplained happens
- If possible set up another time to check what they know as a result of your intervention

---

## Health education and promotion

- The World Health Organisation (WHO) defines health education as 'any combination of learning experiences designed to help individuals and communities improve their health, by increasing their knowledge and influencing their attitudes'.
- Health promotion is defined by WHO as 'the process of enabling people to increase control over, and to improve, their health. It moves beyond a focus on individual behaviour towards a wide range or social and environmental interventions'.
- Increased knowledge and changed behaviour in individuals and communities/populations are the goals of health education and promotion.
- Behaviour change can occur as a result of a person changing what they do (e.g. stopping smoking), by governments making laws that alter many people's behaviours (e.g. banning smoking in

public places) or by communities exerting pressure to change behaviour (e.g. publicising the effects of passive smoking).
- Educating people about their health, encouraging them to lead healthier lifestyles and feel in control of their health and alterations to it are essential features of nursing.
- All nurses, whatever their practice setting, will be involved in educating patients and their families/carers about health, and ways to improve their health or maintain a healthy lifestyle. These can range from education about medication to how to increase exercise and reduce weight.
- Some nurses, largely public health nurses and occupational health nurses, will take part in developing local and national policy on health improvements or creating healthy workplaces, hospitals and schools.

*Adult Nursing at a Glance*, First Edition. Andrée le May. © 2015 John Wiley & Sons, Ltd. Published 2015 by John Wiley & Sons, Ltd.
Companion website: www.ataglanceseries.com/nursing/adult

# 23 Discharge planning

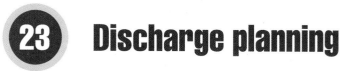

## Essential components of discharge planning in hospital

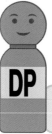

**DP**

- Start to plan discharge as soon as feasible
- Involve the patient and family/carers as soon as possible
- Discuss with the multi-disciplinary team, make a joint, agreed discharge plan and set an Expected Date for Discharge (EDD). Ensure a key worker is appointed if the patient has complex needs
- Explain care needed after discharge to the patient and their family/carers: agree the discharge plan and EDD with them
- Communicate with community teams/social services and others as appropriate to arrange care package and other support
- Monitor patient's progress and review plan regularly: update EDD if necessary
- Communicate any change in the plan to all involved (especially the patient and their family!)
- Closer to the time of discharge ensure that all relevant letters/summaries are prepared and sent to the GP and other teams
- Ensure drugs are prescribed and ready for the patient to take away
- Ensure any equipment or supplies needed at home are available or ordered for delivery with an expected delivery date
- Check transport arranged and out-patient department aware of patient's discharge (if required)
- Give the patient written information about their care following discharge and ensure that they and their family/carers know who (and how) to contact for advice once they leave hospital
- Make sure all documentation is completed accurately

## Essential components of discharge planning from community nursing care

**DP**

- Agree with the patient and their family/carers the plan for likely discharge at the start of the care package
- If long-term nursing care has been provided by the community nursing team and transfer to another facility (e.g. a nursing home) is required, accurate details of the patient's care, preferences and requirements should be collated and passed on

*Adult Nursing at a Glance*, First Edition. Andrée le May. © 2015 John Wiley & Sons, Ltd. Published 2015 by John Wiley & Sons, Ltd.
Companion website: www.ataglanceseries.com/nursing/adult

# Discharge planning

- Planning a person's discharge from nursing care starts during their initial assessment when care is being planned and agreed.
- For patients having surgery or any other planned procedure discharge planning will start during their pre-assessment visit.
- Discharge planning always occurs in partnership with the patient and their family/carers as well as other members of the multi-disciplinary team.
- In primary care, discharge from nursing care is usually negotiated between the patient, their family/carers and the nursing team/nurse.
- In hospital wards, patients are often given an expected date of discharge (EDD) once their medical condition has been stabilised. Having an EDD helps all members of the multi-disciplinary team, the patient and their family/carers plan ahead.
- Discharge planning is usually led by a senior member in the nursing team or the patient's key worker.
- A person's discharge from any care environment should be coordinated, efficiently undertaken and, where appropriate, ensure the smooth passage of a person's care from one service to another.
- Hospitals, particularly, are likely to have discharge policies to guide discharge planning. Some wards will have their own tailored policy. Other healthcare settings may also have policies and you should seek them out – if there are none follow the essential components detailed above.
- Inadequate discharge planning can result in patients and their families/carers being unprepared for the realities of returning home from hospital or transferring to another care environment (e.g. a nursing or residential home) or receiving unsuitable care.
- Poor discharge planning from hospital may mean that patients have to stay in hospital longer or are re-admitted or recover less well.
- Discharge planning should take into account all the aspects of a comprehensive assessment (e.g. the physical, psychological, social, emotional, spiritual and cultural dimensions). It will also, for some people, be necessary to discuss economic and environmental factors e.g. housing, benefits, and return-to-work, alongside daily routines such as shopping and cooking during this process.
- Referral to members of the multi-disciplinary team for assessment should be made as soon as possible.
- Some patients may decide to discharge themselves from hospital against medical advice and this needs to be reported appropriately and recorded.
- Some people will have particular care needs following discharge from hospital or transfer between services. This group includes people who are elderly, who are dying, whose condition is unpredictable, who live alone, who require equipment they are not yet familiar with, those who are homeless or live in poor housing conditions and those with learning difficulties or ongoing health problems.

# Principles of effective discharge planning

1 The discharge plan is agreed in partnership with the patient, their family/carers and the multi-disciplinary team.

2 The patient and family/carers are fully informed of the plan and help shape it.

3 A named nurse/key worker is appointed to coordinate a patient's discharge from any healthcare service.

4 All relevant documents are updated and information is transferred to all appropriate services in time to ensure continuity of care is maintained.

5 Relevant services are introduced into the care package at the right time to ensure continuity of care.

6 The patient is discharged from care/transferred from one service to another as anticipated.

7 Success is monitored.

8 Deviations from the plan are identified and corrected.

## 24 Evaluation

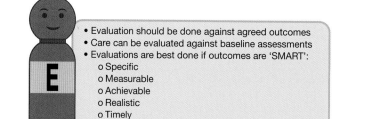

- Evaluation should be done against agreed outcomes
- Care can be evaluated against baseline assessments
- Evaluations are best done if outcomes are 'SMART':
  o Specific
  o Measurable
  o Achievable
  o Realistic
  o Timely

## Evaluation

- Evaluation is about judging how effective nursing has been.
- Evaluation and monitoring are closely linked.
- Evaluation is used here to refer to an assessment of a completed episode of care, whereas monitoring is seen as a continuous evaluative exercise which iterates with assessment.
- At a broad level, evaluation centres on determining if a patient's condition has improved, remained stable or deteriorated.
- At a more specific level, the achievement (or not) of each patient-centred goal set during the assessment process should be evaluated.
- Each goal should have an accompanying measurable outcome (e.g. the patient will walk 20 minutes each day) that can be evaluated.

- Understanding why a patient does not reach goals is important to planning future care both for the patient and others.
- Understanding what has helped a patient to reach goals, but was not part of the care plan, is also useful.
- A patient's and their family's/carer's satisfaction with care can also be evaluated.
- The results of evaluations should be recorded in the care plan or nursing notes and communicated to others in the multi-disciplinary team as required.
- Evaluations should be discussed within the nursing team or the multi-disciplinary team in order to improve care or celebrate successful care.

*Adult Nursing at a Glance*, First Edition. Andrée le May. © 2015 John Wiley & Sons, Ltd. Published 2015 by John Wiley & Sons, Ltd.
Companion website: www.ataglanceseries.com/nursing/adult

# 25 Research and service development

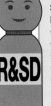

To do this effectively you need to be able to assess the rigour of research and its usefulness for practice.
Start by deciding if there is a good fit between the research question being answered in the study and your practice question.
If there is a good fit then assess how rigorously the research was conducted before deciding to use it by asking a few questions:
- Were the research design and methods appropriate for answering the research question?
- Were there enough participants in the study to justify the findings?
- Were threats to validity, reliability and credibility taken into account?
- Have the results been analysed appropriately?
- Do the results answer the research question?
- Are limitations clearly discussed?
- Are the conclusions based on the results and are they justified?

## Research and service development

Using research findings to underpin practice is important because it means:
- You can give the most up-to-date and appropriate research based care to patients and their families/carers.
- You can use research findings about working practices (e.g. how to communicate effectively in multi-disciplinary teams) to create environments within which the best care possible can be delivered.
- You can use research findings to justify decisions.
- You can use research findings to argue for better resources or different ways of doing things rather than relying on hunches or doing what has always been done.

- You can use research findings to improve the working environment and thereby improve care, as this environment impacts not only on the health and wellbeing of staff but also of patients and their families/carers.
- You can use research findings to help you to think differently and be more creative in your practice.
- You can use research findings to develop nursing services, in combination with identified service needs and good practice, as well as individual patient care.

Research findings melded with the views and experiences of patients and carers and staff are useful in the development of services.

Having a research base helps to improve nursing as a profession.

More information is available in Section 3.

*Adult Nursing at a Glance*, First Edition. Andrée le May. © 2015 John Wiley & Sons, Ltd. Published 2015 by John Wiley & Sons, Ltd.
Companion website: www.ataglanceseries.com/nursing/adult

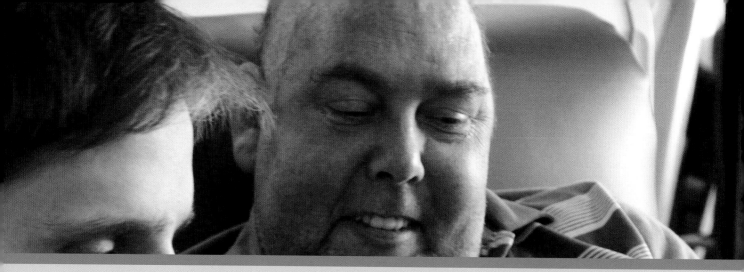

# Chapters

# Nursing people with common disorders

Don't forget to visit the companion website for this book at www.ataglanceseries.com/nursing/adult to do some practice MCQs on these topics.

# 26 Nursing people with cardiovascular disorders

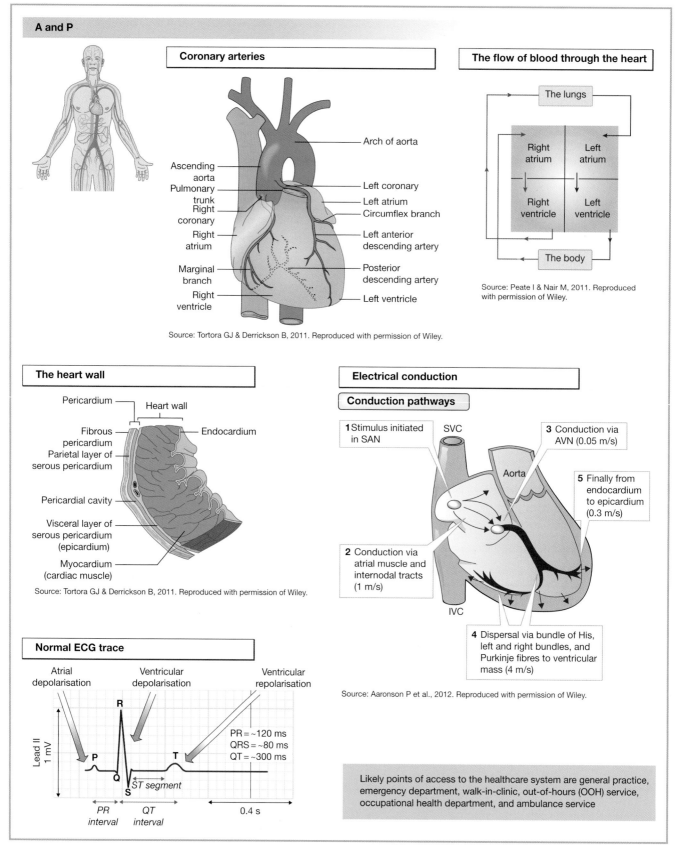

## A and P

### Coronary arteries

Arch of aorta
Ascending aorta
Pulmonary trunk
Right coronary
Right atrium
Marginal branch
Right ventricle

Left coronary
Left atrium
Circumflex branch
Left anterior descending artery
Posterior descending artery
Left ventricle

Source: Tortora GJ & Derrickson B, 2011. Reproduced with permission of Wiley.

### The flow of blood through the heart

The lungs

Right atrium — Left atrium
Right ventricle — Left ventricle

The body

Source: Peate I & Nair M, 2011. Reproduced with permission of Wiley.

### The heart wall

Pericardium
Heart wall
Fibrous pericardium
Parietal layer of serous pericardium
Pericardial cavity
Visceral layer of serous pericardium (epicardium)
Myocardium (cardiac muscle)
Endocardium

Source: Tortora GJ & Derrickson B, 2011. Reproduced with permission of Wiley.

### Electrical conduction

#### Conduction pathways

1 Stimulus initiated in SAN
SVC
3 Conduction via AVN (0.05 m/s)
Aorta
5 Finally from endocardium to epicardium (0.3 m/s)
2 Conduction via atrial muscle and internodal tracts (1 m/s)
IVC
4 Dispersal via bundle of His, left and right bundles, and Purkinje fibres to ventricular mass (4 m/s)

Source: Aaronson P et al., 2012. Reproduced with permission of Wiley.

### Normal ECG trace

Atrial depolarisation
Ventricular depolarisation
Ventricular repolarisation

R
P
Q
S
T
ST segment

PR = ~120 ms
QRS = ~80 ms
QT = ~300 ms

Lead II 1 mV

PR interval
QT interval
0.4 s

Likely points of access to the healthcare system are general practice, emergency department, walk-in-clinic, out-of-hours (OOH) service, occupational health department, and ambulance service

# Key facts

- The cardiovascular system comprises the heart and blood vessels.
- Disorders of the cardiovascular system can result in acute or chronic conditions.
- Disorders of this system are called cardiovascular disease (CVD).
- The main disorders of the heart are associated with blockage of the coronary arteries, heart muscle damage, altered electrical activity, valve disease or infection.
- The main disorders of the blood vessels result from atheroma, dysfunctional venous valves and aneurysm.
- Hypertension is an important contributor to several cardiovascular disorders.
- Over 80% of CVD deaths are in low- and middle-income countries (WHO, 2013).

# Common cardiovascular disorders

- Hypertension
- Coronary heart disease
- Acute coronary syndromes (unstable angina and heart attack)
- Chronic coronary syndromes
- Heart failure
- Valve diseases
- Arrhythmias
- Aneurysm
- Peripheral vascular disease.

Each is covered in the following pages.

# A and P

- The heart is a four-chambered organ situated between the lungs in the thoracic cavity.
- The heart is surrounded by the protective pericardium.
- The four chambers of the heart are the right and left ventricles and the right and left atria. The atria are smaller than the ventricles.
- The chambers work as two pumps – the right ventricle and right atrium (right heart pump) and the left ventricle and left atrium (left heart pump).
- The right pump receives deoxygenated blood from the body into the right atrium via the superior vena cava, the inferior vena cava and the coronary sinus. Blood flows through the tricuspid valve into the right ventricle. The right ventricle then pumps blood into the pulmonary circulatory system via the pulmonary arteries to the lungs.
- The left pump receives oxygenated blood from the lungs into the left atrium via four pulmonary veins. Blood flows through the bicuspid valves to the left ventricle and is then pumped via the aorta into the systemic circulatory system and the rest of the body.
- The right ventricle wall is thinner and less muscular than the left ventricle. Pumping blood into the pulmonary circulatory system requires less effort than pumping to the systemic circulatory system.

- The atria and ventricles are divided by a wall/septum to ensure that deoxygenated and oxygenated blood does not mix.
- The heart comprises specialised heart muscle known as the myocardium.
- The activity of the myocardium is controlled by a series of nerve cells that make up the conduction system of the heart. This conduction system ensures that the chambers contract and relax in the right sequence.
- The conduction system of the heart includes the sinoatrial node (SAN) (the pacemaker), the atrioventricular node (AVN) (controls delivery of the action potential to the ventricles) and Purkinje fibres which ensure the rapid transport of action potentials through the ventricle walls.
- The cardiac cycle refers to the heart's mechanical activity.
- Pressure changes during the cardiac cycle make the heart valves open and close so blood flows through the heart. Blood moves from higher pressure to lower pressure.
- Systole refers to the contraction of a heart chamber.
- Diastole refers to the relaxation of a heart chamber.
- Heart rate is controlled by hormones (adrenalin from the adrenal medulla and thyroxine from the thyroid gland) and the autonomic nervous system (via the cardiovascular centre in the medulla oblongata).
- Resting heart rate is influenced by fitness, age, gender and temperature.

# Essentials of best practice

Nursing someone with any cardiovascular disorder requires you to be aware of all of the essentials of best practice. These will be expanded for each of the disorders listed above in the subsequent pages.

Assessment of the cardiovascular system involves monitoring:

- Heart rate and pulse
- Blood pressure
- Skin colour and temperature
- Urine output
- Central venous pressure
- Mental state
- Respiratory function.

See Chapter 27 for more details.

## Patient information

There are several patient support groups and charities focusing on cardiovascular disorders. You can find most of them on the Self Help UK website www.self-help.org.uk.

Some useful ones are:

The British Heart Foundation www.bhf.org.uk.
The Arrhythmia Alliance www.arrhythmiaalliance.org.uk.
Cardiomyopathy Association www.cardiomyopathy.org.
You will also find very helpful patient-centred fact sheets at www.patient.co.uk/.

# 27 Signs, symptoms, assessment and emergencies

## Important assessments of cardiovascular system (based on Dougherty and Lister, 2011)

Assessment of the cardiovascular system involves monitoring:
- Pulse – count rate (normal range 55–90/min); feel rhythm (normally regular sequence) and amplitude (strength) for 60 seconds
- Apical beat – listen with stethoscope: compare rate with radial pulse in patients with atrial fibrillation
- Blood pressure (BP) – normal range 110–140 mmHg systolic/70–90 mmHg diastolic. Taken electronically or manually
- Electrocardiogram (ECG) – shows electrical activity of heart: 12 lead usually in hospital: ambulatory in community
- Pulse oximetry – electronic probe positioned on end of finger – gives pulse rate and oxygen saturation (normal 95–100%)
- Skin colour and condition (e.g. flushed, pallor, cyanosis: dry, cold, warm, sweaty, clammy)
- Central venous pressure (if appropriate)
- Respiratory function (Chapter 37): (the MRC Breathlessness Scale may be useful)
- Urine output
- Mental state: anxiety, level of confusion (incorrect responses to questions) or new disorientation related to self, time and/or place.
- Level of consciousness (the Glasgow Coma Scale may be used)
- Distress and fatigue

Find out more about the patient's lifestyle, e.g. diet, exercise, alcohol consumption and smoking

Find out more about their family history in relation to cardiovascular disease.

## Box 27 Medical Research Council (MRC) Dyspnoea Scale

| Grade | Degree of breathlessness related to activities |
|-------|-----------------------------------------------|
| 1 | Not troubled by breathlessness except on strenuous exercise |
| 2 | Short of breath when hurrying or walking up a slight hill |
| 3 | Walks slower than contemporaries on level ground because of breathlessness, or has to stop for breath when walking at own pace |
| 4 | Stops for breath after walking about 100 m or after a few minutes on level ground |
| 5 | Too breathless to leave the house, or breathless when dressing or undressing |

## Causes of shock

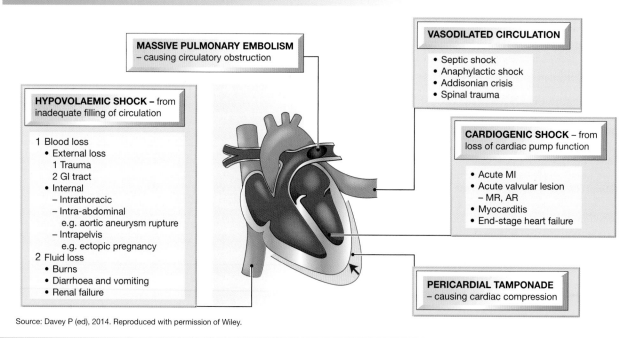

**MASSIVE PULMONARY EMBOLISM**
– causing circulatory obstruction

**VASODILATED CIRCULATION**
- Septic shock
- Anaphylactic shock
- Addisonian crisis
- Spinal trauma

**HYPOVOLAEMIC SHOCK –** from inadequate filling of circulation

1 Blood loss
- External loss
  1 Trauma
  2 GI tract
- Internal
  – Intrathoracic
  – Intra-abdominal
    e.g. aortic aneurysm rupture
  – Intrapelvis
    e.g. ectopic pregnancy
2 Fluid loss
- Burns
- Diarrhoea and vomiting
- Renal failure

**CARDIOGENIC SHOCK –** from loss of cardiac pump function
- Acute MI
- Acute valvular lesion
  – MR, AR
- Myocarditis
- End-stage heart failure

**PERICARDIAL TAMPONADE**
– causing cardiac compression

Source: Davey P (ed), 2014. Reproduced with permission of Wiley.

*Adult Nursing at a Glance*, First Edition. Andrée le May. © 2015 John Wiley & Sons, Ltd. Published 2015 by John Wiley & Sons, Ltd.
Companion website: www.ataglanceseries.com/nursing/adult

# Common signs and symptoms

There are a wide range of signs and symptoms related to cardiovascular disorders. They include:

- Pain/discomfort: localised in chest or radiating to, for example, neck, jaw, arm (usually left). Chest tightness.
- Pain in limbs due to claudication/peripheral ischaemia.
- Abdominal pain, nausea, vomiting.
- Dizziness (and fainting).
- Shortness of breath.
- Sweating/clammy skin.
- Cyanosis or pallor.
- Palpitations.
- Peripheral oedema.
- Tiredness, fatigue and exhaustion.
- Agitation.
- Confusion and disorientation (due to hypoxia).
- Fear (some people have feelings of impending doom).
- Altered heart rate, rhythm, BP.
- Pyrexia.

# Cardiovascular emergencies

Recognising and responding to sudden deteriorations in a patient's condition is vital. Two situations where rapid intervention can be life-saving are cardiac arrest and shock.

## Cardiac arrest is a medical emergency

The cardiac arrest may occur if there is, for example:

- myocardial infarction;
- left ventricular failure;
- shock;
- brain injury.

If a cardiac arrest occurs you will need to start basic life support (BLS) immediately (Section 1) and call for medical assistance or an emergency ambulance.

Cardiac arrest will be accompanied by respiratory arrest.

**Your knowledge of BLS should be regularly updated. You can find out the latest information by looking at the Resuscitation Council's website** www.resus.org.uk.

## Shock is a medical emergency

Shock shows itself by hypoperfusion and reduced tissue oxygenation. Reduced tissue oxygenation causes aerobic metabolism to change to anaerobic resulting in lactic acidosis or metabolic acidosis (serum pH decreased).

Shock is associated with multi-system failure and high mortality.

There are several different types of shock (cardiogenic, obstructive, distributive and hypovolaemic). All have consequences for the cardiovascular system.

Management varies depending on the type of shock but the aim of treatment is always to maximise perfusion of vital organs. People at risk of shock include those with:

- chest pain (or post-MI);
- cardiac arrhythmias;
- infections (including those acquired in hospital);
- multiple trauma;
- severe burns;
- haemorrhage (e.g. GI tract, post-operative or post-partum);
- multiple allergies (having tests with a contrast medium).

Common signs and symptoms of shock which nurses need to be aware of and act on immediately are:

- low systolic BP <90 mmHg;
- alterations to heart rate (e.g. rapid weak thready pulse in cardiogenic shock; bounding pulse in distributive shock);
- increased respiratory rate;
- cool (sweaty) skin;
- cyanosis;
- dizziness, agitation, lethargy;
- confusion;
- low urine output;
- obvious loss of blood (e.g. post-op, GI tract bleed);
- excessive diarrhoea or vomiting;
- pain (review analgesia);
- abnormal blood gases and electrolytes;
- unresponsive hypoglycaemia.

Check assessment against Early Warning System. Call for immediate help, stay with the patient and monitor closely.

Ongoing nursing care will depend largely on medical treatment and the patient's condition but will include:

✓ Accurate, frequent monitoring of vital signs (+ECG) and oxygen saturation
✓ Accurate monitoring of fluid intake and output
✓ Accurate assessment and monitoring of level of consciousness
✓ Accurate assessment, monitoring and treatment of pain
✓ Care of infusions and urinary catheter and infection control
✓ Administration of prescribed medications and oxygen
✓ Skilled, reassuring communication with the patient and their family and carers
✓ Rapid communication of deterioration to the medical team

# 28 Nursing people with hypertension

**Primary care**

**Prevalence:** 1 in 3 adults (2 in 3 people over 65)

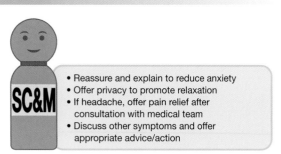

**A&M**
- Ensure BP recording devices checked and calibrated
- Monitor as directed in treatment plan – monthly, annually
- Make sure environment quiet
- Measure BP with patient seated and arm outstretched and supported
- Monitor co-morbidities e.g. kidney function (dip-test for protein in urine and haematuria)

**HE&P**
- Lifestyle advice can make all the difference
- Sometimes no medication is needed following alterations
- Review weight against height. Review calorie intake if overweight
- Review waist measurements (>94 cm (37 inches) in men: >80 cm (31 inches) in women = risk of CVD and hypertension)
- Review diet – increase fruit and vegetables (5-a-day): cut down salt (don't add to food and cut out processed food): reduce fat intake – switch to low fat
- Review exercise – encourage increase in brisk walking, cycling or dancing to 30 mins most days (make exercise part of usual routine, e.g. get off bus one stop earlier and walk the last bit of journey)
- Review smoking and alcohol consumption: cut down or cut out
- Cut down on caffeine
- Offer advice about local support groups

**Consequences of hypertension**

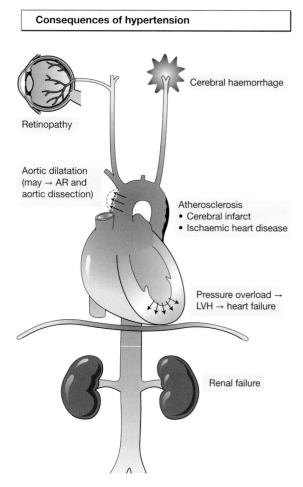

Retinopathy

Cerebral haemorrhage

Aortic dilatation (may → AR and aortic dissection)

Atherosclerosis
- Cerebral infarct
- Ischaemic heart disease

Pressure overload → LVH → heart failure

Renal failure

Source: Davey P (ed), 2014. Reproduced with permission of Wiley.

**Ward care**

**SC&M**
- Reassure and explain to reduce anxiety
- Offer privacy to promote relaxation
- If headache, offer pain relief after consultation with medical team
- Discuss other symptoms and offer appropriate advice/action

**A&M**
- Monitor for other symptoms
- Contact doctor if headache (or worsening headache), visual alteration, confusion – these may be early signs of cerebrovascular disease
- Review by doctor if systolic 180 or above

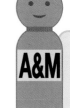

Likely points of access to the healthcare system are general practice, and walk-in-clinic

*Adult Nursing at a Glance*, First Edition. Andrée le May. © 2015 John Wiley & Sons, Ltd. Published 2015 by John Wiley & Sons, Ltd.
Companion website: www.ataglanceseries.com/nursing/adult

# Key facts

- Blood pressure (BP) is a measure of the force exerted by the blood on the blood vessel walls due to the contraction of the heart.
- BP = cardiac output (CO) x systemic vascular resistance (SVR)
- Normal BP ranges between 110–140 mmHg systolic and 70–85 mmHg diastolic.
- BP naturally increases with age and varies with emotion, positioning and other factors.
- Abnormal BP is described as hypotension (low BP – systolic <100 mmHg) or hypertension (high BP – sustained at higher than 140/90 mmHg).
- Hypertension can develop when artery walls lose elasticity and smaller blood vessels narrow.
- Hypertension can be divided into essential (primarily associated with genetic and lifestyle factors but no single known cause) and secondary hypertension (due to other identifiable causes, e.g. renal dysfunction).
- Hypertension is usually asymptomatic and picked up at a health check.
- Some people's BP is higher when measured by a health professional (white coat effect) due to anxiety.
- Hypertension is an important contributor to several cardiovascular disorders.
- Several lifestyle factors are associated with hypertension, for example being overweight, excess alcohol consumption, smoking, lack of exercise, high salt intake.
- Hypertension may run in families.
- Hypertension is treated with lifestyle changes and/or drugs.

# Effects of hypertension

- Cerebrovascular disease
- Vascular disease
- Left ventricular hypertrophy
- Renal failure
- Visual impairment due to retinal haemorrhage.

# A and P

Two readings are taken when measuring BP – systolic pressure and diastolic pressure. Systolic pressure is the pressure when the left ventricle contracts and the blood enters the aorta. Diastolic pressure is when the aortic valve closes and blood flows from the aorta to smaller vessels. Aortic pressure is at its lowest at this time and reflects the resistance of the blood vessels.

BP fluctuates during the day (diurnal variation) – usually being highest in the morning.

# Diagnosis

Usually 24-hour ambulatory monitoring of BP instigated by the GP.
Some people will record their BP at home and keep a diary.

# Associated screening tests

Blood – check cholesterol and other lipids.
Urine – check for protein/blood (kidney function).
ECG – heart function.

# At risk groups

- People over 65 years of age.
- People of African-Caribbean and South Asian origin.
- People with a family history.
- People who are obese.

# Essentials of best practice

Providing the right sort of nursing care for people with hypertension depends on the context within which they are being cared for. Most people will have their blood pressure monitored and stabilised at the GP's practice. This work will usually be carried out by the practice nurse and will largely entail

✓ Accurate assessments and regular monitoring
✓ Communication with the healthcare team, patient and family
✓ Risk assessment and management
✓ Health education and promotion
✓ Evaluation

When hypertension is extreme (>180/110 mmHg) or becomes hard to control, a person may be referred to a consultant physician and nursing care may then involve nurses working in the outpatient department (OPD) or on medical/surgical wards if the hypertension is secondary to another cause or a co-morbidity of another presenting illness. Nursing care in the OPD is likely to be similar to that provided by the practice nurse. If a patient's hypertension requires hospitalisation care may also need to focus on

✓ Symptom control and management
✓ Accurate assessments and regular monitoring
✓ Discharge planning

# Treatment

Lifestyle modification.
Drugs (e.g. ACE (angiotensin converting enzyme) inhibitors, beta blockers, angiotensin II antagonists, calcium-channel blocker, diuretics) depending on age and ethnic origin.

---

**Patient information**

British Hypertension Society www.bhsoc.org.
Blood Pressure Association www.bloodpressureuk.org.
British Heart Foundation www.bhf.org.uk.
You will also find very helpful patient-centred fact sheets at www.patient.co.uk/.

# 29 Nursing people with coronary heart disease (stable angina)

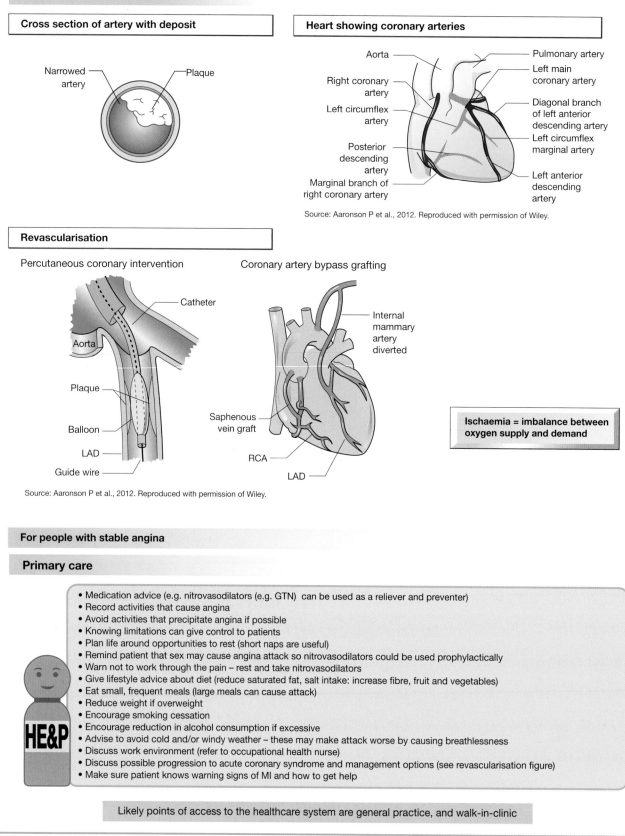

## A and P

### Cross section of artery with deposit

Narrowed artery

Plaque

### Heart showing coronary arteries

Aorta

Right coronary artery

Left circumflex artery

Posterior descending artery

Marginal branch of right coronary artery

Pulmonary artery

Left main coronary artery

Diagonal branch of left anterior descending artery

Left circumflex marginal artery

Left anterior descending artery

Source: Aaronson P et al., 2012. Reproduced with permission of Wiley.

## Revascularisation

### Percutaneous coronary intervention

Catheter

Aorta

Plaque

Balloon

LAD

Guide wire

### Coronary artery bypass grafting

Internal mammary artery diverted

Saphenous vein graft

RCA

LAD

Source: Aaronson P et al., 2012. Reproduced with permission of Wiley.

**Ischaemia = imbalance between oxygen supply and demand**

## For people with stable angina

### Primary care

HE&P

- Medication advice (e.g. nitrovasodilators (e.g. GTN) can be used as a reliever and preventer)
- Record activities that cause angina
- Avoid activities that precipitate angina if possible
- Knowing limitations can give control to patients
- Plan life around opportunities to rest (short naps are useful)
- Remind patient that sex may cause angina attack so nitrovasodilators could be used prophylactically
- Warn not to work through the pain – rest and take nitrovasodilators
- Give lifestyle advice about diet (reduce saturated fat, salt intake: increase fibre, fruit and vegetables)
- Eat small, frequent meals (large meals can cause attack)
- Reduce weight if overweight
- Encourage smoking cessation
- Encourage reduction in alcohol consumption if excessive
- Advise to avoid cold and/or windy weather – these may make attack worse by causing breathlessness
- Discuss work environment (refer to occupational health nurse)
- Discuss possible progression to acute coronary syndrome and management options (see revascularisation figure)
- Make sure patient knows warning signs of MI and how to get help

Likely points of access to the healthcare system are general practice, and walk-in-clinic

*Adult Nursing at a Glance*, First Edition. Andrée le May. © 2015 John Wiley & Sons, Ltd. Published 2015 by John Wiley & Sons, Ltd.
Companion website: www.ataglanceseries.com/nursing/adult

# Key facts

- The coronary arteries provide the heart with important nutrients and oxygen to enable effective pumping.
- Coronary Heart Disease (CHD) is a collective name for diseases affecting the health of the heart muscle.
- CHD is linked to coronary atherosclerosis (narrowing of the blood vessels' lumen due to the accumulation of atheroma) and resultant ischaemia or infarction.
- If a piece of atheroma breaks away from the artery wall a blood clot forms around it leading to blockage of a coronary artery. This causes damage to the myocardium as nutrients and oxygen cannot reach the heart muscle.
- Having CHD can increase your chances of having a heart attack (myocardial infarction (MI)).
- Angina and MI are the most common presentations of symptomatic CHD. Symptomatic CHD can be described as a spectrum with stable angina (exertional) at the less severe end and MI at the most severe.
- CHD is a significant cause of death in men and women: 1 in 5 deaths in men: 1 in 7 deaths in women.
- Unstable angina and heart attacks are also referred to as Acute Coronary Syndrome (ACS).

# Risk factors

- High blood pressure
- High blood cholesterol levels
- Family history of CHD
- Smoking
- Physical inactivity
- Overweight
- Poor diet – high in fat and low in fibre
- Excessive alcohol consumption
- Diabetes.

# Angina

- Angina occurs when the coronary arteries are narrowed by atheroma, meaning that insufficient blood reaches the heart muscle when any extra effort is needed for example for greater activity than normal.
- Angina presents as episodic chest pain or discomfort which may spread to the arms, left shoulder, neck, jaw and sometimes stomach.
- Angina can occur on exertion, on a cold day, after food or if the patient is upset.

- Angina pain is usually relieved after a few minutes by rest or taking nitrovasodilators (e.g. glycerine trinitrate (GTN) tablet or spray under tongue).
- Pharmacological management may include β-blockers or calcium-channel blockers (CCB) coupled with short acting nitrovasodilators.
- Long-term management may require revascularisation, for example a stent or coronary artery bypass graft (CABG).
- Angina can be stable, variant or unstable.
- Stable angina is predictable and controlled with drugs.
- Variant angina is uncommon: caused by severe occlusive spasm of one or more coronary artery.
- Unstable angina is when symptoms first develop and there is uncertainty about differentiating between angina and MI, when stable angina worsens or changes from its usual pattern and/or when treatment is not effective.
- Unstable angina is part of ACS.
- Angina is diagnosed by considering the history of symptoms and their relief, blood tests for cholesterol, ECGs and exercise ECGs as well as other invasive cardiac tests, for example coronary angiography.

# Essentials of best practice

Providing the right sort of nursing care for people with CHD depends on the severity of their presenting symptoms and their diagnosis. For people with stable angina the practice nurse will largely be responsible for:

✓ Accurate assessments and regular monitoring
✓ Communication with the healthcare team, patient and family
✓ Risk assessment and management
✓ Symptom control and management
✓ Health education and promotion
✓ Evaluation

For people who are more seriously ill with unstable angina or an MI, specialist nursing care in either a coronary care unit or cardiology ward will be necessary.

## Patient information

British Heart Foundation www.bhf.org.uk.
You will also find very helpful patient-centred fact sheets at www.patient.co.uk/.

# 30 Nursing people with CHD (acute coronary syndromes)

## CCU care for patient admitted with ACS

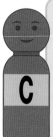

**A&M**

- Most life threatening problems occur in the first 48 hours after admission, so careful assessment and monitoring in CCU is required
- Assess pain levels, nausea and anxiety: give medications/oxygen as prescribed and monitor effects
- Aim to keep patient pain free (nausea may be a side effect of diamorphine)
- Assess level of knowledge about condition
- Explain interventions, equipment and plans and reassure
- ECG monitoring will be continuous in early phase to detect worsening MI or arrhythmia: report changes
- Observe for signs of cardiac failure and report changes
    - o increased heart rate (NB: pain may also cause tachycardia)
    - o fall in blood pressure
    - o decreasing blood oxygen saturation
    - o restlessness
    - o breathlessness
    - o falling pulse pressure
- Monitor IVI, fluid intake and output (NB: renal function and cardiac output are related: low urine output could be sign of cardiogenic shock)
- Monitor bowel movements and prevent constipation – extra straining will result in extra work for heart
- Monitor temperature. May be elevated for first 48 hours. Prolonged elevation may be linked to pericarditis
- Assess extent to which patient needs help with activities of daily living: in acute phase discourage exertion and promote rest – confine to bed/bed area
- As recovery progresses determine with patient suitable activity levels and monitor effects of resumption of activity
- Liaise with ward to ensure smooth transfer when patient's condition is stable

## Ward care for patient transferred from CCU with ACS

**C**

- Reassure patient following admission to ward as move from CCU may cause anxiety
- Explain immediate danger is over and make time to discuss patient's and family's/friend's fears and feelings about ACS
- Answer questions honestly – or refer to someone who can have a more informed conversation (doctor, chaplain, more senior nurse/specialist nurse)
- Always use easily understood explanations and where appropriate give leaflets to support information
- Give patient information about patient and self-help groups (e.g. British Heart Foundation)

**DP**

- Make sure cardiac rehabilitation programme is arranged and patient and family know about this
- Get rehabilitation nurse/coordinator/specialist nurse to visit prior to discharge to discuss immediate recommended activity levels at home
- Ensure medications required at home are ready: explain how to use them
- Check discharge letters are written and sent appropriately
- Check patient and family know how to get advice in emergency
- Remind the patient to discuss condition with GP, practice nurse and, if appropriate, occupational health nurse/doctor

- Talk about patient's and family's concerns and tailor advice to suit their needs
- Explain rehabilitation plans during ward stay and following discharge – gentle build-up of activity alternating with rest
- Talk about resuming usual activities following discharge home (e.g. exercise and sex)
- Reassure patient that angina and shortness of breath may occur after discharge
- Explain use of rest and nitrovasodilators for angina
- Give advice about stopping smoking and diet modification
- Advise patient and family that some people feel depressed or anxious after MI and suggest early appointment with GP if this is the case
- Discuss cardiac rehabilitation programmes and check patient is referred (programmes provide advice about e.g. activity levels and lifestyle modification, psychological support and staged exercise programmes)

**HE&P**

### ECG trace typical of myocardial infarction

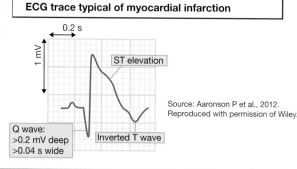

0.2 s

1 mV

ST elevation

Q wave:
>0.2 mV deep
>0.04 s wide

Inverted T wave

Source: Aaronson P et al., 2012.
Reproduced with permission of Wiley.

Likely points of access to the healthcare system are general practice, out-of-hours (OOH) service, emergency department, and ambulance service

*Adult Nursing at a Glance*, First Edition. Andrée le May. © 2015 John Wiley & Sons, Ltd. Published 2015 by John Wiley & Sons, Ltd.
Companion website: www.ataglanceseries.com/nursing/adult

# Key facts

- Unstable angina (UA) and heart attacks (myocardial infarctions (MI)) are referred to as Acute Coronary Syndromes (ACS) and are medical emergencies.
- Their common pathology is sudden total/near total blockage of a coronary vessel usually due to atherosclerotic plaque rupture leading to an intracoronary thrombus. (See Chapter 26 for Coronary artery diagram.)
- The blockage may be episodic or transient (UA) or complete resulting in reduced blood flow or complete blockage and the death of some of the myocardium (MI).
- Presentation and treatment depends on where the blockage is and whether it is complete or partial.
- MIs are either ST elevation myocardial infarctions (STEMI) or non-ST segment elevation myocardial infarctions (NSTEMI). Both are acute MIs but managed differently.
- STEMI = sustained elevation of the ST segments of ECG indicating a large area of myocardium death (probably full thickness of ventricular wall). Elevated troponins (troponins are proteins found in heart muscle: damage causes specific troponins to leak out into the blood stream).
- NSTEMI = less myocardial damage so may not cause ST elevation but elevated troponins present. May be other ECG changes, for example ST depression or T-wave inversion.
- UA = ACS symptoms but no ST elevation/raised troponins.
- UA results in ischaemia but no destruction of myocardium.
- ECG changes other than ST elevation may be present.
- MIs can occur in people with or without a history of angina.
- Accurate diagnosis is essential for correct management.
- MI is managed within a coronary care unit/ cardiology ward.

# Common signs and symptoms of MI

- Pain usually at rest: unrelieved by nitrovasodilators.
- Pain is continuous and lasts longer than 15 minutes.
- Pain described as crushing, tight or constricting.
- Pain may radiate to arms and neck.
- Rarely pain only in the neck and jaw: sometimes no pain at all.
- Fear.
- Sometimes shortness of breath.
- Change in heart rate (usually tachycardia), rhythm and BP.
- Change in level of consciousness.
- Pallor and/or sweaty or clammy skin.
- Nausea and vomiting.
- Cyanosis.

# Diagnosis and medical management

- Diagnosis is made by examination, history taking, 12-lead ECGs to identify STEMI/ NSTEMI /UA, blood tests to assess myocardial damage (e.g. troponins T and I).
- In the acute phase management focuses on symptom control (pain relief usually with diamorphine, anti-emetics to reduce nausea and oxygen if hypoxic), improving blood flow to the heart and reducing demand for oxygen by rest and drug therapy.

- STEMI treatment focuses on reperfusion/revascularisation either pharmacological (thrombolysis) or by Percutaneous Coronary Intervention (PCI) (balloon catheter passed into coronary artery, balloon inflated to open narrowed vessel, stent inserted).
- NSTEMI and UA treated pharmacologically, for example antiplatelet therapy (e.g. aspirin), anti-thrombin therapy (e.g. low molecular weight heparin). β-blockers and nitrates may be used. Both conditions can progress to STEMI.
- Following the acute phase attention focuses on education, rehabilitation and secondary prevention (e.g. long-term aspirin and statin use) and cardiac interventions (e.g. revascularisation).

# Risk factors

- High blood pressure
- High blood cholesterol levels
- Family history of CHD
- Smoking
- Physical inactivity
- Overweight
- Poor diet – high in fat and low in fibre
- Excessive alcohol consumption
- Diabetes.

# Essentials of best practice

Providing highly skilled nursing care for people with MI is critical to their recovery. Many different nurses may be involved in a person's care pathway depending on where the patient presents with symptoms (e.g. practice nurses, occupational health nurses, nurses working in walk-in clinics and emergency departments). Practice nurses and occupational health nurses may be the first people consulted in the early stages of MI when assessment, reassurance and rapid referral to the ED are essential. They may also be responsible for ongoing monitoring and health education and promotion once the patient is discharged from hospital. Once admitted to hospital – either to a coronary care unit or cardiology ward, nursing care will entail:

✓ Accurate assessments and regular monitoring
✓ Symptom control and management
✓ Communication with the healthcare team, patient and family
✓ Risk assessment and management
✓ Health education and promotion
✓ Evaluation
✓ Discharge planning

# Complications

Cardiac arrest, arrhythmias, hypoxia, cardiogenic shock, emboli.

---

**Patient information**

British Heart Foundation www.bhf.org.uk.
You will also find very helpful patient-centred fact sheets at www.patient.co.uk/.

# 31 Nursing people with arrhythmias

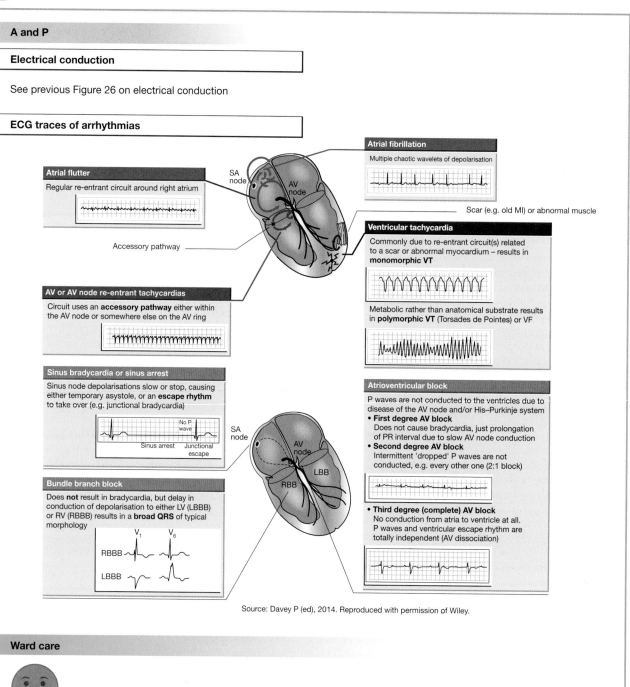

## A and P

### Electrical conduction

See previous Figure 26 on electrical conduction

### ECG traces of arrhythmias

**Atrial flutter**
Regular re-entrant circuit around right atrium

**Atrial fibrillation**
Multiple chaotic wavelets of depolarisation

Scar (e.g. old MI) or abnormal muscle

Accessory pathway

**AV or AV node re-entrant tachycardias**
Circuit uses an **accessory pathway** either within the AV node or somewhere else on the AV ring

**Ventricular tachycardia**
Commonly due to re-entrant circuit(s) related to a scar or abnormal myocardium – results in **monomorphic VT**

Metabolic rather than anatomical substrate results in **polymorphic VT** (Torsades de Pointes) or VF

**Sinus bradycardia or sinus arrest**
Sinus node depolarisations slow or stop, causing either temporary asystole, or an **escape rhythm** to take over (e.g. junctional bradycardia)

No P wave

Sinus arrest  Junctional escape

**Atrioventricular block**
P waves are not conducted to the ventricles due to disease of the AV node and/or His–Purkinje system
- **First degree AV block**
  Does not cause bradycardia, just prolongation of PR interval due to slow AV node conduction
- **Second degree AV block**
  Intermittent 'dropped' P waves are not conducted, e.g. every other one (2:1 block)

**Bundle branch block**
Does **not** result in bradycardia, but delay in conduction of depolarisation to either LV (LBBB) or RV (RBBB) results in a **broad QRS** of typical morphology

RBBB

LBBB

- **Third degree (complete) AV block**
  No conduction from atria to ventricle at all. P waves and ventricular escape rhythm are totally independent (AV dissociation)

Source: Davey P (ed), 2014. Reproduced with permission of Wiley.

## Ward care

**A&M**
- Observe patient's condition and monitor symptoms: report deteriorations
- Monitor ECG: report arrhythmias and any alterations
- Assess patient's knowledge of condition and provide appropriate information
- Provide reassurance and explanation about medical interventions
- Monitor pulse and BP to assess cardiac output
- Assess impact on family, keep them informed of management and answer questions

Likely points of access to the healthcare system are general practice, out-of-hours (OOH) service, emergency department, and ambulance service

*Adult Nursing at a Glance*, First Edition. Andrée le May. © 2015 John Wiley & Sons, Ltd. Published 2015 by John Wiley & Sons, Ltd.
Companion website: www.ataglanceseries.com/nursing/adult

## Key facts

- Normal heart rhythm is called sinus rhythm. The normal number of heart beats in sinus rhythm is between 60 and 100 at rest. If this regular rhythm is greater than 100 it is sinus tachycardia: if slower than 60 it is sinus bradycardia.
- Arrhythmias are abnormal heart beats caused by irregularities in the electrical conduction system of the heart. They cause an irregular pulse. They can be seen on ECG tracings as disturbance in the usual PQRST wave.
- Arrhythmias can cause alterations in heart rate, myocardial oxygen requirement and blood flow.
- Arrhythmias can either be fast (tachyarrhythmia) or slow (bradyarrhythmia).
- Tachyarrhythmias include atrial flutter, atrial fibrillation, ventricular tachycardia and ventricular fibrillation.
- Bradyarrhythmias include sinus bradycardia or sinus arrest, bundle branch block and atrioventricular block.
- Minor arrhythmias are common and usually unproblematic. Sometimes these are due to extra (ectopic) heart beats followed by a slight pause before the next beat. People might feel this as a palpitation.
- Sometimes people confuse palpitations with arrhythmias. Palpitations are when a person is aware of their heart beating rather than its rhythm. Palpitations are not always associated with changes in heart rhythm and not felt in bradyarrhythmias.
- Some arrhythmias can compromise cardiac function and cause sudden death such as ventricular tachycardia or ventricular fibrillation.
- Although serious arrhythmias can be asymptomatic, patients often experience arrhythmias as dizziness, feeling faint or fainting (syncope), shortness of breath, chest pain, headache, or being unable to sustain usual levels of activity.

## Diagnosis

- Physical examination
- History taking
- 12-lead ECGs.

## Essentials of best practice

A patient may develop an arrhythmia whilst in hospital or be admitted with one. Every nurse should be able to recognise a normal ECG pattern and deviation from it. The consequences of arrhythmias vary and often one arrhythmia can progress to a more serious type – for example atrial flutter to atrial fibrillation or ventricular tachycardia to ventricular fibrillation – so careful assessment and monitoring of ECGs is vital together with close observation for symptoms (see Appendix).

Nursing care centres on monitoring the patient's condition, their response to treatment of the arrhythmia and any underlying conditions such as CHD. Nursing care will largely focus on

- ✓ Accurate assessments and regular monitoring
- ✓ Communication with the healthcare team, patient and family
- ✓ Risk assessment and management
- ✓ Health education and promotion
- ✓ Evaluation
- ✓ Discharge planning

## Complications

Cardiac arrest, emboli depending on arrhythmia.

---

**Patient information**

British Heart Foundation www.bhf.org.uk.
You will also find very helpful patient-centred fact sheets at www.patient.co.uk/.

---

# 32 Nursing people with valve disease

## A and P

### Heart and valves

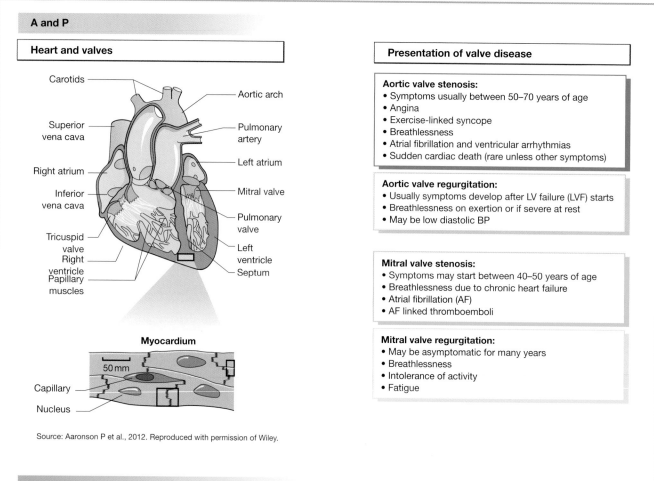

- Carotids
- Aortic arch
- Superior vena cava
- Pulmonary artery
- Left atrium
- Right atrium
- Mitral valve
- Inferior vena cava
- Pulmonary valve
- Tricuspid valve
- Left ventricle
- Right ventricle
- Septum
- Papillary muscles

**Myocardium**

- 50 mm
- Capillary
- Nucleus

Source: Aaronson P et al., 2012. Reproduced with permission of Wiley.

### Presentation of valve disease

**Aortic valve stenosis:**
- Symptoms usually between 50–70 years of age
- Angina
- Exercise-linked syncope
- Breathlessness
- Atrial fibrillation and ventricular arrhythmias
- Sudden cardiac death (rare unless other symptoms)

**Aortic valve regurgitation:**
- Usually symptoms develop after LV failure (LVF) starts
- Breathlessness on exertion or if severe at rest
- May be low diastolic BP

**Mitral valve stenosis:**
- Symptoms may start between 40–50 years of age
- Breathlessness due to chronic heart failure
- Atrial fibrillation (AF)
- AF linked thromboemboli

**Mitral valve regurgitation:**
- May be asymptomatic for many years
- Breathlessness
- Intolerance of activity
- Fatigue

## Ward care

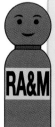

- Patients may be admitted to the ward feeling very breathless and frightened: ensure patients can be seen by and can call nurses
- Nutritional status may be compromised: assess risk of malnourishment and consult dietician: nutritional state should be improved if possible before surgery
- Tiredness may be problematic because of interrupted sleep due to breathlessness: discuss positioning and napping
- Activity may be restricted due to breathlessness: risk of VTE so encourage passive leg exercises and deep breathing
- After surgery strenuous exercise and driving should be avoided until the sternum heals
- Discuss return to work: determine likely risks and refer to occupational health nurse or GP
- Discuss care of replacement valve: if mechanical valve anticoagulation is necessary and needs monitoring
- If anti-coagulants prescribed advise about food interactions, e.g. grapefruit
- Discuss the need to tell dentists and other doctors about valve replacement and possible prophylactic antibiotics
- Discuss activity levels and sex: remember to remind patient to avoid putting strain on sternum

Likely points of access to the healthcare system are general practice, out-of-hours (OOH) service, emergency department, and ambulance service

*Adult Nursing at a Glance*, First Edition. Andrée le May. © 2015 John Wiley & Sons, Ltd. Published 2015 by John Wiley & Sons, Ltd.
Companion website: www.ataglanceseries.com/nursing/adult

# Key facts

- The heart valves can malfunction.
- Most commonly problems affect the aortic and mitral valves.
- Valve disease can be grouped into incompetence/regurgitation or stenosis.
- Regurgitation is when the valve cannot close properly (i.e. is incompetent) and there is leakage behind the valve. This occurs commonly in the aortic and mitral valves. It is rare to find this in the tricuspid and pulmonary valves.
- Stenosis is when the valves become stiffened and the cusps fuse together so the opening of the valve is narrowed. This narrowing (stenosis) means that there is backflow through the valve into the heart chamber that expelled the blood. This may occur in the tricuspid, mitral or aortic valves.
- Regurgitation is commonly linked to age-related degeneration, infective endocarditis, inflammatory diseases (e.g. systemic lupus erythematosus (SLE), rheumatoid arthritis and ankylosing spondylitis) and CHD.
- Stenosis may be a result of childhood rheumatic fever, particularly in the mitral valve, and age-related degeneration in the aortic valve. Congenital valve problems may also cause stenosis.
- Aortic stenosis and aortic regurgitation mean that the left ventricle has to work harder to pump blood out of the heart and this causes left ventricular (LV) hypertrophy. LV hypertrophy can eventually lead to myocardial dysfunction, arrhythmias and heart failure.
- Mitral valve stenosis is almost entirely related to childhood rheumatic fever; another cause may be SLE.
- Mitral valve regurgitation can be caused by mitral valve stenosis or by stretching the valve ring when LV is dilated as it is in left heart failure.
- Mitral valve disease can lead to heart failure.

# A and P

- The heart consists of four chambers – the atria and the ventricles. Blood enters and leaves each chamber of the heart through separate one-way valves, which open and close reciprocally (i.e. one closes before the other opens) to ensure that the flow of blood is in one direction only.
- Two sets of valves are responsible for doing this: the atrioventricular (AV) valves and the semi-lunar valves.
- There are two AV valves: the tricuspid valve (three cusps) and the bicuspid (two cusps) or mitral valve.
- The tricuspid valve lies between the right atrium and right ventricle. The bicuspid/mitral valve lies between the left atrium and left ventricle.
- There are also two other important valves – the semi-lunar valves. These are the aortic valve and the pulmonary valve. They have three cusps each. The aortic valve is between the aorta and the left ventricle. The pulmonary valve is between the pulmonary artery and the right ventricle. These valves are important in maintaining the one way circulation of blood between the heart and the lungs and the heart and the body.
- Blood leaves the left ventricle through the aortic valve into the aorta.
- Blood leaves the right ventricle for the lungs through the pulmonary valve into the pulmonary artery.

# Diagnosis

- Physical examination
- History taking
- Echocardiogram
- ECG
- Chest x-ray.

# Treatment

Usually surgical replacement of the dysfunctional valve either with a mechanical or biological valve. Pharmacological control may be considered (e.g. diuretics, Angiotensin-Converting Enzyme (ACE) inhibitors).

# Essentials of best practice

Nursing care centres on supporting the person and their family through surgical replacement of the valve or other invasive procedures, carefully monitoring their post-intervention condition as you would do for anyone who has had surgery and providing them with sound advice about their recovery and cardiac rehabilitation. Although people may present with symptoms of valve disease in primary care their main interactions with nurses are likely to be in hospital. Nursing care will largely focus on:

✓ Accurate assessments and regular monitoring
✓ Communication with the healthcare team, patient and family
✓ Risk assessment and management
✓ Health education and promotion
✓ Evaluation
✓ Discharge planning

# Complications

Cardiac arrest, emboli related to arrhythmia, heart failure.

---

**Patient information**

British Heart Foundation www.bhf.org.uk.
You will also find very helpful patient-centred fact sheets at www.patient.co.uk/.

# 33 Nursing people with heart failure

## Underlying causes of heart failure

| Primary defect | Examples |
| --- | --- |
| Myocardial dysfunction | Ischaemic heart disease, Diabetes mellitus Pregnancy, congenital cardiomyopathies Myocardial disease e.g. amyloidosis |
| Volume overload | Aortic or mitral valve regurgitation |
| Pressure overload | Aortic stenosis, hypertension |

| Primary defect | Examples |
| --- | --- |
| Impaired filling | Reduced ventricular compliance: hypertension, hypertrophy, fibrosis Constrictive pericarditis: rheumatic heart disease Cardiac tamponade: excess fluid pressure in pericardial space |
| Arrhythmias | Atrial fibrillation |
| High output | Thyrotoxicosis, arteriovenous shunts, anaemia |

Source: Aaronson P et al., 2012. Reproduced with permission of Wiley.

## Primary care

**A&M**

- Discuss symptoms and draw up individualised plan to minimise them: consider fatigue reduction, reducing breathlessness, enhancing nutritional status (use MUST scale or similar), mobility and associated restrictions on activities of daily living
- Discuss and monitor medication regime, side-effects and adherence: consider using daily dose pill box and encourage reminders from relatives/friends if forgetful
- Monitor effectiveness of plan either by re-visit or telephone or email
- Check for pressure ulcers and red areas: give advice about pressure relief: refer to OT for equipment or community nurses
- Give the patient the contact details of local charities to help with equipment borrowing (e.g. wheelchairs, commodes) and transport
- Remind person about passive exercises and deep breathing: discuss frequency and need for help with leg exercises
- Refer to specialist community HF team if available
- Consider referral to specialised exercise programme (and associated support)
- Make sure you have an up-to-date weight in order to assess changing fluid retention and nutritional status
- Monitor heart rate and rhythm and ankle oedema regularly and report alterations or general deterioration of condition to GP

**C**

- Accurate assessment and monitoring requires clear and simple communication which is also reassuring
- Supplement verbal communication with written information
- Make sure that the patient knows how to get in touch with you
- Consider getting the patient to write a symptom diary to discuss at their next visit
- If you suspect depression, discuss this and make a referral to the GP
- Try to put patients and their families in touch with support groups to provide psychological, practical and social support
- Make sure immediate healthcare team is aware of condition and plans for care
- Refer for expert advice and support from multi-disciplinary heart failure team

## Ward care

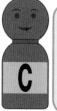

**A&M**

- Monitor levels of breathlessness and associated respiratory distress: give medication and oxygen as prescribed and monitor effect
- Stay near patient and explain care and anticipated effects of care
- Position patient in bed or upright chair to ease breathlessness and promote comfort
- Monitor pulse, blood pressure and respiratory rate
- Monitor fluid intake (may be restricted) and output (commode or urinal near bed): be alert to diminishing urine output
- Monitor sputum quantity and characteristics (e.g. frothy): apply nasopharyngeal suction if necessary
- Advise about sleeping sitting up and adjust pillows accordingly or find suitable chair to sleep in: discuss napping and sleep habits
- Assess and monitor nutritional status (use MUST scale or equivalent) and refer to dietician if necessary
- Weigh every day, at the same time and on the same scales and record: report alterations
- Avoid constipation – aperients may be needed due to restricted fluids and also poor nutritional intake
- Reduce activity levels but ensure passive exercises and deep breathing encouraged because of risk of emboli

Likely points of access to the healthcare system are general practice, out-of-hours (OOH) service, emergency department, and ambulance service

*Adult Nursing at a Glance*, First Edition. Andrée le May. © 2015 John Wiley & Sons, Ltd. Published 2015 by John Wiley & Sons, Ltd.
Companion website: www.ataglanceseries.com/nursing/adult

# Key facts

- Heart failure (HF) is a serious, potentially fatal, clinical syndrome which impacts on multiple systems.
- HF results from the inability to maintain adequate cardiac output.
- HF can have many different causes but always manifests in the same pathophysiology, signs and symptoms.
- HF can be acute or chronic. Acute HF is a sudden loss of cardiac function, for example secondary to ACS, causing pulmonary oedema and cardiogenic shock: can resolve with treatment.
- When HF is a long-term condition, management rather than cure is the objective of care.
- Chronic heart failure (CHF) is complex and progressive: CHF is due to insufficient cardiac output to meet demands of the body.
- Chronic heart failure is a common problem for older people accounting for at least 5% of admissions to medical and elderly care wards.
- People living with heart failure are likely to frequently visit their GP so much care is provided in primary care.

# A and P

- A common cause of HF is impaired ventricular contraction, for example due to damaged myocardium. HF can involve either ventricle by itself or both.
- Left heart failure (LHF) results in the build-up of blood returning from the lungs in the left ventricle and atrium and congestion of the lungs. This causes breathlessness (which worsens when lying down), fatigue and an enlarged heart.
- Right heart failure (RHF) means that de-oxygenated blood from the body (systemic) cannot efficiently be pumped to the lungs. This causes congestion in the systemic circulatory system resulting in fluid retention in the legs (oedema) and, if severe, ascites.
- RHF may be because of lung problems, embolism or valve disease but most likely because of the presence of LHF.

# Diagnosis

- Physical examination
- History taking
- Echocardiogram
- ECG
- Chest x-ray.

# Treatment

Treat underlying cause and any arrhythmias.
Dietary restrictions.
Pharmacological: e.g. diuretics, ACE inhibitors, Angiotensin II receptor antagonists, digoxin.

# Essentials of best practice

Chronic heart failure is extremely debilitating and frightening. Since it impacts on many systems you might expect patients to experience a range of symptoms including some of the following: breathlessness and copious frothy sputum, ascites, anorexia, nausea, constipation, oedema (ankle and sacrum), disorientation, fatigue, poor wound healing and risk of pressure ulcers, diminished urinary output, cyanosis and cold feet and hands. Nursing largely focuses on the management of medications and addressing symptoms in line with the patient's wishes.

Although people may be admitted to hospital with varying degrees of heart failure much of the care for those with HF is undertaken in primary care. Nursing care will largely focus on:
✓ Accurate assessments and regular monitoring
✓ Communication with the healthcare team, patient and family
✓ Health education and promotion
✓ Symptom control and management

# Complications

- Thromboembolism (DVT and PE)
- Atrial fibrillation
- Ventricular arrhythmias (syncope and sudden death)
- Progressive pump failure requiring heart transplantation.

## Patient information

British Heart Foundation www.bhf.org.uk.
You will also find very helpful patient-centred fact sheets at www.patient.co.uk/.

# 34 Nursing people with aneurysms

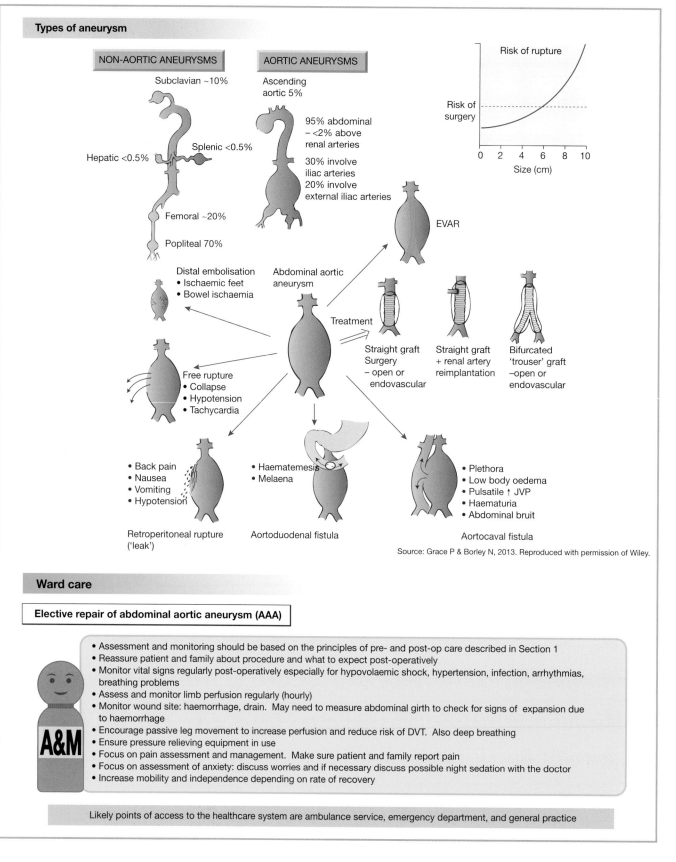

## Types of aneurysm

**NON-AORTIC ANEURYSMS**

Subclavian ~10%

Hepatic <0.5%

Splenic <0.5%

Femoral ~20%

Popliteal 70%

**AORTIC ANEURYSMS**

Ascending aortic 5%

95% abdominal – <2% above renal arteries

30% involve iliac arteries
20% involve external iliac arteries

Risk of rupture

Risk of surgery

Size (cm)

Distal embolisation
• Ischaemic feet
• Bowel ischaemia

Abdominal aortic aneurysm

EVAR

Treatment

Straight graft Surgery – open or endovascular

Straight graft + renal artery reimplantation

Bifurcated 'trouser' graft –open or endovascular

Free rupture
• Collapse
• Hypotension
• Tachycardia

• Back pain
• Nausea
• Vomiting
• Hypotension

Retroperitoneal rupture ('leak')

• Haematemesis
• Melaena

Aortoduodenal fistula

• Plethora
• Low body oedema
• Pulsatile ↑ JVP
• Haematuria
• Abdominal bruit

Aortocaval fistula

Source: Grace P & Borley N, 2013. Reproduced with permission of Wiley.

## Ward care

### Elective repair of abdominal aortic aneurysm (AAA)

**A&M**

• Assessment and monitoring should be based on the principles of pre- and post-op care described in Section 1
• Reassure patient and family about procedure and what to expect post-operatively
• Monitor vital signs regularly post-operatively especially for hypovolaemic shock, hypertension, infection, arrhythmias, breathing problems
• Assess and monitor limb perfusion regularly (hourly)
• Monitor wound site: haemorrhage, drain.  May need to measure abdominal girth to check for signs of expansion due to haemorrhage
• Encourage passive leg movement to increase perfusion and reduce risk of DVT.  Also deep breathing
• Ensure pressure relieving equipment in use
• Focus on pain assessment and management.  Make sure patient and family report pain
• Focus on assessment of anxiety: discuss worries and if necessary discuss possible night sedation with the doctor
• Increase mobility and independence depending on rate of recovery

Likely points of access to the healthcare system are ambulance service, emergency department, and general practice

*Adult Nursing at a Glance*, First Edition. Andrée le May. © 2015 John Wiley & Sons, Ltd. Published 2015 by John Wiley & Sons, Ltd.
Companion website: www.ataglanceseries.com/nursing/adult

# Key facts

- An aneurysm is a permanent local dilatation of an artery.
- The affected artery may be 1.5 times its normal diameter.
- Aneurysms can occur in the abdominal aorta, and the iliac, femoral and popliteal arteries. Cerebral and thoracic aneurysms are less common.
- Abdominal aortic aneurysms (AAA) are the most common.
- AAA screening can be done by ultrasound.
- AAA is more common in men than women.
- AAA screening is available to men over 65.
- AAA may be present if there are other vascular diseases.
- If AAA is present then careful monitoring is needed to enable intervention to be planned electively.
- Treatment = endovascular aneurysm repair (EVAR) (e.g. stent insertion) or surgical repair with graft: no medical treatment possible.
- If repair is successful then there is a good prognosis.
- A high degree of mortality (around 85%) is associated with ruptured AAA.

# Risk factors

- Smoking
- Atherosclerosis
- Hypertension
- Hyperlipidaemia.

# Diagnosis

- Usually asymptomatic
- History/presentation – pulsating mass: local organ pain due to pressure from aneurysm
- Ultrasound
- CT scan.

# Essentials of best practice

The mention of the word aneurysm will be frightening and patients and their families will need reassurance and psychological support. For those whose aneurysms have been detected at screening or before rupture careful monitoring and assessment will occur as an outpatient prior to elective surgery or EVAR. For those with sudden rupture of an aneurysm emergency surgery is necessary. In the case of ruptured AAA nursing care will focus on stabilising BP largely by infusion of blood expanders, medication administration and preparation for emergency surgery.

For people admitted for elective repair of aneurysms, nursing care will revolve around pre-operative preparation and post-operative care. Post-operative care will largely focus on:

✓ Accurate assessments and regular monitoring
✓ Communication with the healthcare team, patient and family
✓ Discharge planning

Specialist vascular nurses should be consulted if available.

# Complications

Thromboembolism (DVT and PE).

| Patient information |
| --- |
| British Heart Foundation www.bhf.org.uk. The Circulation Foundation www.circulationfoundation.org.uk. You will also find very helpful patient-centred fact sheets at www.patient.co.uk/. |

# 35 Nursing people with peripheral vascular disease

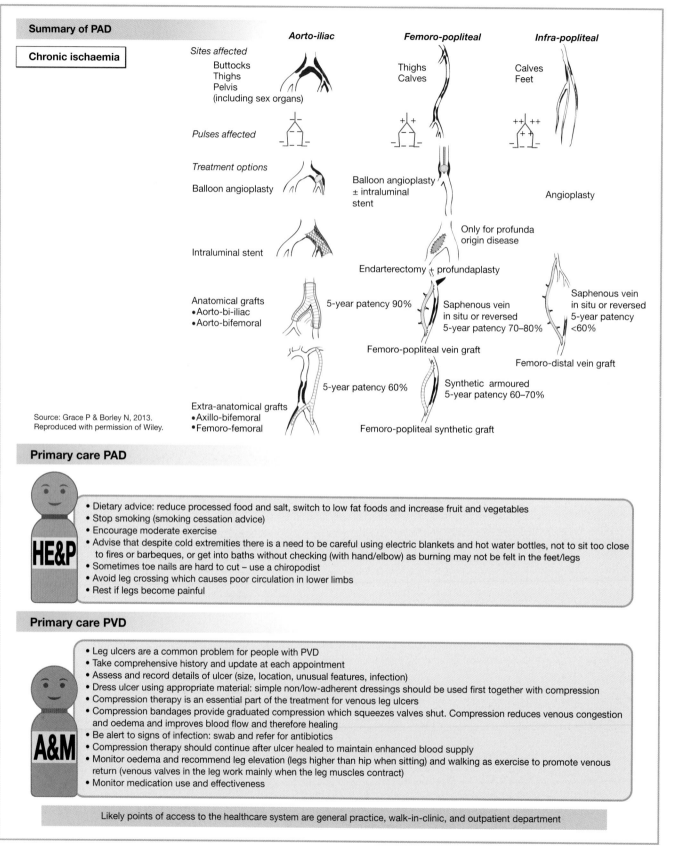

**Summary of PAD**

Chronic ischaemia

**Aorto-iliac** | **Femoro-popliteal** | **Infra-popliteal**

*Sites affected*
Buttocks
Thighs
Pelvis
(including sex organs)

Thighs
Calves

Calves
Feet

*Pulses affected*

*Treatment options*
Balloon angioplasty

Balloon angioplasty
± intraluminal
stent

Angioplasty

Intraluminal stent

Only for profunda
origin disease

Endarterectomy + profundaplasty

Anatomical grafts
• Aorto-bi-iliac
• Aorto-bifemoral

5-year patency 90%

Saphenous vein
in situ or reversed
5-year patency 70–80%

Femoro-popliteal vein graft

Saphenous vein
in situ or reversed
5-year patency
<60%

Femoro-distal vein graft

5-year patency 60%

Synthetic armoured
5-year patency 60–70%

Extra-anatomical grafts
• Axillo-bifemoral
• Femoro-femoral

Femoro-popliteal synthetic graft

Source: Grace P & Borley N, 2013.
Reproduced with permission of Wiley.

## Primary care PAD

**HE&P**

- Dietary advice: reduce processed food and salt, switch to low fat foods and increase fruit and vegetables
- Stop smoking (smoking cessation advice)
- Encourage moderate exercise
- Advise that despite cold extremities there is a need to be careful using electric blankets and hot water bottles, not to sit too close to fires or barbeques, or get into baths without checking (with hand/elbow) as burning may not be felt in the feet/legs
- Sometimes toe nails are hard to cut – use a chiropodist
- Avoid leg crossing which causes poor circulation in lower limbs
- Rest if legs become painful

## Primary care PVD

**A&M**

- Leg ulcers are a common problem for people with PVD
- Take comprehensive history and update at each appointment
- Assess and record details of ulcer (size, location, unusual features, infection)
- Dress ulcer using appropriate material: simple non/low-adherent dressings should be used first together with compression
- Compression therapy is an essential part of the treatment for venous leg ulcers
- Compression bandages provide graduated compression which squeezes valves shut. Compression reduces venous congestion and oedema and improves blood flow and therefore healing
- Be alert to signs of infection: swab and refer for antibiotics
- Compression therapy should continue after ulcer healed to maintain enhanced blood supply
- Monitor oedema and recommend leg elevation (legs higher than hip when sitting) and walking as exercise to promote venous return (venous valves in the leg work mainly when the leg muscles contract)
- Monitor medication use and effectiveness

Likely points of access to the healthcare system are general practice, walk-in-clinic, and outpatient department

*Adult Nursing at a Glance*, First Edition. Andrée le May. © 2015 John Wiley & Sons, Ltd. Published 2015 by John Wiley & Sons, Ltd.
Companion website: www.ataglanceseries.com/nursing/adult

# Key facts

- Peripheral vascular disease includes arterial and venous disease.
- Arterial and venous disease can occur separately or together.
- Peripheral arterial disease (PAD) is commonly caused by arteriosclerosis.
- In PAD reduction in blood flow to peripheral tissues results in acute or chronic ischaemia.
- PAD affects 10% of the population over 65 years of age in the Western world.
- Peripheral venous disease (PVD) occurs because of obstruction (e.g. thrombus or thrombophlebitis) or venous valve incompetence.
- Leg ulcers are associated with both PAD and PVD.

# Risk factors for peripheral vascular disease

- Smoking
- Atherosclerosis
- Hypertension
- Hyperlipidaemia
- Diabetes mellitus
- Family history.

# Diagnosis

- History/presenting signs and symptoms
- Ultrasound.

# Presentation PAD

*Chronic*:
- Claudication = aching pain in leg after walking: relieved by rest.
- Cold peripheries.
- Capillary refill time prolonged.
- Rest pain at night.
- Absent pulses depending on location of diseased artery.
- Arterial ulcers (over pressure points – heels, toes).
- Erectile dysfunction.

*Acute*:
- Pain – sudden and severe.
- Pallor/mottling.
- Cold limb.
- Pins and needles or paralysis.
- Pulses altered – weak/absent.

# Presentation PVD

*Chronic*:
- Oedema (foot to calf).
- Warm peripheries.
- Brownish/red colour; maybe cyanosis; often mottled.
- Varicose veins visible.
- Ulcers (ankles).
- Heavy legs, feel full.

*Acute*:
- Pain minimal, but tender along course of inflamed vein.

# Essentials of best practice

## PAD

Nursing care will largely focus on both lifestyle advice and medication monitoring for those with non-disabling PAD or pre- and post-operative care for those requiring surgery (e.g. balloon angioplasty and stent insertion, bypass surgery, surgical embolectomy, amputation). Nursing will be given either in primary care or hospital care. In primary care, nursing will focus on:
✓ Accurate assessments and regular monitoring
✓ Health education and promotion
✓ Symptom control and management
In ward care, nursing will depend on the procedure being carried out but will focus primarily on:
✓ Accurate assessments and regular monitoring
✓ Discharge planning
✓ Symptom control and management

## PVD

Nursing care, from practice nurses or community nurses, will largely focus on assessing and monitoring progress and ulcer management. Some ulcers will not heal and will require grafting in hospital. In all instances nursing care will involve:
✓ Accurate assessments and regular monitoring
✓ Health education and promotion
✓ Symptom control and management
Specialist vascular nurses should be consulted if available.
See also wound care in Section 1.

# Complications

Coronary heart disease for those with PAD: pulmonary embolism and deep vein thrombosis in those with PVD.

---

**Patient information**

The Circulation Foundation www.circulationfoundation.org.uk. You will also find very helpful patient-centred fact sheets at www.patient.co.uk/.

# 36 Nursing people with respiratory disorders

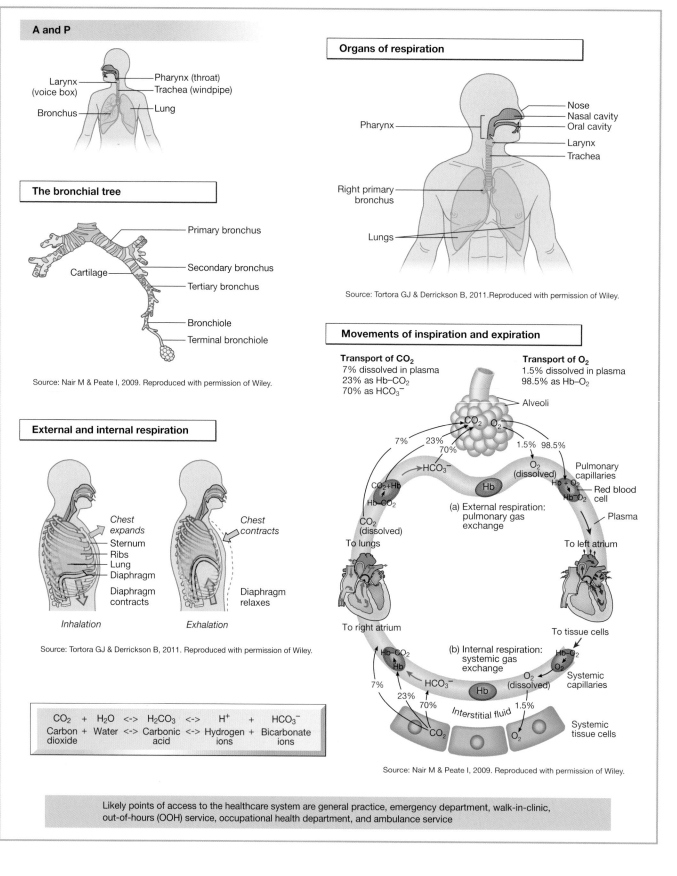

## A and P

Larynx (voice box)
Pharynx (throat)
Trachea (windpipe)
Bronchus
Lung

## The bronchial tree

Primary bronchus
Secondary bronchus
Cartilage
Tertiary bronchus
Bronchiole
Terminal bronchiole

Source: Nair M & Peate I, 2009. Reproduced with permission of Wiley.

## External and internal respiration

Chest expands
Sternum
Ribs
Lung
Diaphragm
Diaphragm contracts

*Inhalation*

Chest contracts
Diaphragm relaxes

*Exhalation*

Source: Tortora GJ & Derrickson B, 2011. Reproduced with permission of Wiley.

$$CO_2 + H_2O \longleftrightarrow H_2CO_3 \longleftrightarrow H^+ + HCO_3^-$$

Carbon + Water <-> Carbonic <-> Hydrogen + Bicarbonate
dioxide          acid        ions       ions

## Organs of respiration

Nose
Nasal cavity
Oral cavity
Pharynx
Larynx
Trachea
Right primary bronchus
Lungs

Source: Tortora GJ & Derrickson B, 2011. Reproduced with permission of Wiley.

## Movements of inspiration and expiration

**Transport of $CO_2$**
7% dissolved in plasma
23% as $Hb-CO_2$
70% as $HCO_3^-$

**Transport of $O_2$**
1.5% dissolved in plasma
98.5% as $Hb-O_2$

Alveoli
7%  23%  70%
1.5%  98.5%
$HCO_3^-$
$CO_2 + Hb$
$O_2$ (dissolved)
Hb
$Hb-CO_2$
Hb
$Hb-O_2$
$CO_2$ (dissolved)
To lungs

(a) External respiration: pulmonary gas exchange

Pulmonary capillaries
Red blood cell
Plasma
To left atrium

To right atrium
To tissue cells

$Hb-CO_2$
Hb
7%
$HCO_3^-$
23%
70%
$CO_2$

(b) Internal respiration: systemic gas exchange

$Hb-O_2$
$O_2$
$O_2$ (dissolved)
1.5%
Interstitial fluid

Systemic capillaries
Systemic tissue cells

Source: Nair M & Peate I, 2009. Reproduced with permission of Wiley.

Likely points of access to the healthcare system are general practice, emergency department, walk-in-clinic, out-of-hours (OOH) service, occupational health department, and ambulance service

*Adult Nursing at a Glance*, First Edition. Andrée le May. © 2015 John Wiley & Sons, Ltd. Published 2015 by John Wiley & Sons, Ltd.
Companion website: www.ataglanceseries.com/nursing/adult

# Key facts

- Cells need oxygen to survive: they produce carbon dioxide as a waste gas.
- The respiratory system ensures that sufficient oxygen is transported to cells and excess carbon dioxide is removed. This process is called respiration.
- Respiration has four components: (1) pulmonary ventilation (breathing); (2) external respiration; (3) transport of gases; (4) internal respiration.
- Respiration involves two body systems working together – the respiratory system and the circulatory system.
- The respiratory system is responsible for pulmonary ventilation (air getting in (inhalation) and out (exhalation) of the lungs) and external respiration ($O_2$ diffusing from the lungs to haemoglobin and $CO_2$ diffusing from the blood to the lungs and being exhaled).
- The circulatory system (blood, blood vessels and the heart) is responsible for the transport of gases from the lungs to the body and internal respiration (the delivery of $O_2$ to the cells for metabolism and the collection of waste $CO_2$ from them).
- The respiratory system comprises the upper respiratory tract and the lower respiratory tract.
- The respiratory system – alongside the kidneys and chemical buffers in the blood – helps to maintain the body's acid-base balance by the expulsion and retention of $CO_2$.
- The amount of $CO_2$ exhaled should equal the $CO_2$ produced in cell metabolism to maintain the acid-base balance.
- Disorders of the respiratory system can result in acute or chronic conditions.
- Spirometry and peak expiratory flow rate (PEFR) assess lung function. Blood tests also assess lung function.

# Common respiratory disorders

- Respiratory failure
- Respiratory tract infections
- Asthma
- Chronic Obstructive Pulmonary Disease.

Each is covered in the following pages.

Common signs and symptoms associated with respiratory disorders are presented in Chapter 37.

# A and P

- The upper respiratory tract comprises the nose, nasal cavity, mouth, oral cavity and pharynx.
- The lower respiratory tract comprises the larynx, trachea, and the bronchi, bronchioles, alveoli in the two lungs.
- The lungs are divided into regions called lobes (three in the right, two in the left) and each lobe is divided into lobules. Each lung holds within it a primary bronchus. Every lobe is served by a secondary bronchus which splits into tertiary bronchi and then a network of bronchioles (known as branching of the bronchial tree) each culminating in a terminal bronchiole.

- The terminal bronchiole leads to respiratory bronchioles.
- Each respiratory bronchiole ends in an alveolar duct that terminates in a series of alveoli clustered together as alveolar sacs. External respiration occurs in the one cell thick alveoli.
- Each lung is surrounded by two thin protecting membranes – parietal and visceral pleura: pleural fluid lubricates the gap between them, reducing friction during breathing. The lungs and pleura are protected by the thoracic cage.
- The heart lies in the space (mediastinum) between the lungs.
- Breathing rate and depth are controlled by respiratory centres in the brain stem (pons and medulla oblongata). These normally alter breathing according mainly to the level of carbon dioxide, but also to some extent oxygen, present in the body. These levels trigger (or drive) breathing.
- Air flows into the lungs because of a pressure gradient between the atmosphere and the lungs. Inhalation occurs if pressure in the atmosphere is greater than in the lungs and exhalation occurs when pressure in the lungs is greater than the atmosphere.
- The respiratory (diaphragm, internal and external intercostals) and abdominal muscles alter that pressure gradient.
- The alveoli export $CO_2$ from the body and import $O_2$ across a thin membrane served by a rich capillary system.
- $O_2$ diffuses across the alveolar–capillary membrane into blood returning, oxygenated, in pulmonary *veins* to the heart.
- Waste $CO_2$ from the cells is brought in de-oxygenated blood by the venous system to the heart, which then pumps it to the alveoli via the pulmonary *arterial* system. (NB: all the other arteries in the body carry *oxygenated* blood.)
- $CO_2$ diffuses across the alveolar–capillary membrane because its partial pressure is higher in the blood than in the alveoli.
- $O_2$ diffuses across the alveolar–capillary membrane because its partial pressure is higher in the alveoli than in the blood.

# Essentials of best practice

Nursing someone with any respiratory disorder requires you to pay attention to all the essentials of best practice. These will be expanded on in the subsequent pages for each of the disorders listed above. Chapter 37 details assessment of the respiratory system, common signs and symptoms and respiratory emergencies.

## Patient information

There are several patient support groups and charities focusing on respiratory disorders. You can find most of them on the Self Help UK website www.self-help.org.uk.
Some useful ones are:
The British Lung Foundation www.blf.org.uk.
Asthma UK www.asthma.org.uk/.
You will also find very helpful patient-centred fact sheets at www.patient.co.uk.

# 37 Signs, symptoms, assessment and emergencies

## Important assessments of respiration (based on Dougherty and Lister, 2011)

- Airway assessment – check for obstructions (e.g. vomit, tongue, foreign bodies): ask a conscious patient a question – if they answer their airway is likely to be unobstructed
- Breathing assessment
  - o colour of skin and mucous membranes (check for cyanosis – central and peripheral: cyanosis can be seen if oxygen saturations drop to 85–90%: pallor may suggest anaemia or shock)
  - o indications of laboured breathing, e.g. use of accessory muscles (abdominal, sternomastoid and scalene – look at neck during inspiration to see contraction of sternomastoid muscle). Nasal flaring may be present and a patient may breathe through pursed lips
  - o rhythm, rate and depth of breathing: Normal rate 12–18 breaths/minute: expiration lasts about twice as long as inspiration: monitor carefully patients with rates of 24 breaths/minute and seek medical advice immediately if rates increase to 27 breaths/minute or decrease to 8 breaths/minute. Check if breathing is deep/shallow or changed from a previous pattern
  - o breathlessness can be assessed using the MRC Dyspnoea Scale
  - o the shape and expansion of the chest. Look for deviations from the normal shape of the chest and also check that expansion is equal on both sides of the chest. Report deviations
  - o if a patient cannot complete a sentence without becoming breathless call for immediate advice
- Non-invasive assessment of the oxygen saturation of arterial blood ($SpO_2$) by pulse oximetry. The range of normal oxygen saturation is 95–100%. (NB people with chronic respiratory conditions will have a lower range which is normal for them.) Oxygen saturation should be kept above 94% in acutely ill adults *and between 88–92% for people at risk or with hypercapnia.* **These levels should always be checked with the doctor or senior nurse before monitoring begins.**
  The pulse oximeter (a probe consisting of one light emitting diode opposite one light detector) is attached to a patient's finger, ear or toe. In hypoxaemia, the probe measures the blueness of the blood. To be effective the light needs to easily pass through the tissue – so choose tissue that is not thickened, like hard skinned finger tips, or difficult for light to pass through, like nails with varnish or nicotine stained fingers. Position the pulse oximeter away from excessive artificial light or sunlight as this will alter its readings. Inaccurate readings may be obtained from patients with particular conditions (e.g. carbon monoxide poisoning or poor perfusion)
- Sputum: assess amount, smell, consistency and colour. You should ask if a patient's sputum has changed recently. Ask if any blood has been present too
- Assess a patient's level of confusion (incorrect responses to questions) or new disorientation related to self, time and/or place
- Assess the patient's level of consciousness. The Glasgow Coma Scale may be used
- Assessment of distress and fatigue should be made
- Lung function is assessed by spirometry and peak expiratory flow rate measurement. (Spirometry measures how much air is blown out of the lungs and how quickly. Results of spirometry show the severity of airflow obstruction. Peak Expiratory Flow Rate (PEFR) is a measure of the maximum speed that air can be exhaled via the mouth, it measures airway resistance)
- Find out if the patient smokes and details of their smoking pattern and history of cessation
- Find out if any respiratory problems impact on the patient's ability to perform activities of daily living

---

### Box 37  Medical Research Council (MRC) Dyspnoea Scale

| Grade | Degree of breathlessness related to activities |
|---|---|
| 1 | Not troubled by breathlessness except on strenuous exercise |
| 2 | Short of breath when hurrying or walking up a slight hill |
| 3 | Walks slower than contemporaries on level ground because of breathlessness, or has to stop for breath when walking at own pace |
| 4 | Stops for breath after walking about 100 m or after a few minutes on level ground |
| 5 | Too breathless to leave the house, or breathless when dressing or undressing |

*Adult Nursing at a Glance*, First Edition. Andrée le May. © 2015 John Wiley & Sons, Ltd. Published 2015 by John Wiley & Sons, Ltd.
Companion website: www.ataglanceseries.com/nursing/adult

# Common signs and symptoms

- Altered respiratory rate: slowed or quickened
- Altered heart rate
- Pyrexia
- Malaise (feeling under the weather)
- Breathlessness (see MRC Dyspnoea Scale)
- Changed breathing noises (e.g. stridor)
- Wheeze
- Chest tightness
- Leaning forward to help breathing
- Cough – dry/productive
- Sputum altered in any way
- Blood present in sputum
- Agitation
- Confusion and disorientation (due to hypoxia)
- Tiredness, fatigue and exhaustion
- Pain
- Fear
- Cyanosis or pallor
- Inability to speak in full sentences.

# Respiratory emergencies

Recognising and responding to sudden deteriorations in a patient's condition is vital. Two situations where rapid intervention can be life-saving are respiratory arrest and tension pneumothorax.

## Respiratory arrest is a medical emergency

The respiratory system may stop working if there is:
- Airway obstruction (foreign body or tongue).
- Severe lung disease (pneumonia, severe airway obstruction e.g. in asthma, COPD exacerbations or end-stage COPD).
- Left ventricular failure.
- Brain injury (e.g. stroke, drug overdose).

Any of these may cause a respiratory arrest. If a respiratory arrest occurs you will need to start basic life support (BLS) immediately.

Respiratory arrest will usually lead to cardiac arrest.

## Tension pneumothorax is a medical emergency

A pneumothorax is when air leaks into the pleural space. There are various types of pneumothorax but the most rapidly life-threatening is a tension pneumothorax. In this instance the leak creates a one-way valve drawing air into the pleural space which cannot escape. The increased volume of air in the pleural space causes an increase in pressure above atmospheric pressure resulting in compression of the lung and movement of the mediastinum and heart towards the opposite side (a mediastinal shift). This reduces cardiac filling and output.

Tension pneumothorax results in severe dyspnoea, tracheal deviation (movement), tachycardia and hypotension. If unrecognised and untreated, death will occur.

Treatment is by aspiration and the insertion of a chest tube and an underwater-sealed chest drain. (The underwater-sealed drain acts as a one-way valve allowing air to escape from the pleural cavity during expiration but not to be drawn back since the end of the tube is covered with water.) Care should be taken to keep these drains below the level of the patient's chest so that water doesn't enter the pleural cavity.

A tension pneumothorax may result from trauma, asthma or chronic lung disease such as COPD.

**Your knowledge of BLS should be regularly updated. You can find out the latest information by looking at the Resuscitation Council's website www.resus.org.uk.**

# 38 Nursing people with respiratory failure

## Type I and Type II respiratory failure

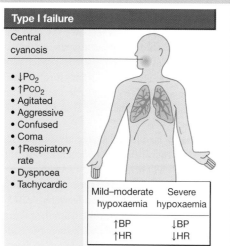

### Type I failure

Central cyanosis

- $\downarrow PO_2$
- $\uparrow PCO_2$
- Agitated
- Aggressive
- Confused
- Coma
- $\uparrow$Respiratory rate
- Dyspnoea
- Tachycardic

| Mild–moderate hypoxaemia | Severe hypoxaemia |
|---|---|
| $\uparrow$BP | $\downarrow$BP |
| $\uparrow$HR | $\downarrow$HR |

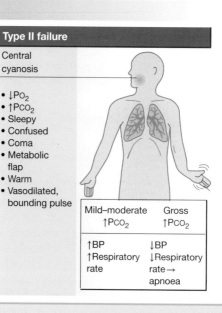

### Type II failure

Central cyanosis

- $\downarrow PO_2$
- $\uparrow PCO_2$
- Sleepy
- Confused
- Coma
- Metabolic flap
- Warm
- Vasodilated, bounding pulse

| Mild–moderate $\uparrow PCO_2$ | Gross $\uparrow PCO_2$ |
|---|---|
| $\uparrow$BP | $\downarrow$BP |
| $\uparrow$Respiratory rate | $\downarrow$Respiratory rate $\rightarrow$ apnoea |

Source: Davey P (ed), 2014.
Reproduced with permission of Wiley.

## Oxygen therapy
- The aim of oxygen therapy is to treat or prevent hypoxia (lack of oxygen in body tissues)
- Oxygen is delivered in concentrations higher than ambient air
- Care needs to be taken to administer the correct amount of oxygen depending on whether respiratory failure is Type I or Type II
- Giving the wrong dosage of oxygen can have serious consequences for patients
- It is essential that you explain about oxygen therapy to the patient since their cooperation is needed to achieve the best result
- Oxygen therapy should be prescribed with target saturation ranges based on a patient's clinical condition
- Oxygen delivery devices (low flow/high flow systems) deliver oxygen
- Oxygen should be administered through the correct delivery system which should be selected for each patient
- Low flow, variable performance devices are nasal cannulae or simple semi-rigid plastic face masks
- High flow, fixed performance devices are masks with a Venturi barrel (Venturi-type masks)
- Oxygen should be humidified if flow rates are above 4 l/min or there is nasal discomfort/dryness
- A dry mouth can result from oxygen therapy so regular mouth care should be given
- Patients will find it difficult to talk so make sure alternatives, e.g. pen and paper, are available

**A&M**

## Oxygen therapy
- Careful, regular monitoring is essential
- Regular pulse oximetry readings should be taken to determine if prescribed oxygen therapy is achieving target saturation
- Oxygen flow rate and method of delivery need to be documented
- Continue to make the full range of respiratory assessments (see Chapter 37)

## Continuous Positive Airway Pressure (CPAP)
- CPAP uses a tightly fitting mask and flow generator to deliver a positive pressure of oxygen which keeps the airways open throughout the respiratory cycle
- CPAP increases functional residual capacity (FRC) of the lungs by preventing full exhalation (the amount of gas not exhaled is measured in centimetres of water pressure ($cmH_2O$)
- CPAP therapy is usually set between 5–15 $cmH_2O$
- CPAP promotes the use of more alveoli (recruitment) in external respiration (gaseous exchange) so improving oxygenation
- Careful explanation of how this system works is needed as it relies on the patient's cooperation
- Tight mask fitting is critical to the effectiveness of this treatment: leaks will limit the usefulness of CPAP

**A&M**

## Using Continuous Positive Airway Pressure (CPAP) (usually in HDU or ITU)
- Careful monitoring of arterial blood gases (ABGs) is important
- Continue to make the full range of respiratory assessments (see Chapter 37)

Likely points of access to the healthcare system are general practice, emergency department, walk-in-clinic, out-of-hours (OOH) service, and ambulance service

# Key facts

- Respiratory failure means that the body's cells do not receive adequate amounts of oxygen for survival and/or cannot offload enough $CO_2$.
- Respiratory failure is defined by abnormal levels of arterial oxygen (low) or carbon dioxide (high).
- There are two types of respiratory failure: Type I (hypoxaemia) and Type II (hypercapnia with hypoxaemia).
- Hypoxaemia refers to lack of oxygen in arterial blood due to a failure of oxygenation ($PaO_2 < 8\,kPa$).
- Hypercapnia refers to excess carbon dioxide in arterial blood due to a failure of respiration ($PaCO_2 > 6\,kPa$).
- Respiratory failure can be acute, chronic or acute-on-chronic.
- Respiratory failure can result from, for example, underlying lung pathology, respiratory muscle weakness or exhaustion or depressed breathing as in drug overdose.
- Excess $CO_2$ reduces $O_2$ binding to haemoglobin in the lungs increasing the chance of hypoxaemia.
- Excess $CO_2$ in Type II respiratory failure can disturb the acid-base balance.
- (NB: If arterial blood pH deviates from its normal range of 7.35–.45 an acid-base imbalance results, which is known as an acidosis (<7.35) or alkalosis (>7.45).)
- Respiratory acidosis occurs when excessive arterial $CO_2$ in Type II respiratory failure causes arterial blood pH to fall below 7.35.
- Potential respiratory failure can sometimes be averted. Nurses should be alert for early warning signs of respiratory failure and call for medical advice as soon as possible.
- If left untreated the patient's condition will deteriorate resulting in coma and death.
- Diagnosis is made by the measurement of arterial blood gases (measuring pH is also important).
- Patients with respiratory failure should be monitored in a high dependency area (respiratory rate, ECG, pulse oximetry, BP, arterial blood gas analysis, Glasgow Coma Scale).

# A and P

- If too much $CO_2$ is retained, the respiratory control centre in the brain stem stimulates faster, deeper breathing in an attempt to blow off the excess. If sufficient $CO_2$ cannot be expired it builds up in the body. (If $CO_2$ levels are too low – e.g. from hyperventilation – the respiratory centre makes the breathing slower & shallower so $CO_2$ accumulates.) $O_2$ levels can also affect respiration by similar feedback loops (high $O_2$ leading e.g. to slowed breathing).
- Adequate alveolar ventilation ($V_A$, the amount of air reaching the alveoli) and perfusion ($Q$, the amount of blood flow through pulmonary capillaries) are needed for normal gaseous exchange. This is assessed by the $V_A : Q$ ratio. Problems with either can cause hypoxaemia and/or hypercapnia.
- $CO_2$ produced by cell metabolism is transported in blood to the lungs in haemoglobin and as dissolved gas, but mainly as carbonic acid, which forms bicarbonate and hydrogen ions, which recombine to form water and carbon dioxide to be expired from the alveoli. This process normally helps maintain the blood pH (the hydrogen-ion concentration in solution) and any alteration to this finely balanced equilibrium, such as hypercapnia, can change the acid-base balance. Normally the pH of arterial blood is slightly alkaline. Changed levels of carbon dioxide alter the pH which in turn affects many other bodily systems and homeostatic mechanisms, and so can quickly become life-threatening.

# Hypoxaemia

Hypoxaemia can result from hypoventilation (e.g. drug overdose), diffusion impairment (e.g. pulmonary fibrosis together with exercise), ventilation-perfusion imbalance (e.g. in COPD or pneumonia), low inspired oxygen tension (e.g. at high altitude). See above for signs and symptoms. Treatments include oxygen therapy to promote saturation of haemoglobin. Continuous Positive Airway Pressure (CPAP) or intubation and mechanical ventilation may be necessary. (*Care should be taken when nursing patients with COPD and chronic hypoxia since they rely on reduced $O_2$ rather than higher $CO_2$ to drive respiration (hypoxic drive): giving oxygen may remove the drive and stop them breathing.*)

# Hypercapnia

Hypercapnia can result from defective central control of breathing (e.g. drug overdose), Guillain Barré syndrome, myasthenia gravis, chest wall disease (kyphoscoliosis), some neuromuscular diseases and primary lung disease (e.g. COPD) or any other cause of severe hypoxia. See above for signs and symptoms. Treatments and care should focus on the underlying condition. Oxygen therapy may be prescribed. Position alteration, chest physiotherapy and deep breathing may be useful. Non-invasive or invasive artificial ventilation may be needed.

# Early warning signs of respiratory failure

- Restlessness.
- Confusion.
- Increased rate of breathing with greater effort and use of respiratory and abdominal muscles.
- Changed pattern of breathing.
- Flaring of the nostrils.
- Pale or cyanosed, clammy skin.

# Essentials of best practice

Providing highly skilled, vigilant nursing care is essential for people with respiratory failure. This will include:

- ✓ Accurate assessment and regular monitoring
- ✓ Communication with the healthcare team, patient and family
- ✓ Risk assessment and management
- ✓ Evaluation
- ✓ Discharge planning

## Patient information

You will find very helpful patient-centred fact sheets at www.patient.co.uk/.

# Nursing people with respiratory infections

**Primary care**

**Consult a doctor or nurse if you:**
- Develop a severe headache
- Vomit
- Have difficulty breathing or your breathing is faster than usual
- Become more breathless than usual
- Turn blue around the lips and the skin below your mouth
- Or your family/carer notice that you are becoming confused or your speech is slurred
- Feel extremely tired
- Get pains in your chest particularly associated with breathing
- Cough up blood
- Have difficulty swallowing or are drooling
- Cannot complete a sentence without becoming breathless – call for immediate advice

**HE&P**

Source: Davey P (ed), 2014.
Reproduced with permission of Wiley.

**CURB-65 criteria for severity of pneumonia**

1 point for each of the following:

**C**onfusion

**U**rea (>7 mmol/l)

**R**espiratory rate (>30/min)

**B**lood pressure (systolic BP <90 or diastolic BP <60 mmHg)

**65** age ≥ 65 years

Risk of ITU admission or death:
- 0 :   0.7%
- 1 :   3.2%
- 2 : 13.0%
- 3 : 17.0%
- 4 : 41.5%
- 5 : 57.0%

Likely points of access to the healthcare system are general practice, emergency department, walk-in-clinic, out-of-hours (OOH) service, occupational health department, and ambulance service

*Adult Nursing at a Glance*, First Edition. Andrée le May. © 2015 John Wiley & Sons, Ltd. Published 2015 by John Wiley & Sons, Ltd.
Companion website: www.ataglanceseries.com/nursing/adult

# Key facts

- Infections of the respiratory system are divided into two: upper respiratory tract infections and lower respiratory tract infections.
- Respiratory tract infections are usually caused by viruses, bacteria or fungi.
- Antibiotics may be prescribed for bacterial infections and should be taken as directed.
- Upper respiratory tract infections include the common cold, pharyngitis, laryngitis, bronchitis and sinusitis.
- Most upper respiratory tract infections are short lived and self-limiting. Symptoms include sneezing, nasal blockage, congestion and discharge, fever, sore throat, cough, sputum and headache.
- For upper respiratory tract infections, self-care advice (take antipyretics and mild analgesics (e.g. paracetamol), keep warm, avoid unnecessary contact with people, rest, drink enough fluids to not feel thirsty and eat normally) is provided by the GP, practice nurse or pharmacist.
- Lower respiratory tract infections affect the lung. Pneumonia is a common infection of the lower respiratory tract.
- Information about how to recognise a deteriorating condition and when to call for medical assistance should be given (above).

# Pneumonia

- Pneumonia is an acute, infective respiratory illness of the lungs.
- Pneumonia can be caused by viruses, bacteria or fungi.
- There are four main types:
  - community acquired pneumonia;
  - hospital acquired (nosocomial) pneumonia;
  - aspiration pneumonia;
  - pneumonia in immunocompromised people.
- Fever, cough, chest pain and breathlessness are common symptoms. Some people also have headaches, confusion, myalgia and malaise.
- Most people with community acquired pneumonia are cared for at home.
- It is important to be able to recognise deterioration in a patient's condition. The C(U)RB-65 scale (above) is used to do this. One point is allocated to the presence of each criterion – the higher the score the more serious the condition.
- Treatment may include antibiotics, oxygen therapy, intravenous fluid therapy and nutritional support. Physiotherapy may also be necessary.
- Vaccination is available against pneumonia and is advised for all people over 65 years of age or with long-term respiratory conditions.

# Pneumonia: essentials of best practice

The nursing care of patients with pneumonia, whether in primary care or in hospital, needs to be observant and vigilant. Care focuses on monitoring temperature, pulse, respirations and blood pressure, administering oxygen as prescribed, helping with activities of daily living, ensuring adequate fluid intake and nutrition, relieving breathlessness through positioning (leaning forward in bed on the bed table supported by pillows or just sitting forward in a chair),

helping a person to expectorate sputum with or without the assistance of the physiotherapist. A patient's condition can deteriorate rapidly and this, if it happens, needs swift attention.

# Tuberculosis (TB)

- TB is a disease caused by *Mycobacterium tuberculosis*.
- TB is a notifiable (in the UK) communicable disease which poses a major global health problem.
- TB is found in the lungs (pulmonary) and in other parts of the body (extra-pulmonary) such as the lymph nodes, CNS, bones and joints.
- TB is spread by respiratory droplets.
- TB can affect a person of any age. TB is more likely to affect immunocompromised people.
- Symptoms include night sweats, fever and a productive cough. People with advanced TB may also have loss of appetite, weight loss and haemoptysis.
- Treatment includes combinations of drugs (usually four) over 6 months. Adherence to these long-term drug regimens can be difficult for some patients.
- TB can be resistant to drugs. This is known as multi-drug resistant TB (MDR-TB).
- Infection control is critical in minimising the spread of TB.
- Contact tracing is also important in reducing TB's spread.
- Childhood immunisation is the most effective preventative measure against TB.

# Tuberculosis: essentials of best practice

Nursing people with TB can span community and hospital care. Initially a patient is most likely to be nursed at home: only if their condition worsens will they be admitted to hospital. Nursing care at home primarily focuses on education about medication regimes and adherence to them and infection control. If a person is admitted to hospital, strict infection control procedures will be put in place until treatment is shown to be effective. Specialist TB nurses will advise about care and contact tracing. Prevention of TB is important and health visitors, midwives, school nurses and practice nurses have a key role in ensuring that infants and children are immunised.

# Essentials of best practice

When nursing anyone with a respiratory infection attention should be paid to:
- ✓ Accurate assessment and regular monitoring
- ✓ Communication with the healthcare team, patient and family
- ✓ Symptom control and management
- ✓ Discharge planning

---

**Patient information**

You will find very helpful patient-centred fact sheets at www.patient.co.uk/.

# 40 Nursing people with asthma

## Primary care

### Asthma management

Effective asthma management is about enabling the patient to feel confident in understanding asthma, how it affects them and how it can best be managed by them. Patient education is a critical element of successful asthma management.
Patient education should focus on:
- Explaining asthma, symptoms and potential triggers
- Working out with the patient their own triggers and how to avoid them
- Explaining how medication works to relieve or prevent acute attacks and checking the effectiveness of the current regime
- Teaching and (re)-checking inhaler technique and peak flow monitoring (a peak flow diary)
- Discussing how to detect and manage general deterioration (discussing peak flow monitoring and a stepped approach to care may be useful)
- Discussing how to recognise *and* react to asthma attacks: this is vital as attacks can be life-threatening
- Constructing a personalised self-management action plan with the patient which includes:
    o details of what medicine should be taken, how much and when
    o how to tell when symptoms are getting worse and what to do about it
    o emergency information on what to do during an asthma attack
    (Asthma UK has a useful template)
Regularly reviewing a patient's self-management of their asthma and updating their action plan and knowledge are critical to successful asthma management.

**HE&P**

### Methods of delivering bronchodilators

**Dry powder device**
For routine use

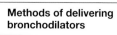

Window

**Spacer devices**
Useful in the elderly or very young
- Less coordination needed
- Lower pharyngeal deposition of drug

cr

**Nebuliser treatment**
Useful if sick
- Less coordination needed
- ? vapourises

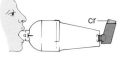

To mask or T piece

Drug solution

Oxygen or compressed air

Source: Davey P (ed), 2014.
Reproduced with permission of Wiley.

### Management of chronic asthma

**Step 1**
Relief bronchodilators as required

**Step 2**
Step 1 + regular inhaled steroid

**Step 3**
Inhaled steroid + long-acting β-agonist or LTRA or oral slow-release theophylline

**Step 4**
High-dose inhaled steroid + long-acting β-agonist + trial of other bronchodilators

**Step 5**
Oral steroid in lowest dose to maintain control

**Step 6**
Step down after 3–6 months stability

Source: Davey P (ed), 2014.
Reproduced with permission of Wiley.

### Levels of severity

| | In between attacks | Moderate | Severe | Life threatening |
|---|---|---|---|---|
| | Normal exam Normal lung function tests | PEFR <65% predicted ↓ Admit to hospital | PEFR <50% Pulse rate >110 Respiratory rate >25 Can't complete sentences Wheezy chest Alert → mild confusion | PEFR <33% Bradycardia Exhaustion Can't talk at all Silent chest Confusion → coma |
| $PO_2$ | | ↓ | ↓↓ | ↓↓↓ |
| $PCO_2$ | | ↓ | → | ↑ |
| pH | | Ⓝ or ↑ | Ⓝ | ↓ |
| | | | | **Alert ITU** |

Source: Davey P (ed), 2014.
Reproduced with permission of Wiley.

Likely points of access to the healthcare system are general practice, emergency department, walk-in-clinic, out-of-hours (OOH) service, occupational health department, and ambulance service

*Adult Nursing at a Glance*, First Edition. Andrée le May. © 2015 John Wiley & Sons, Ltd. Published 2015 by John Wiley & Sons, Ltd.
Companion website: www.ataglanceseries.com/nursing/adult

# Key facts

• Asthma is hard to define, but Asthma UK says: 'When a person with asthma comes into contact with something that irritates their airways (an asthma trigger), the muscles around the walls of the airways tighten so that the airways become narrower and the lining of the airways becomes inflamed and starts to swell. Sometimes, sticky mucus or phlegm builds up, which can further narrow the airways. These reactions cause the airways to become narrower and irritated - making it difficult to breath and leading to symptoms of asthma.'

• The symptoms of asthma are cough, wheeze, chest tightness and breathlessness. A person with asthma may have one or more of these.

• Clinically asthma is said to be present if a combination of cough, wheeze or breathlessness occurs with *variable* airflow obstruction. Airway obstruction is reversible.

• People with a family history of asthma, eczema or allergies are more likely to develop asthma.

• Asthma is a chronic condition with acute exacerbations.

• Asthma can be divided into three groups – extrinsic, intrinsic, and occupational.

• Extrinsic asthma is common in childhood and largely triggered by allergens (e.g. dust mites, animal hair/fur, pollen). Allergens are inhaled and absorbed by the bronchial mucosa triggering an inflammatory reaction which results in bronchial muscle spasm, oedema and secretion of thick mucus. Asthma attacks may lessen with age and good management.

• Intrinsic asthma develops later in life and is less likely to be caused by allergens. Intrinsic asthma may respond less well to treatment than extrinsic asthma.

• Occupational asthma is caused by workplace allergens. (Workplace allergens and particulates can also cause other serious lung diseases such as asbestosis and other lung fibroses.)

• Exercise, cold air, high atmospheric ozone (e.g. in thunder storms), viral infections and emotional stress can also trigger asthma attacks. Rarely asthma attacks can be caused by aspirin.

• Diagnosis is made by lung function tests which may show airflow obstruction. Serial peak flow measurements may show a pattern of morning dips and night time peaks of PEFR. Peak flow measurements are important markers of severity once asthma has been diagnosed.

• Being unable to complete a sentence in one breath is a serious warning sign – call for immediate medical help.

• Asthma symptoms are controllable. Management of asthma focuses on keeping a patient free from symptoms on the minimum of medication.

• Asthma management takes place largely in primary care.

• Poor control of asthma may result in poor lung function. For some people airflow obstruction may become irreversible.

• Risk factors for death from asthma include poor treatment compliance and admissions to ITU/hospital despite treatment with steroids.

• Everyone with asthma should have a personalised asthma action plan (see Asthma UK for a template).

# Essentials of best practice

Most nursing care for patients with asthma will be undertaken in primary care by practice nurses who regularly monitor a patient's medication regimes, lung function and attack frequency. If a patient's asthma is not well controlled the practice nurse will consult the GP and advise a review. Practice nurses will provide advice about medications and inhaler techniques, avoidance of triggers, recognising the severity of asthma attacks and knowing when to seek medical help.

If a patient is admitted to hospital with a severe asthma attack, highly skilled, observant nursing is needed: a patient's condition can quickly deteriorate and severe asthma attacks can be life-threatening. In this instance the aim of treatment is to minimise hypoxia and reduce bronchoconstriction and airway inflammation. Treatment with oxygen therapy, corticosteroids and nebulised bronchodilators delivered via an oxygen supply will be started immediately.

Nursing should incorporate the following essentials of best practice:

✓ Accurate assessment and regular monitoring (see Chapter 37)

✓ Communication with the healthcare team, patient and family

✓ Discharge planning in conjunction with specialist respiratory nurses

The guidance on oxygen therapy outlined in Chapter 37 should be adhered to.

## Patient information

Asthma UK www.asthma.org.uk.
The British Lung Foundation www.blf.org.uk.
The Asthma UK Adviceline is open Monday to Friday from 9 am to 5 pm. The number to call is 0800 121 62 44.
You will also find very helpful patient-centred fact sheets at www.patient.co.uk/.

# 41 Nursing people with COPD

## Primary care

### COPD management combines health education and promotion with symptom control

Management of COPD is about lifestyle change and medication adherence.
- Everyone with COPD should have a self-management plan
- Stopping smoking is of the greatest importance: smoking cessation advice and support should be given
- Pulmonary rehabilitation reduces the effects of COPD and improves quality of life. Discuss referral to local courses
- Often people with COPD use just the upper part of their chest and less air enters and leaves the lungs than is possible: this means that more energy is used in breathing. Teaching people to use their diaphragms can help. Referral to a physiotherapist who can teach breathing exercises will help reduce the work of breathing and increase effectiveness
- Taking more general exercise (up to 20 minutes a day) will improve patients' COPD symptoms and help them to feel better. This may be hard at first because exercise causes breathlessness: if this happens, stopping, recovering and then continuing is advised
- Eating well is important – dietary advice should be given and weight reviewed (both overweight and underweight). Referral to a dietician might be needed
- Discuss medication use and inhaler technique. Most drugs used to treat COPD are given via inhalers
- It is important to discuss exacerbations (flare-ups) and what, if anything promotes them so that triggers can be avoided
- Flare-ups usually cause worsened breathlessness and cough (with or without sputum). Sputum may be thicker or its colour may change suggesting an infection. Inhalers may seem less effective. Fever, generally feeling off colour or tired may also be some of the first symptoms experienced
- Antibiotics and oral steroids may be prescribed to take in emergency if a flare-up occurs. Remember to remind patients to finish the course of antibiotics if they start one even if they feel better and their symptoms improve
- Sometimes drugs may not suit patients, so ask them to come back if they have side-effects or their symptoms do not improve
- Remind the patient about vaccinations for pneumonia and flu
- Sometimes people with COPD feel anxious or depressed: ask the patient to come and see you or the doctor if they feel this way – reassurance or just talking about their problems can help
- People with COPD sometimes need extra oxygen if they fly. Oxygen levels in planes are normally lower than in the air we breathe. If a patient's COPD is moderate or severe oxygen levels should be checked before flying. Airlines can advise on the availability of oxygen during flights – contacting them in advance is necessary
- Some people with COPD may be eligible for government support. Contact with the relevant local benefits office may be needed

## COPD escalator

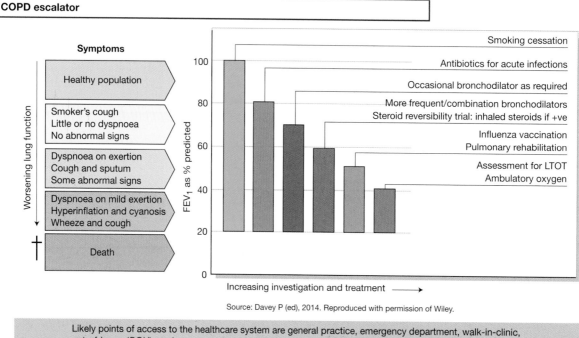

Source: Davey P (ed), 2014. Reproduced with permission of Wiley.

Likely points of access to the healthcare system are general practice, emergency department, walk-in-clinic, out-of-hours (OOH) service, occupational health department, and ambulance service

*Adult Nursing at a Glance*, First Edition. Andrée le May. © 2015 John Wiley & Sons, Ltd. Published 2015 by John Wiley & Sons, Ltd.
Companion website: www.ataglanceseries.com/nursing/adult

# Key facts

• Chronic Obstructive Pulmonary Disease (COPD) is a chronic, slowly progressing disorder characterised by fixed or partially reversible airway obstruction.
• There is no cure for COPD but skilled management of symptoms can slow its progress. Lifestyle changes and medication can improve health and wellbeing.
• COPD affects 1 in 8 middle-aged and older adults in the UK and accounts for around 5% of UK deaths each year.
• COPD is most common in industrialised countries and inner cities, in people who have worked in jobs where they have been exposed to noxious substances and in older people.
• Cigarette smoking can result in COPD: smoking cessation is strongly advised and can considerably improve COPD. Many people with COPD have never smoked.
• Chronic bronchitis, emphysema and bronchiectasis are included under the umbrella of COPD. Chronic undiagnosed, untreated or poorly controlled asthma may lead to COPD.
• Symptoms of COPD include cough and shortness of breath particularly on exertion. Sputum may also be present.
• COPD causes hypoxaemia, hypercapnia and polycythaemia (raised red blood cell count).
• People with COPD become exhausted from the work of breathing and as a consequence find activities of daily living hard to do.
• Diagnosis is made by physical examination, history taking and spirometry which is important for an accurate diagnosis.
• The severity of COPD is defined by the degree of airflow obstruction (Forced Expiratory Volume in 1 s (FEV1)). Flow in and out of the lungs is impeded.
• Long-term oxygen therapy (LTOT) may be prescribed for people with chronic hypoxaemia. LTOT is low dose oxygen given for around 16 hours each day usually overnight. (NB: A high percentage of $O_2$ may reduce respiratory drive.)
• Pulmonary rehabilitation (exercise training, breathing control, disease education, nutritional advice and social/psychological support) can improve symptoms and a person's quality of life.
• An exacerbation of COPD means that a person's symptoms worsen. This may be linked to a respiratory tract infection or other triggers such as air pollution. COPD often worsens in the winter.
• Caring for a patient with COPD requires input from the multidisciplinary team. Nursing input will vary depending on the patient's needs but is likely to involve nurses working in primary and community care, specialist respiratory nurses, nurses working in acute respiratory wards and HDUs and in palliative care.
• The drive to breath in some people with COPD may shift from carbon dioxide to hypoxaemia. Care should always be taken when giving oxygen to people with COPD as increasing oxygen levels can remove their drive for respiration and provoke respiratory failure.
• Vaccination against pneumonia and annual influenza vaccinations are strongly advised.

# The effects of COPD

COPD can result in depression, anxiety, isolation, malnutrition as a result of breathlessness and reduced appetite, exercise intolerance and poor quality of life. Respiratory failure may be a long-term consequence of COPD. Nurses should consider these when planning care with a patient and their family/carers. Family and carers may also feel depressed, anxious, exhausted and isolated.

# Essentials of best practice

The aim of nursing is to reduce symptoms and the effects of COPD and increase a patient's quality of life. Most nursing care for patients with COPD will be undertaken in primary care by practice nurses and community nurses. Practice nurses and GPs will regularly monitor a patient's condition. Practice nurses will help patients to identify early warning signs and symptoms associated with a worsening condition, and advise about what to do and when to seek medical help. Community nurses will be involved in the management of people having an exacerbation of COPD or with worsening COPD and the long-term management of those requiring LTOT. Care assistants working alongside nurses in primary care and the community will also have a role in helping a person with COPD to maintain their usual activities of daily living. Visits to specialist respiratory nurses in community clinics or out-patient departments may also be necessary. Pulmonary rehabilitation should be recommended to people with COPD who score above 3 on the MRC Dyspnoea Scale (see Chapter 37). People having acute exacerbations of COPD can be cared for at home by respiratory specialist nurses. Once well the patient will be discharged back to the care of the GP and primary and community nurses.

If a patient is admitted to hospital with a severe exacerbation of COPD highly skilled, observant nursing is required. Exacerbation of COPD can lead to either Type I or Type II respiratory failure. Nurses need to be alert to signs and symptoms of respiratory failure (see Chapter 38). Medical treatment may include bronchodilators, antibiotics and oral corticosteroids. Prescribed oxygen therapy should be used in conjunction with arterial blood gas (ABG) monitoring and pulse oximetry. Physiotherapy will be important too.

Nursing, whether at home or in hospital, should incorporate the following essentials of best practice:
✓ Accurate assessment and regular monitoring (see Chapter 37)
✓ Communication with the healthcare team, patient and family
✓ Symptom control and management
✓ Health Education and Promotion
✓ Discharge planning

---

**Patient information**

The British Lung Foundation www.blf.org.uk.
Breathe Easy groups run by the British Lung Foundation provide support for people with COPD and their carers.
You will also find very helpful patient-centred fact sheets at www.patient.co.uk/.
Smoking cessation help can be got from www.smokefree.nhs.uk/.

# 42 Nursing people with digestive disorders

## A and P

### The digestive system

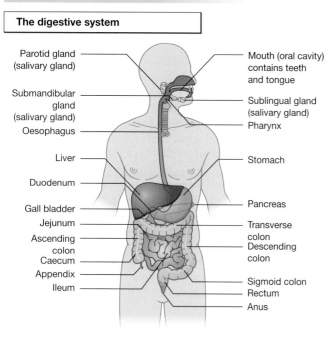

Parotid gland (salivary gland)
Submandibular gland (salivary gland)
Oesophagus
Liver
Duodenum
Gall bladder
Jejunum
Ascending colon
Caecum
Appendix
Ileum

Mouth (oral cavity) contains teeth and tongue
Sublingual gland (salivary gland)
Pharynx
Stomach
Pancreas
Transverse colon
Descending colon
Sigmoid colon
Rectum
Anus

Source: Tortora GJ & Derrickson B, 2011. Reproduced with permission of Wiley.

### Peristalsis

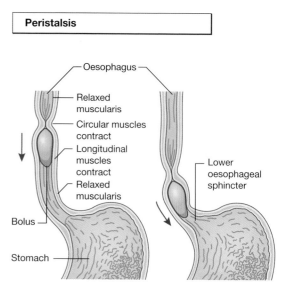

Oesophagus
Relaxed muscularis
Circular muscles contract
Longitudinal muscles contract
Relaxed muscularis
Bolus
Stomach
Lower oesophageal sphincter

Anterior view of frontal sections of peristalsis in oesophagus

Source: Tortora GJ & Derrickson B, 2011. Reproduced with permission of Wiley.

### Summary of the role of the digestive system hormones

| Hormone | Origin | Target | Action | Stimulus |
|---|---|---|---|---|
| Gastrin | Stomach | Stomach | Increases gastric gland secretion of hydrochloric acid<br>Gastric emptying | Presence of protein in the stomach |
| Secretin | Duodenum | Stomach | Inhibits gastric gland secretion<br>Inhibits gastric motility | Acidic and fatty chyme in the duodenum |
| | | Pancreas | Increases pancreatic juice secretion<br>Promotes cholecystokinin action | |
| | | Liver | Increases bile secretion | |
| Cholecystokinin | Duodenum | Pancreas | Increases pancreatic juice secretion | Chyme in the duodenum |
| | | Gall bladder | Stimulates contraction | |
| | | Hepatopancreatic sphincter | Relaxes – entry to duodenum open | |

Source: Peate I & Nair M, 2011. Reproduced with permission of Wiley.

Likely points of access to the healthcare system are general practice, emergency department, walk-in-clinic, out-of-hours (OOH) service, occupational health department, and ambulance service

*Adult Nursing at a Glance*, First Edition. Andrée le May. © 2015 John Wiley & Sons, Ltd. Published 2015 by John Wiley & Sons, Ltd.
Companion website: www.ataglanceseries.com/nursing/adult

# Key facts

- The digestive system (or gastrointestinal system) starts in the mouth and ends at the anus.
- This system breaks food down, mechanically and chemically, into nutrients and waste. The body uses nutrients for growth and repair and energy.
- The digestive system operates through five processes: ingestion, propulsion, digestion, absorption and elimination.
- Ingestion is the process of taking food and fluid into the digestive system through the mouth.
- Propulsion is the movement of food and fluid through the system.
- Digestion is the process of breaking food down, mechanically by chewing or chemically by enzymes or acid.
- Absorption is when the products of digestion and excess water leave the system and enter the blood and lymph systems for distribution to the body.
- Elimination is when waste from digestion is excreted as faeces through the anus.
- The main organs of digestion are the mouth, pharynx, oesophagus, stomach, small intestine and large intestine. These organs are assisted by accessory organs: the salivary glands, liver, pancreas and gall bladder.

# Common digestive disorders

- Infections
- Gastro-oesophageal reflux disease (GORD)
- Gastritis
- Peptic ulcers
- Malabsorption
- Irritable bowel syndrome
- Inflammatory bowel disease
- Diverticular disease
- Appendicitis
- Haemorrhoids
- Hepatitis
- Gall stones
- Cholecystitis
- Pancreatitis.

Each is covered in the following pages. See Chapter 43 for common signs and symptoms associated with digestive disorders.

# A and P

- The upper digestive tract comprises the mouth, pharynx, oesophagus and stomach. These organs are involved in the ingestion, propulsion and digestion of food and fluids.
- The small intestine is involved in absorption and the large intestine in elimination.
- Food starts its journey through the digestive system in the mouth where it is broken down mechanically by the teeth and lubricated by saliva. This process prepares the food for swallowing.
- Saliva, containing bactericidal lysozyme, moistens the mouth keeping it clean and healthy. Alterations to saliva predispose a person to mouth ulcers and infections.

- The salivary glands secrete salivary amylase, an enzyme that starts the breakdown of carbohydrate molecules to maltase.
- Once the food has been chewed sufficiently and moistened it leaves the mouth as a bolus and enters the oropharynx. This is known as the voluntary phase of swallowing.
- The pharyngeal phase of swallowing comes next. This reflex action, coordinated by the medulla oblongata, is triggered by the presence of food: it causes the contraction of pharyngeal muscles which ensures the closure of the nasopharynx and the trachea enabling food to move into the oesophagus (oesophageal phase) rather than the respiratory system.
- Waves of muscular contraction (peristalsis) move the bolus down the oesophagus to the stomach. This passage is helped by thick lubricating mucus secreted by the oesophageal mucosa.
- Once in the stomach food is mixed with gastric juices: bacteria are killed and protein breakdown begins. The mix of food and gastric juices is called chyme.
- Chyme leaves the stomach via the pyloric sphincter entering the six-metre long small intestine. The chyme is mixed with intestinal juices secreted by the cells lining the small intestine, pancreatic juices from the pancreas and bile from the liver. These together enable the absorption of nutrients.
- Nutrients are primarily absorbed in the small intestine.
- The small intestine comprises three parts (the duodenum, jejunum and ileum).
- Food residue moves from the ileum into the large intestine via the ileocaecal valve. Most of the remaining water is absorbed in the large intestine together with some vitamins, minerals and electrolytes. Food residue passes through the large intestine becoming more solid and is eventually eliminated through the anus as faeces.
- Faeces contains fibre, water, fatty acids, epithelial cells, microbes and stercobilin (from bilirubin breakdown).
- If food residue passes through the large intestine too quickly excess water is not absorbed resulting in diarrhoea: if it passes through too slowly, too much water is absorbed, resulting in constipation.
- The digestive system secretes various hormones (see above).

# Essentials of best practice

Digestive disorders range from mild to severe. Nursing someone with a digestive disorder may take place in the community, the GP surgery, the ED or OOH service or in a hospital ward. The essentials of best practice required to care for common digestive disorders are covered in the subsequent pages. In addition Chapter 43 details assessment of the digestive system, common signs and symptoms and emergencies of the digestive system.

## Patient information

There are several patient support groups and charities focusing on digestive disorders. You can find most of them on the Self Help UK website http://www.self-help.org.uk.
You will also find very helpful patient-centred fact sheets at www.patient.co.uk/.

# 43 Signs, symptoms, assessment and emergencies

## Important assessments of the digestive system (based on Dougherty and Lister, 2011 and O'Brien, 2012)

Making a nursing assessment of a patient with a digestive system disorder should focus on four areas – nausea and vomiting (Section 1), nutrition, swallowing and elimination (below).

- Nutrition
  - o Start with assessing the patient's oral health: ask the patient about their usual routines and if anything has altered
  - o Check if any medications have caused problems with their oral health – soreness, ulcers, taste changes
  - o Check if their lips are pink, moist and intact: a dry mouth and cracked lips might suggest dehydration
  - o Check if their gums are pink and without signs of infection or bleeding
  - o Check that dentures, if worn, are available and if any teeth have crowns or bridgework (particularly if going for anaesthesia)
  - o Ask about usual pattern of eating and drinking and if these have been disrupted and how
  - o Ask about alcohol consumption (and smoking)
  - o Ask if a patient has any problems with any functional aspects of their upper digestive system – chewing, swallowing, heartburn
  - o Ask if they have any pain/discomfort (e.g. bloating) associated with eating or the organs of the digestive system
  - o Ask if their appetite has changed or taste/weight altered in any way
  - o Ask if they have food intolerances or allergies
  - o Use a nutritional screening tool (e.g. MUST)
- Swallowing
  - o Ask the patient (or their family/carer) if they have problems swallowing
  - o Observe for swallowing difficulties or indications that a problem might be present (e.g. you might see drooling, poor control of food when it's in the mouth, coughing, choking, repeated throat clearing, a wet sounding voice)
  - o Refer to the speech and language therapy team for a swallowing assessment if the patient has difficulties and the dietician for modifications to their diet
  - o Discuss in the nursing/multi-disciplinary team the most appropriate form of nutritional support if problems are suspected but an assessment cannot be made immediately
- Elimination
  - o Ask about usual bowel habits and any deviation from these, for example diarrhoea or constipation or a change in normal routines
  - o If patient has a suspected infection stool specimens may need to be taken
  - o Urine testing for ketones and glucose is also important. The presence solely of ketones can indicate inadequate food intake. Glucose plus ketones may suggest diabetes

Whenever there is deviation from a person's usual patterns, report these changes to a senior colleague or doctor: or advise the patient to

A&M

# Common signs and symptoms

Malaise (feeling under the weather)

Pyrexia

Abdominal cramps

Diarrhoea

Constipation

Loss of appetite

Dry skin due to dehydration

Confusion and disorientation due to dehydration

Nausea

Vomiting

Regurgitation

Heartburn

Difficulty swallowing

Weight loss

Discomfort/pain

Bloating

Fear

Anxiety

Blood in faeces.

# Emergencies: digestive system

Recognising and responding to sudden deteriorations in a patient's condition is vital. Two situations where rapid intervention can be life-saving are gastrointestinal bleeding (below) and shock (Section 1).

# Gastrointestinal bleeding

Bleeding from the gastrointestinal (GI) tract can occur via the mouth or via the anus.

Haematemesis (vomiting blood) is usually caused by problems of the upper GI tract. The blood may be fresh, but altered blood may also be vomited; this looks like brown coffee grounds because the blood has been changed by intestinal acid and enzymes.

Malaena is the passage of thick, sticky, black, treacle-like, offensively smelly stools containing altered blood: this may be caused by problems anywhere from the oesophagus to the colon. Solid dark stool that tests positive to occult blood (not visible) is not malaena.

Bright red blood in stools or on toilet paper is usually associated with anorectal problems. Darker red blood sometimes mixed with clots in stools is linked to problems higher up the GI tract.

Gastrointestinal bleeding may be minor requiring investigation and appropriate treatment or major requiring rapid intervention to prevent death due to hypovolaemic shock. Major gastrointestinal bleeding is associated with peptic ulcer disease (PUD), varices (oesophageal and gastric), gastritis, diverticular disease and angiodysplasia in the colon (small vascular malformation seen in older people).

# Essentials of best practice

Major GI tract bleeding is a medical emergency. Call for help immediately.

GI tract bleeding is very frightening both for the patient and their family (and also for health professionals!). Keeping a calm manner and explaining clearly and simply what is happening is essential.

• In some instances bleeding may be expected. If this is the case regular, frequent monitoring of pulse, blood pressure, respiratory rate and oxygen saturation should be made to try to detect haemorrhage early. Deviations from normal should be reported immediately and documented.

• Also monitoring level of consciousness in those at risk is important. Family and nurses, because they spend the most time with patients, may be the first to recognise small alterations which could be useful early warning signs of a worsening condition.

• If a patient is having a major bleed, observations of pulse, blood pressure, respiratory rate, oxygen saturation and level of consciousness need to be made every 15 minutes. Pulse and respirations will be rapid, blood pressure will be low, and oxygen saturation will be lower than normal. Confusion or agitation may be present. Skin will be cold and clammy.

• It is important to remember the principles of CPR whilst dealing with major gastrointestinal bleeding (Section 1) – a patient's condition can deteriorate suddenly. Keep Airway, Breathing and Circulation in your mind at all times.

• If a patient has profuse haematemesis, suction may be needed to keep their airway clear.

• Fluid resuscitation is a key element of the management of major GI tract bleeding.

• Estimate/measure blood loss (and keep a record of it) since the amount of blood lost will guide management.

• Help with gaining access for IV line may be needed.

• Monitor IVI, blood transfusion and other medications being administered (e.g. vasoconstriction agents) and treatments (e.g. a balloon tamponade tube may have been inserted nasogastrically to try to stop bleeding).

• Monitor hourly output from urinary catheter if inserted. (Or insert catheter at first opportunity.) Report any reduction in urine production or no urine or mismatch between intake and output. Under perfusion of the kidneys will lead to kidney failure.

• Prepare the patient for emergency endoscopy and treatment or other surgery as appropriate (Section 1).

Family and carers need support during this time too. Careful, simple explanations should be given. After a bleed has been controlled successfully patients (and their families/carers) may want to discuss with you what happened and how likely a recurrence may be.

# 44 Nursing people with infections of the digestive system

## Food poisoning

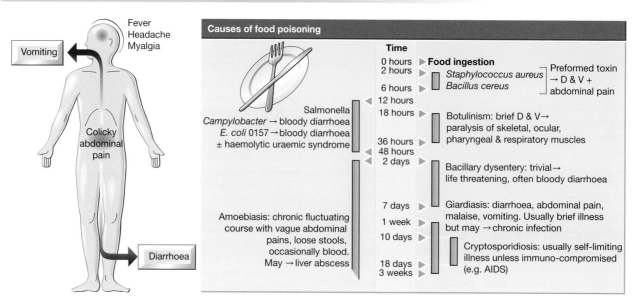

Fever
Headache
Myalgia

Vomiting

Colicky abdominal pain

Diarrhoea

**Causes of food poisoning**

**Time**

| Time | |
|---|---|
| 0 hours | ▶ **Food ingestion** |
| 2 hours | *Staphylococcus aureus* ⎫ Preformed toxin |
| 6 hours | *Bacillus cereus* ⎭ → D & V + abdominal pain |
| 12 hours | ◀ |
| 18 hours | ▶ Botulism: brief D & V → paralysis of skeletal, ocular, pharyngeal & respiratory muscles |

Salmonella
Campylobacter → bloody diarrhoea
E. coli 0157 → bloody diarrhoea
± haemolytic uraemic syndrome

36 hours ▶
48 hours ◀
2 days ◀ ▶ Bacillary dysentery: trivial → life threatening, often bloody diarrhoea

7 days ▶ Giardiasis: diarrhoea, abdominal pain, malaise, vomiting. Usually brief illness but may → chronic infection
1 week ▶
10 days ▶

Cryptosporidiosis: usually self-limiting illness unless immuno-compromised (e.g. AIDS)

Amoebiasis: chronic fluctuating course with vague abdominal pains, loose stools, occasionally blood. May → liver abscess

18 days ▶
3 weeks ▶

Source: Davey P (ed), 2014. Reproduced with permission of Wiley.

## Primary care

**Advice to patients on recognising signs of deterioration or concern and when to consult a doctor or nurse**

- Mild/moderate dehydration: advise to drink more than usual (usual = 2 litres/day PLUS 200 ml for every time you have diarrhoea). Consider taking over-the counter rehydration medication (e.g. dioralyte) and consult doctor/practice nurse if experiencing:
  o Tiredness
  o Dizziness/feeling light headed
  o Headache
  o Muscle cramps
  o Passing smaller amounts of urine than usual
  o Dry mouth and tongue
  o Irritability
  o Sunken eyes
- Severe dehydration is a medical emergency:
  o Rapid heart rate
  o Being confused (this might only be recognised by other people)
  o Weakness
  o Producing very little urine
  o Coma
- Blood in diarrhoea or vomit
- Persistent high fever
- Infections caught abroad
- If condition worsens
- If patient is elderly, pregnant, immuno-compromised or has an underlying health problem

**HE&P**

Likely points of access to the healthcare system are general practice, emergency department, walk-in-clinic, out-of-hours (OOH) service, occupational health department, and ambulance service

*Adult Nursing at a Glance*, First Edition. Andrée le May. © 2015 John Wiley & Sons, Ltd. Published 2015 by John Wiley & Sons, Ltd.
Companion website: www.ataglanceseries.com/nursing/adult

# Key facts

• Infections of the digestive system are usually spread through human-to-human contact, food or water. They can be either acute or chronic.

• Acute gastroenteritis (infection of the intestines) typically presents as diarrhoea with or without vomiting and is accompanied by abdominal pain, pyrexia, headache and myalgia. Onset is usually sudden.

• Gastroenteritis is most commonly caused by viruses or bacteria.

• Viral infections include those from noroviruses and are easily spread through contact with unwashed hands and/or surfaces.

• Most cases of acute gastroenteritis settle with little intervention. Patients are treated in primary care and advised about hydration, rehydration medication (e.g. dioralyte) and cross-infection. If symptoms persist a stool specimen should be sent for analysis so that treatment can be tailored to the cause.

• Antibiotics may be prescribed against bacterial gastroenteritis if symptoms persist.

• Patients needing hospitalisation are likely to be older, dehydrated, exhausted or have an infection caused by a more serious causative agent (e.g. *E. coli* O157 or *clostridium botulinum*). Intravenous fluids and antibiotics may be needed.

• Chronic gastroenteritis may be caused by giardiasis, gastrointestinal tuberculosis or amoeba. Treatment is usually with medication. Attention should be drawn to rehydration.

# Essentials of best practice

The nursing care of patients with food poisoning or gastrointestinal infections, whether in primary care or in hospitals, focuses on rehydration, symptom control and infection control. The following essentials of best practice are at the core of this care:

✓ Accurate assessment and regular monitoring
✓ Communication with the healthcare team, patient and family
✓ Health education and promotion
✓ Symptom control and management
✓ Discharge planning

## Patient information

You will find very helpful patient-centred fact sheets at www.patient.co.uk/.

# 45 Nursing people with gastro-oesophageal reflux disease

## Complications of reflux

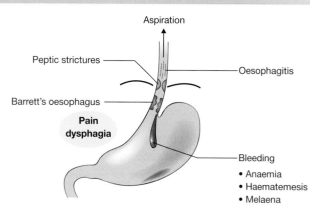

Aspiration

Peptic strictures —

Oesophagitis

Barrett's oesophagus —

**Pain dysphagia**

Bleeding
- Anaemia
- Haematemesis
- Melaena

Source: Davey P (ed), 2014. Reproduced with permission of Wiley.

## Primary/Hospital care

| Advice to patients on minimising the effects of gastro-oesophageal reflux |

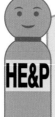

HE&P

- Lifestyle advice: patients should be advised to avoid food and drink known to cause reflux (e.g. fatty foods, tomatoes, alcohol, chocolate and coffee) as well as individual triggers. Anyone who is overweight should be encouraged to lose weight. Anyone who smokes should be encouraged to stop and advised about self-help options. Eat smaller more frequent meals
- Being in certain positions can exacerbate GORD and patients should be advised to avoid lying flat or bending forwards after food. Raising the head of the bed by about 20 cm can make a difference: BUT using more pillows than usual can increase pressure on the abdomen and may worsen GORD
- Medication regimens should be discussed and adherence monitored. Often long-term medication is needed. Any problems with medication should be discussed with the GP

Likely points of access to the healthcare system are general practice, emergency department, walk-in-clinic, out-of-hours (OOH) service, occupational health department, and ambulance service

# Key facts

• Gastro-oesophageal reflux disease (GORD) is common in the Western world and affects between 20–40% of the population.
• GORD commonly presents with heartburn, effortless regurgitation, belching and sometimes nausea. These symptoms can be linked to particular positions, for example bending forwards/lying down. Intermittent pain on swallowing may also be present. Chest pain may occur so angina needs to be ruled out before a diagnosis of GORD can be made.
• Be aware of dismissing chest pain as an exacerbation of established GORD when it is really an MI.
• Lifestyle factors, for example smoking, obesity, stress, fatty foods, pastry, alcohol and chocolate can exacerbate symptoms.
• Diagnosis is made by history taking, upper gastrointestinal endoscopy and if symptoms are persistent manometry and pH recording to select patients for anti-reflux surgery.
• Management is primarily through lifestyle changes and medication (e.g. antacids, proton pump inhibitors (PPIs), prokinetics, $H_2$-receptor antagonists ($H_2$RAs)): surgery may be necessary for those with hiatus hernias (e.g. laparoscopic antireflux surgery (LARS)).
• Hiatus hernias are when the stomach protrudes into the chest through a defect in the diaphragm.

# A and P

GORD is associated with ineffective closing of the lower oesophageal sphincter. This results in reflux of the stomach's contents into the oesophagus. The acid gastric contents cause abrasion to the oesophagus and the classic symptoms of burning and discomfort found in patients with GORD.

# Essentials of best practice

The nursing care of patients with GORD focuses on health education and promotion (see above).

For patients requiring surgery, the principles of pre- and postoperative care described in Section 1 should be adhered to. Special preparation may be needed for some procedures and these may vary according to local practice.

The following essentials of best practice are important:

✓ Accurate assessment and regular monitoring
✓ Communication with the healthcare team, patient and family
✓ Health education and promotion
✓ Symptom control and management
✓ Discharge planning

---

**Patient information**

You will find very helpful patient-centred fact sheets at www.patient.co.uk/ and NHS choices www.nhs.uk/Conditions/.

# 46 Nursing people with stomach disorders

## The stomach

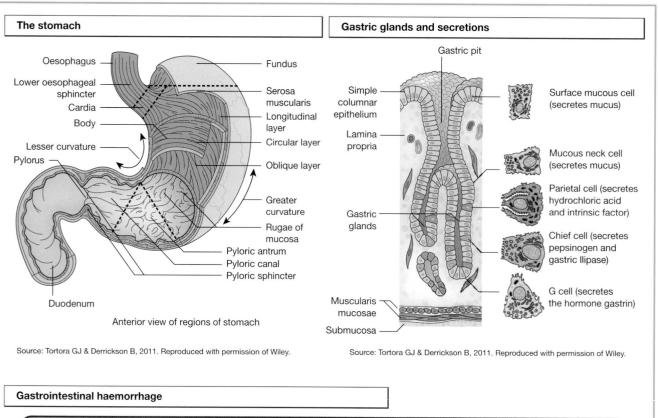

Oesophagus
Lower oesophageal sphincter
Cardia
Body
Lesser curvature
Pylorus

Fundus
Serosa muscularis
Longitudinal layer
Circular layer
Oblique layer
Greater curvature
Rugae of mucosa
Pyloric antrum
Pyloric canal
Pyloric sphincter

Duodenum

Anterior view of regions of stomach

Source: Tortora GJ & Derrickson B, 2011. Reproduced with permission of Wiley.

## Gastric glands and secretions

Gastric pit

Simple columnar epithelium
Lamina propria

Gastric glands

Muscularis mucosae
Submucosa

Surface mucous cell (secretes mucus)

Mucous neck cell (secretes mucus)

Parietal cell (secretes hydrochloric acid and intrinsic factor)

Chief cell (secretes pepsinogen and gastric lipase)

G cell (secretes the hormone gastrin)

Source: Tortora GJ & Derrickson B, 2011. Reproduced with permission of Wiley.

## Gastrointestinal haemorrhage

Major GI tract bleeding is a medical emergency. Call for help immediately.

GI tract bleeding is very frightening both for the patient and their family (and also for health professionals!). Keeping a calm manner and explaining clearly and simply what is happening is essential.

- In some instances bleeding may be expected. If this is the case, regular, frequent monitoring of pulse, blood pressure, respiratory rate and oxygen saturation should be made to try to anticipate haemorrhage. Deviations from normal should be reported immediately and documented
- Also monitoring level of consciousness in those at risk is important. Family and nurses, because they spend the most time with patients, may be the first to recognise small alterations which could be useful early warning signs of a worsening condition
- If a patient is having a major bleed, observations of pulse, blood pressure, respiratory rate, oxygen saturation and level of consciousness need to be made every 15 minutes. Pulse and respirations will be rapid, blood pressure will be low, and oxygen saturation will be lower than normal. Confusion or agitation may be present. Skin will be cold and clammy
- It is important to remember the principles of CPR whilst dealing with major gastrointestinal bleeding (Section 1) – a patient's condition can deteriorate suddenly. Keep Airway, Breathing and Circulation in your mind at all times
- If a patient has profuse haematemesis, suction may be needed to keep their airway clear
- Fluid resuscitation is a key element of the management of major GI tract bleeding
- Estimate/measure blood loss (and keep a record of it) since the amount of blood lost will guide management
- Help with gaining access for IV line may be needed
- Monitor IVI, blood transfusion and other medications being administered (e.g. vasoconstriction agents) and treatments (e.g. a balloon tamponade tube may have been inserted nasogastrically to try to stop bleeding)
- Monitor hourly output from catheter if inserted. (Or insert catheter at first opportunity.) Report any reduction in urine production or no urine or mismatch between intake and output. Under perfusion of the kidneys will lead to kidney failure
- Prepare the patient for emergency endoscopy and treatment or other surgery as appropriate (Section 1)

Family and carers need support during this time too; careful, simple explanations should be given. After a bleed has been controlled successfully patients (and their families/carers) may want to discuss with you what happened and how likely a recurrence may be. If a patient has died as a result of the bleed their family and carers will need empathic support and information (Section 1)

Likely points of access to the healthcare system are general practice, emergency department, walk-in-clinic, out-of-hours (OOH) service, occupational health department, and ambulance service

*Adult Nursing at a Glance*, First Edition. Andrée le May. © 2015 John Wiley & Sons, Ltd. Published 2015 by John Wiley & Sons, Ltd.
Companion website: www.ataglanceseries.com/nursing/adult

## Key facts

• Gastritis and peptic ulceration are common disorders of the stomach and duodenum.

## A and P

The stomach lies in the abdominal cavity. It is joined at one end to the oesophagus and at the other to the duodenum (above). Once in the stomach food is mixed with gastric juices: bacteria are killed and protein breakdown begins. When the stomach is empty the mucosa within the stomach is folded (rugae), when it's full it stretches enabling the stomach to contain around 4 litres of food. The mucosa also contains gastric glands which secrete mucus, hydrochloric acid, intrinsic factor, pepsinogen and gastric lipase and gastrin (above). These are then mixed with water and mineral salts to form gastric juice. Food is mixed with gastric juice to form acidic chyme. Chyme leaves the stomach by the pyloric sphincter entering the six metre long small intestine via the duodenum.

## Gastritis

• Gastritis is an acute or chronic inflammation of the lining of the stomach.
• Acute gastritis can be caused by ingestion of irritants (e.g. aspirin; alcohol) or bacteria (helicobacter pylori).
• Helicobacter pylori is a common cause of chronic gastritis.
• Pain (before or after food), nausea and vomiting are common symptoms associated with acute gastritis.
• Rarely patients experience haematemesis, melaena, weight- loss or iron-deficiency anaemia. Occult blood may be present in faeces.
• Patients with pernicious anaemia, autoimmune disorders, chronic alcoholism, long term use of NSAIDs and peptic ulcers may have chronic gastritis.
• Most people with gastritis are cared for at home by their GP.
• Diagnosis can be made by endoscopy and gastric biopsy. Blood and breath tests are also available for detecting helicobacter pylori.
• Practice nurses may provide advice for patients with gastritis about diet (e.g. avoiding spicy foods and alcohol) and medication.

## Gastritis: essentials of best practice

The nursing care of patients with gastritis focuses on health education and promotion. Encouraging patients to alter their diet to avoid spicy food, alcohol and any other identifiable triggers is important. Medication may be prescribed by the GP if dietary changes are not successful (or helicobacter pylori is found) and advice should be given about adherence to medication and possible side-effects. The importance of avoiding aspirin and over-the-counter NSAIDs should be emphasised. Patients should be reminded to seek urgent medical advice if either symptoms worsen or new signs and symptoms appear (e.g. haematemesis, melaena, weight loss or tiredness).

## Peptic ulceration

• Peptic ulceration can occur in either the stomach (gastric ulcer) or the duodenum (duodenal ulcer).
• Ulcers occur when gastric acid production exceeds normal amounts and causes mucosal damage.
• Helicobacter pylori damage the mucosal defence system and are therefore associated with ulceration.
• Risk factors include the use of gastric irritants such as aspirin and NSAIDs. Smoking is also linked to ulcer development.
• Symptoms associated with peptic ulceration are pain (dyspepsia) and sometimes vomiting: often a patient has no symptoms prior to a gastrointestinal haemorrhage.
• Gastrointestinal haemorrhage is a medical emergency (see Chapter 43).
• Complications of peptic ulceration include vomiting, bleeding (haematemesis/malaena), perforation and peritonitis.
• Treatment includes combinations of drugs to reduce gastric acid, eradicate helicobacter pylori and if unsatisfactory, or the ulcer has perforated, surgery.
• Some gastric ulcers may be early gastric cancer so biopsy is important.

## Peptic ulcers: essentials of best practice

Nursing people with peptic ulceration can span community and hospital care. Management with medication prescribed by the GP may be the first course of treatment for patients with peptic ulceration. This may be complemented by health education and promotion advice from the practice nurse primarily associated with medication adherence and what to do about worsening or new symptoms. Patients will often have diagnostic endoscopies and these may be carried out by specialist nurses as day cases.

Gastrointestinal haemorrhage is an emergency and will require prompt nursing care if a patient is in hospital or prompt advice, if at home, to call for an emergency ambulance (Chapter 43).

If a patient requires surgery, the principles of pre- and post-operative care described in Section 1 should be adhered to.

Surgery is likely to be done as an emergency and the patient (and their family/carers) will be feeling vulnerable and afraid, caring for them will therefore require highly skilled communication as well as attentive, accurate assessment and monitoring.

## Essentials of best practice

When nursing anyone with a disorder of the stomach attention should be paid to:
✓ Accurate assessment and regular monitoring
✓ Communication with the healthcare team, patient and family
✓ Health education and promotion
✓ Discharge planning

### Patient information

You will find very helpful patient-centred fact sheets at www.patient.co.uk.

# 47 Nursing people with intestinal disorders

## The intestines

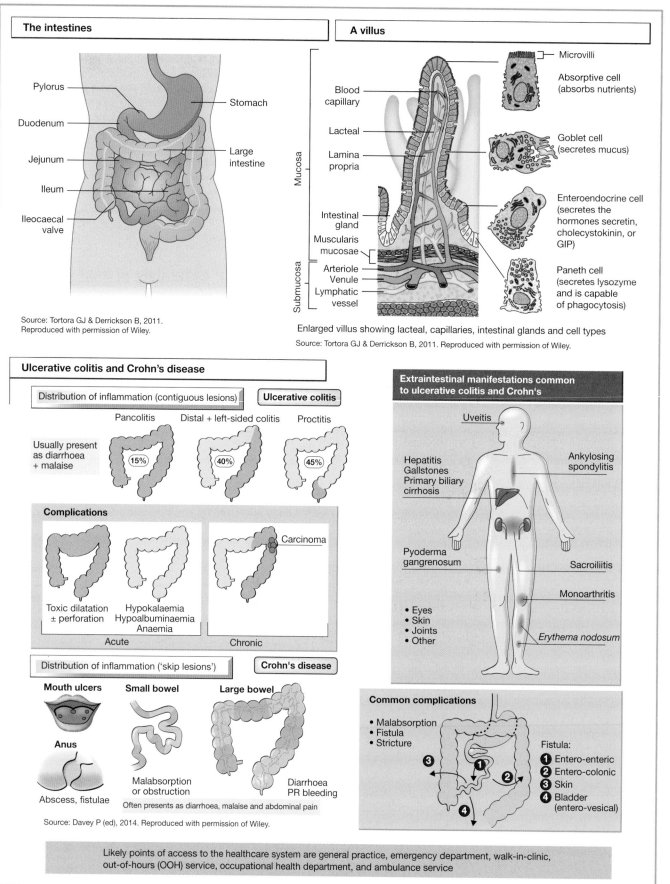

Pylorus
Duodenum
Jejunum
Ileum
Ileocaecal valve
Stomach
Large intestine

Source: Tortora GJ & Derrickson B, 2011.
Reproduced with permission of Wiley.

## A villus

Microvilli

Absorptive cell (absorbs nutrients)

Blood capillary
Lacteal
Lamina propria

Mucosa

Goblet cell (secretes mucus)

Enteroendocrine cell (secretes the hormones secretin, cholecystokinin, or GIP)

Intestinal gland
Muscularis mucosae

Arteriole
Venule
Lymphatic vessel

Submucosa

Paneth cell (secretes lysozyme and is capable of phagocytosis)

Enlarged villus showing lacteal, capillaries, intestinal glands and cell types

Source: Tortora GJ & Derrickson B, 2011. Reproduced with permission of Wiley.

## Ulcerative colitis and Crohn's disease

**Distribution of inflammation (contiguous lesions)**   **Ulcerative colitis**

Pancolitis    Distal + left-sided colitis    Proctitis

Usually present as diarrhoea + malaise

15%    40%    45%

### Complications

Carcinoma

Toxic dilatation ± perforation

Hypokalaemia
Hypoalbuminaemia
Anaemia

Acute

Chronic

**Distribution of inflammation ('skip lesions')**   **Crohn's disease**

**Mouth ulcers**    **Small bowel**    **Large bowel**

**Anus**

Malabsorption or obstruction

Diarrhoea
PR bleeding

Abscess, fistulae

Often presents as diarrhoea, malaise and abdominal pain

Source: Davey P (ed), 2014. Reproduced with permission of Wiley.

## Extraintestinal manifestations common to ulcerative colitis and Crohn's

Uveitis

Hepatitis
Gallstones
Primary biliary cirrhosis

Ankylosing spondylitis

Pyoderma gangrenosum

Sacroiliitis

Monoarthritis

Erythema nodosum

• Eyes
• Skin
• Joints
• Other

### Common complications

• Malabsorption
• Fistula
• Stricture

Fistula:
❶ Entero-enteric
❷ Entero-colonic
❸ Skin
❹ Bladder (entero-vesical)

Likely points of access to the healthcare system are general practice, emergency department, walk-in-clinic, out-of-hours (OOH) service, occupational health department, and ambulance service

*Adult Nursing at a Glance*, First Edition. Andrée le May. © 2015 John Wiley & Sons, Ltd. Published 2015 by John Wiley & Sons, Ltd.
Companion website: www.ataglanceseries.com/nursing/adult

# Key facts

• The small and large intestine can be affected by conditions causing disturbance to the absorption of nutrients, vitamins, mineral, fluids and electrolytes and the elimination of waste.
• These conditions include coeliac disease, irritable bowel syndrome, inflammatory bowel disease and cancer.
• Malabsorption of nutrients results from damage to the absorptive mechanisms of the small intestine (e.g. in coeliac disease gluten allergy triggers an autoimmune reaction which flattens the intestinal villi, and in other bowel conditions resection of large areas may reduce the absorptive capacity of the small intestine), or inflammation (e.g. in Crohn's disease affecting the small intestine), or digestive enzyme deficiency (e.g. in chronic pancreatitis), or acute or chronic infection (e.g. with giardiasis).
• The signs and symptoms of malabsorption include weight loss, tiredness, diarrhoea and steatorrhoea (hard to flush pale offensive stools).
• Irritable Bowel Syndrome (IBS) is a condition affecting the large intestine. IBS is a set of unexplained symptoms (e.g. abdominal distension, abdominal pain, diarrhoea or constipation or fluctuation between diarrhoea and constipation, weight loss, nausea, backache, tiredness).
• Inflammation of the intestine occurs in Inflammatory Bowel Disease (IBD). IBD is divided into ulcerative colitis (UC) and Crohn's disease (CD).
• Disorders of the intestines are largely treated in primary care and the community: here practice nurses, specialist nurses and community nurses have a particular part to play in health education and promotion and symptom control (see diarrhoea and constipation in Section 1). Acute exacerbations of disorders of the intestine may necessitate hospitalisation.

# Ulcerative colitis

UC is the most common form of IBD. UC is characterised by contiguous inflammation of the mucosa of the large intestine from the rectum upwards (colitis): widespread (but relatively superficial) ulceration may occur resulting in chronic diarrhoea (often bloody) and malaise. Rectal bleeding, mucus and pus in stools and the urge to defecate without having any stools to pass (tenesmus) may occur. Extra-intestinal problems such as iritis and skin lesions can develop.

UC usually starts in young adulthood. Cause is unknown but there may be a genetic predisposition to UC. UC is not curable but is treatable with medication and/or surgery. Symptom management is important (Section 1). Most people with UC experience acute episodes interspersed with periods when they are free from symptoms; in 10% of people UC is active all the time whilst others (~10%) can experience long-term remission. A very small number of people will die from UC.

# UC: essentials of best practice

The routine nursing care of patients with UC focuses on health education and promotion and symptom control and management. These are particularly important aspects of care because many of the symptoms of UC (and CD) are perceived as both embarrassing and isolating: minimising symptoms and these feelings will increase a person's sense of wellbeing. Medication will be prescribed by the GP/gastrointestinal specialist and advice should be given about adherence and possible side-effects. Some patients, during acute exacerbations, require hospitalisation for intravenous drug therapy, rehydration, parenteral nutrition, blood transfusion or surgery. Around 20–30% of people require surgery due to perforation, fistulae, abscesses or dilation with the potential for rupture. Regardless of the type of operation undertaken. patients and their family/carers will be anxious about the consequences of surgery (e.g. the formation of a stoma) so careful explanation will be needed – consultation with a stoma nurse specialist should be arranged if a stoma is likely to be formed. If surgery is required adhere to the principles of pre- and post-operative care described in Section 1. Depression may accompany UC.

# Crohn's disease

CD is a chronic inflammatory disease affecting any part of the GI tract from the mouth to the anus. Inflammation in CD is not contiguous as it is in UC. A characteristic pattern of affected and unaffected portions is present – 'skip' lesions. Ulcers are deeper than in UC and sometimes lead to fistulae and abscesses. Symptoms depend on its location. CD often presents with abdominal pain, malaise and diarrhoea. CD is incurable, characterised by remissions and relapses, associated with high morbidity and can result in reduced life expectancy. Treatment is by medication and surgery when complications (e.g. fistulae, abscesses) occur. Nutritional assessment and support is also an essential component of treatment. Extra-intestinal problems include ankylosing spondylitis and uveitis

# CD: essentials of best practice

People with CD often require nursing in hospital. Hospitalisations focus on the intravenous medication, fluid replacement, nutritional support and/or surgery. People admitted to hospital will often by debilitated and anxious. Over half of those with CD will require surgery and as with UC this will cause anxiety associated with the possibility of stoma formation and management (see above). See Section 1 for the principles of pre- and post-operative care.

# Essentials of best practice

When nursing anyone with a disorder of the intestine particular attention should be paid to:
✓ Accurate assessment and regular monitoring
✓ Communication with the healthcare team, patient and family
✓ Health education and promotion
✓ Symptom control and management (see Chapter 8 for essentials of stoma care)

---

**Patient information**

You will find very helpful patient-centred fact sheets at www. patient.co.uk/.
The Gut Trust is a national charity focusing on the self-management of IBS. www.theguttrust.org.
Crohn's and Colitis UK is a national charity focussing on IBD. www.crohnsandcolitis.org.uk.
Coeliac UK provides extensive information about coeliac disease. www.coeliac.org.uk.

# 48 Nursing people with disorders of the intestines and anal canal

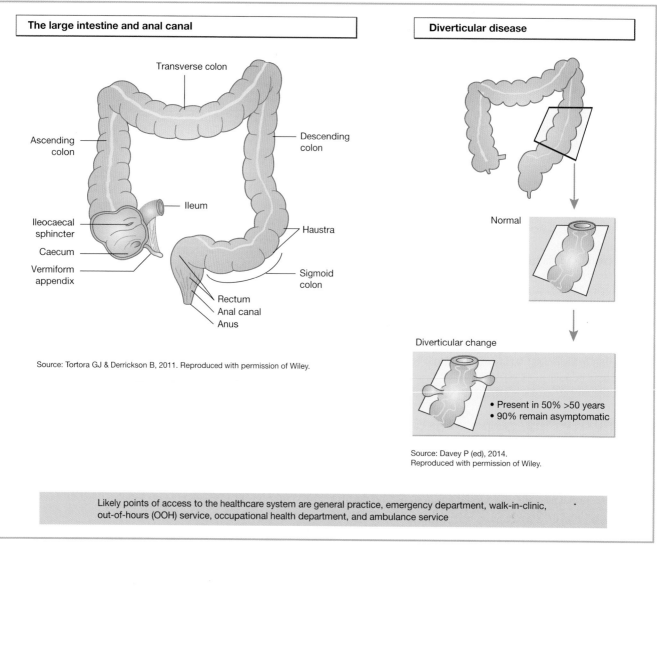

**The large intestine and anal canal**

Transverse colon

Ascending colon

Descending colon

Ileum

Ileocaecal sphincter

Caecum

Vermiform appendix

Haustra

Sigmoid colon

Rectum
Anal canal
Anus

Source: Tortora GJ & Derrickson B, 2011. Reproduced with permission of Wiley.

**Diverticular disease**

Normal

Diverticular change

- Present in 50% >50 years
- 90% remain asymptomatic

Source: Davey P (ed), 2014.
Reproduced with permission of Wiley.

Likely points of access to the healthcare system are general practice, emergency department, walk-in-clinic, out-of-hours (OOH) service, occupational health department, and ambulance service

# Key facts

- Other common problems of the lower intestine and anal canal include diverticular disease, appendicitis and haemorrhoids.
- Diverticular disease is a degenerative change in the colon that causes the formation of out-pouches or pockets of mucosa which push through the muscular wall of the bowel (opposite) and form a diverticulum. Symptoms include constipation, intermittent constipation with intermittent diarrhoea and spasmodic grumbling-type pain. The colon may become inflamed as a result of impaction of faeces in a diverticulum, which in turn can result in infection and abscess formation, pain and fever. This is known as diverticulitis. The diverticulum can erode blood vessels resulting in GI tract bleeding or form fistula with neighbouring organs: they may also perforate causing peritonitis. Treatment depends on the presenting problem but is generally conservative (e.g. avoiding constipation by dietary modification, intravenous fluids and antispasmodic medication) although surgery may be needed. Diverticular disease is more common in older people but is often asymptomatic.
- Appendicitis is an inflammation of the vermiform appendix usually associated with blockage of the lumen. Appendicitis is the most common surgical emergency of the Western world. Removal of the appendix (appendicectomy) can be performed either as open surgery or using a laparoscope. Complications may include perforation, abscess formation and peritonitis. Intravenous antibiotic therapy will be needed if the appendix has perforated.
- Haemorrhoids (piles) are submucosal vascular structures consisting of a dilated venous plexus, a small artery and areolar tissue in the anal canal. Swollen piles result from increased venous pressure from straining to defecate or altered haemodynamics, for example during pregnancy. They can be itchy, bleed or prolapse. Treatment in the first instance consists of using bulk laxatives and eating a high fibre diet to prevent constipation and straining. Injection sclerotherapy, cryosurgery or haemorrhoidectomy may be necessary if bleeding or prolapse occurs.

# Diverticular disease: essentials of best practice

The routine nursing care of people with diverticular disease focuses on health education and promotion and symptom control and management and is predominantly about giving dietary advice. Antispasmodic medication may be prescribed. Patients should be told to avoid stimulant laxatives since increasing the pressure in the colon's muscular wall can cause the development of more diverticula. Hospitalisation may be necessary if pain is severe, dehydration occurs or there is infection. Surgery may be necessary and if so nursing care should be given in line with the principles of pre- and post-operative care detailed in Section 1. As with other inflammatory intestinal conditions fear of stoma formation may be present (Chapter 47).

# Appendicitis: essentials of best practice

Appendicitis is a surgical emergency. Operating before the appendix ruptures and causes peritonitis is the critical concern. People admitted to hospital with appendicitis will be generally fit but acutely ill. Accurate assessment and monitoring is essential to recognise signs of perforation and peritonitis (e.g. increased pain, abdominal rigidity, pyrexia, vomiting, extreme weakness and shock) and report these to senior colleagues or a doctor. If these symptoms persist post-operatively an abdominal abscess may have developed.

See Section 1 for the principles of pre- and post-operative care.

# Haemorrhoids: essentials of best practice

The nursing care of people with haemorrhoids will focus on giving dietary advice (increased fibre, increased fluid intake and increased exercise) to minimise constipation and associated straining and/or pre- and post-operative care if surgery is needed (this is likely to be undertaken as a day case).

See Section 1 for the principles of pre- and post-operative care. Reassurance and prophylactic pain control will be needed post-operatively around the time of the patient's first bowel opening after surgery.

# Essentials of best practice

When nursing anyone with a disorder of the intestine and anal canal attention should be paid to:

✓ Accurate assessment and regular monitoring
✓ Communication with the healthcare team, patient and family
✓ Health education and promotion
✓ Symptom control and management
✓ Discharge planning

---

**Patient information**

You will find very helpful patient-centred fact sheets at www.patient.co.uk/.

# Nursing people with liver disorders

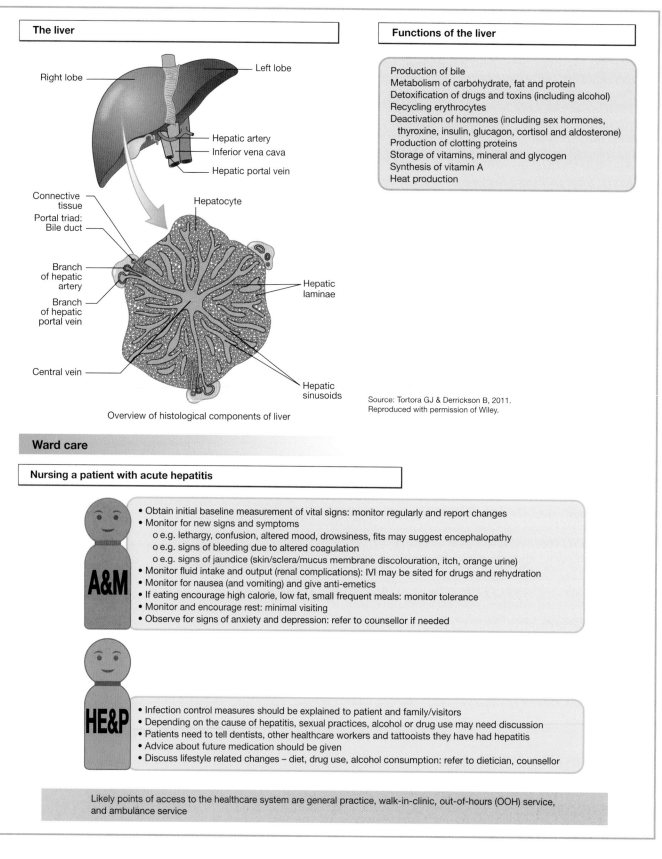

### The liver

Right lobe

Left lobe

Hepatic artery
Inferior vena cava
Hepatic portal vein

Connective tissue
Portal triad:
Bile duct

Branch of hepatic artery

Branch of hepatic portal vein

Central vein

Hepatocyte

Hepatic laminae

Hepatic sinusoids

Overview of histological components of liver

Source: Tortora GJ & Derrickson B, 2011.
Reproduced with permission of Wiley.

### Functions of the liver

Production of bile
Metabolism of carbohydrate, fat and protein
Detoxification of drugs and toxins (including alcohol)
Recycling erythrocytes
Deactivation of hormones (including sex hormones, thyroxine, insulin, glucagon, cortisol and aldosterone)
Production of clotting proteins
Storage of vitamins, mineral and glycogen
Synthesis of vitamin A
Heat production

### Ward care

#### Nursing a patient with acute hepatitis

**A&M**
- Obtain initial baseline measurement of vital signs: monitor regularly and report changes
- Monitor for new signs and symptoms
  - o e.g. lethargy, confusion, altered mood, drowsiness, fits may suggest encephalopathy
  - o e.g. signs of bleeding due to altered coagulation
  - o e.g. signs of jaundice (skin/sclera/mucus membrane discolouration, itch, orange urine)
- Monitor fluid intake and output (renal complications): IVI may be sited for drugs and rehydration
- Monitor for nausea (and vomiting) and give anti-emetics
- If eating encourage high calorie, low fat, small frequent meals: monitor tolerance
- Monitor and encourage rest: minimal visiting
- Observe for signs of anxiety and depression: refer to counsellor if needed

**HE&P**
- Infection control measures should be explained to patient and family/visitors
- Depending on the cause of hepatitis, sexual practices, alcohol or drug use may need discussion
- Patients need to tell dentists, other healthcare workers and tattooists they have had hepatitis
- Advice about future medication should be given
- Discuss lifestyle related changes – diet, drug use, alcohol consumption: refer to dietician, counsellor

Likely points of access to the healthcare system are general practice, walk-in-clinic, out-of-hours (OOH) service, and ambulance service

## Key facts

- The liver, the body's largest gland, is composed of four lobes comprising small hexagonal-shaped lobules (above) which are made up of hepatocytes. Hepatocytes filter, detoxify and process nutrients from the digestive tract. Hepatocytes produce bile as a metabolic byproduct: bile is stored in the gall bladder and used in the duodenum to emulsify fats.
- The liver has many functions (above): damage can have a profound effect. Liver failure is fatal without transplantation.
- Inflammation of the liver is known as hepatitis. It can be acute or chronic.
- Acute hepatitis is caused by viruses or reactions to drugs/toxins or rarely an autoimmune response.
- Hepatitis is sometimes referred to as viral hepatitis and non-viral hepatitis. Viruses cause hepatitis A, B, C, D and E. Non-viral hepatitis is due to drug reactions (drug-induced hepatitis), excessive alcohol consumption (alcohol-induced hepatitis) or autoimmune response (autoimmune hepatitis).
- Viral hepatitis is usually self-limiting with a good prognosis.
- The signs and symptoms of viral hepatitis are usually initial flu-like symptoms (e.g. headache, fever, nasal congestion, sore throat, mild upper abdominal pain and nausea and vomiting) followed by jaundice due to raised bilirubin levels in the blood and the depositing of bile pigments in sclera, skin and mucous membranes. Urine may be orange in colour and stools white due to intrahepatic cholestasis. Jaundice usually resolves in about two weeks with complete recovery. Liver enzymes will be raised.
- Drug-induced hepatitis can result from several drugs. Taking an overdose of paracetamol is a common cause: rapid (<8 hours after ingestion) intravenous administration of an antidote should be given to prevent fatal liver failure.
- In alcohol-induced hepatitis the signs and symptoms are lethargy, diarrhoea, vomiting, malnourishment, malaise, pain in the upper abdomen, fever, an enlarged liver and jaundice.
- Chronic hepatitis is when symptoms of acute hepatitis remain or liver function tests continue to be abnormal 6 months after the initial onset of the illness.
- Chronic hepatitis is usually associated with hepatitis B, C or D, autoimmune hepatitis and alcohol or drug related disease.
- Chronic hepatitis may lead to scarring of the liver (cirrhosis) which, in some people, may lead to liver failure or cancer. Scarring occurs because as the liver recovers from inflammation fibrous tissue and scars form. Cirrhosis reduces normal liver functioning.
- Some people with chronic liver disease may be relatively well (their condition is described as compensated) others may be seriously ill (decompensated).
- Chronic liver disease is associated with reduced liver cell mass, portal vein hypertension causing varices, ascites, encephalopathy (reversible) and jaundice. A patient's condition can deteriorate rapidly because of, for example, GI bleeds, sepsis, and electrolyte disturbance.
- Diagnoses are by clinical examination, history taking, liver function and other blood tests, ultrasonography and biopsy.
- Liver transplantation may be indicated.
- There are vaccines against some forms of viral hepatitis.

## Hepatitis: essentials of best practice

Acute viral hepatitis, without complications, requires little nursing intervention except for advice from the practice nurse. This advice should focus on how to deal with the symptoms of infection (e.g. rest, eat an easily digested light diet of small, high calorie meals and drink extra fluids if feverish). An alternative to paracetamol to reduce pain and pyrexia should be sought: paracetamol should only be taken at doses prescribed by the GP. (NB: advise the patient not to exceed the recommended daily dose.) Anti-emetics may be needed if there is vomiting/nausea. Patients should be reminded to seek medical advice if their symptoms persist for longer than 3–4 weeks, worsen or new signs and symptoms appear (e.g. confusion, altered mood, drowsiness, fits). Advice should also be given about minimising the spread of infection – close contacts (people the person lives with/cooks for/has sex with) should be advised to see their GPs since early vaccination may prevent the disease developing in them. Sometimes people with acute hepatitis require hospitalisation. In these cases nursing care should focus on the presenting signs and symptoms: it will largely focus on:

✓ Accurate assessment and regular monitoring
✓ Health education and promotion
✓ Symptom control and management

## Cirrhosis: essentials of best practice

Nursing care will focus on:

✓ Symptom control and management

and should be tailored to the patient's needs whilst being alert to indications of deterioration (e.g. for encephalopathy – alterations to mood, attention span or altered consciousness and reversal of sleep patterns: e.g. for bleeding from GI tract – monitor vital signs; vomit and stool for blood). If ascites is present, the patient may find mobilising difficult, be breathless (Section 1) and require a sodium free diet and restricted fluid intake: as they are likely to be taking diuretics they will need easy access to a commode or toilet unless catheterised. If cirrhosis is due to alcohol dependency the patient may be anxious about stopping drinking – support and counselling will be needed: drugs will be prescribed to minimise symptoms of alcohol withdrawal. Ruptured varices may create torrential gastro-intestinal bleeding which is a medical emergency (Chapter 43).

## Liver failure: essentials of best practice

End stage liver failure is irreversible. If a liver transplant is not being considered, a discussion about end of life care should be held with the patient and their family/carers (Section 1).

If a liver transplant is an option, care is likely to be transferred to a specialist unit.

---

**Patient information**

You will find very helpful patient-centred fact sheets at www.patient.co.uk/.
The Liver Trust is a national charity focusing on liver disease www.britishlivertrust.org.uk.

# 50 Nursing people with gallstone disease

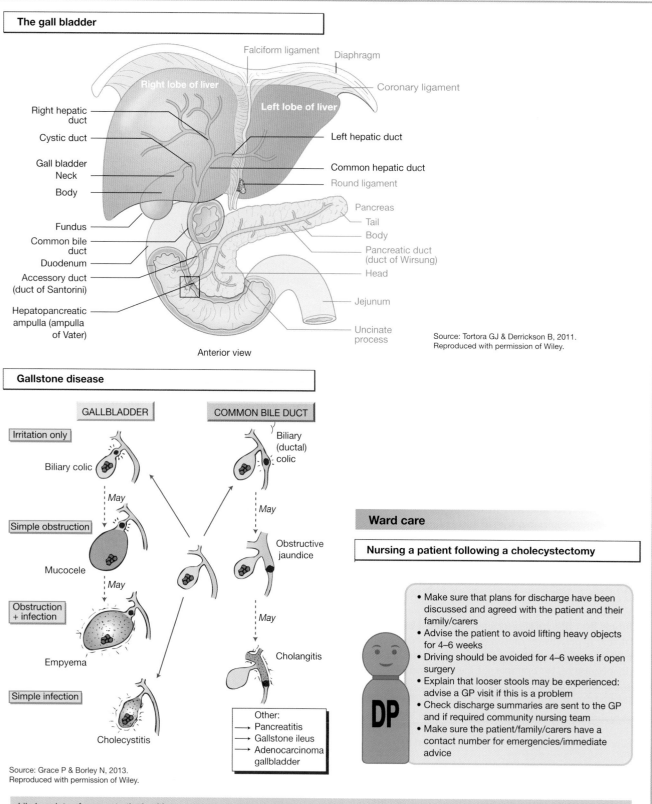

## The gall bladder

Falciform ligament

Diaphragm

Right lobe of liver

Coronary ligament

Left lobe of liver

Right hepatic duct

Cystic duct

Left hepatic duct

Gall bladder
Neck

Common hepatic duct

Body

Round ligament

Pancreas

Tail

Fundus

Body

Common bile duct

Pancreatic duct (duct of Wirsung)

Duodenum

Accessory duct (duct of Santorini)

Head

Jejunum

Hepatopancreatic ampulla (ampulla of Vater)

Uncinate process

Anterior view

Source: Tortora GJ & Derrickson B, 2011.
Reproduced with permission of Wiley.

## Gallstone disease

GALLBLADDER

COMMON BILE DUCT

Irritation only

Biliary colic

Biliary (ductal) colic

*May*

*May*

Simple obstruction

Mucocele

Obstructive jaundice

*May*

Obstruction + infection

Empyema

*May*

Cholangitis

Simple infection

Cholecystitis

Other:
→ Pancreatitis
→ Gallstone ileus
→ Adenocarcinoma gallbladder

Source: Grace P & Borley N, 2013.
Reproduced with permission of Wiley.

## Ward care

### Nursing a patient following a cholecystectomy

DP

- Make sure that plans for discharge have been discussed and agreed with the patient and their family/carers
- Advise the patient to avoid lifting heavy objects for 4–6 weeks
- Driving should be avoided for 4–6 weeks if open surgery
- Explain that looser stools may be experienced: advise a GP visit if this is a problem
- Check discharge summaries are sent to the GP and if required community nursing team
- Make sure the patient/family/carers have a contact number for emergencies/immediate advice

Likely points of access to the healthcare system are general practice, emergency department, out-of-hours (OOH) service, and ambulance service

*Adult Nursing at a Glance*, First Edition. Andrée le May. © 2015 John Wiley & Sons, Ltd. Published 2015 by John Wiley & Sons, Ltd.
Companion website: www.ataglanceseries.com/nursing/adult

# Key facts

- Gallstone disease is more common in women than men.
- Gallstones contain cholesterol or bile pigments or both mixed together. Gallstones can obstruct the bile duct.
- Gallstones may be present in the gall bladder (cholelithiasis). They can be asymptomatic or symptomatic.
- Gallstone disease can affect the gall bladder, the gall bladder and the common bile duct or the pancreas (above).
- The location of the obstruction determines signs, symptoms and treatment.
- Signs and symptoms include pain (sudden and severe or grumbling) in the right upper quadrant of the abdomen (often brought on by fatty food); nausea, vomiting; fever if infection; obstructive jaundice (cholestatic jaundice) with pale stools and orange urine (biliary obstruction).
- Inflammation of the gall bladder is called cholecystitis.
- Gallstones are a major cause of pancreatitis – stones move down the common bile duct and through the hepatopancreatic ampulla.
- Gallstones frequently accompany cancer of the gall bladder.
- If gallstones pass into the small intestine intestinal obstruction may be caused (gallstone ileus).
- Diagnosis is by ultrasonography and endoscopic retrograde cholangiopancreatography (ERCP).
- Management: active monitoring if asymptomatic; lifestyle changes may control initial episodes of biliary colic (reduced fatty diet and small, frequent meals); IV antibiotics to treat infection; ERCP to remove stones in the common bile duct; open, keyhole or laparoscopic surgical removal of the gall bladder (cholecystectomy) (emergency, planned following treatment for cholecystitis or elective following periods of biliary colic and confirmed gallstones).

# A and P

- The gall bladder is a small, green, muscular sac connected to the liver.
- Bile is stored and concentrated in the gall bladder until it is released into the duodenum where it emulsifies fats.
- The gall bladder's muscular walls have many folds in them (rugae) enabling it to stretch to hold large quantities of bile.

- The hormone cholecystokinin (CCK) stimulates the gall bladder to contract. Bile leaves the gall bladder through the cystic duct and moves down the common bile duct into the duodenum through the hepatopancreatic ampulla.
- CCK is secreted from the small intestine into the blood when fatty chyme enters the duodenum.
- CCK also stimulates pancreatic juice to be secreted and the hepatopancreatic sphincter to relax. When this sphincter relaxes bile and pancreatic juice enter the duodenum.

# Cholecystitis: essentials of best practice

Nursing care will focus on:
✓ Accurate assessment and regular monitoring
✓ Symptom control and management
Pain, nausea and vomiting are likely to be the patient's dominant problems (Section 1). Nurses also need to monitor the patient for signs of hypovolaemic shock (due to excessive vomiting, pain) and infection (pyrexia and tachycardia). Careful assessment of fluid balance and response to medication is required. Be attentive for signs of obstructive jaundice (pale stools and orange urine).

Surgical removal of the gall bladder (cholecystectomy) may be needed.

# Cholecystectomy: essentials of best practice

Nursing care will focus on the principles of pre- and post-operative care outlined in Section 1. In addition attention should be paid to:
✓ Discharge planning
Length of time in hospital will depend on the operation performed and any pre-/post-operative complications (e.g. infection).

---

**Patient information**

You will find very helpful patient-centred fact sheets at www.patient.co.uk/.

# 51 Nursing people with pancreatitis

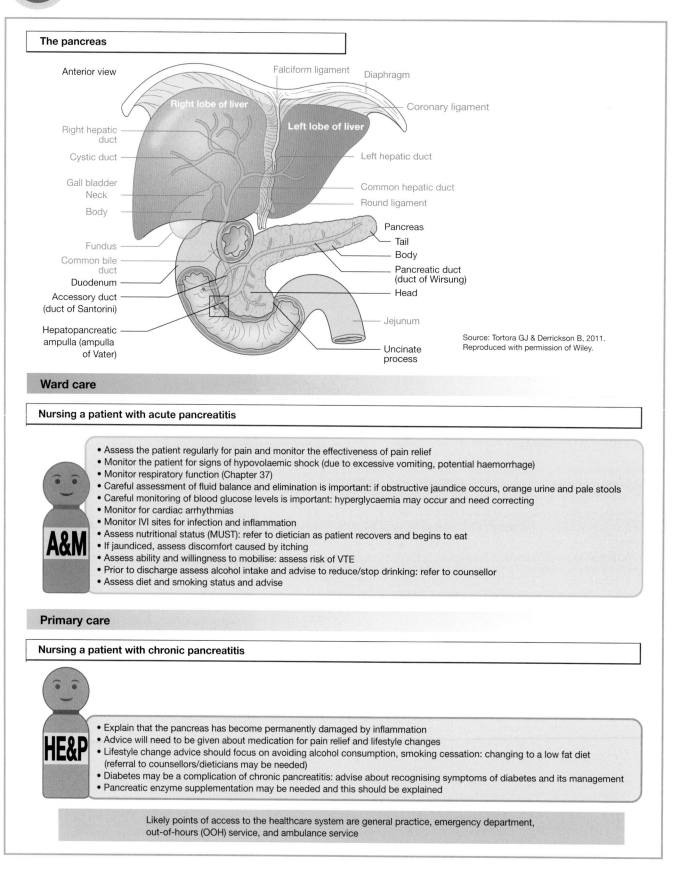

**The pancreas**

Anterior view

Falciform ligament

Diaphragm

Right lobe of liver

Coronary ligament

Left lobe of liver

Right hepatic duct

Cystic duct

Left hepatic duct

Gall bladder
Neck

Common hepatic duct

Body

Round ligament

Fundus

Pancreas

Common bile duct

Tail

Body

Duodenum

Pancreatic duct (duct of Wirsung)

Accessory duct (duct of Santorini)

Head

Hepatopancreatic ampulla (ampulla of Vater)

Jejunum

Uncinate process

Source: Tortora GJ & Derrickson B, 2011. Reproduced with permission of Wiley.

## Ward care

### Nursing a patient with acute pancreatitis

**A&M**

- Assess the patient regularly for pain and monitor the effectiveness of pain relief
- Monitor the patient for signs of hypovolaemic shock (due to excessive vomiting, potential haemorrhage)
- Monitor respiratory function (Chapter 37)
- Careful assessment of fluid balance and elimination is important: if obstructive jaundice occurs, orange urine and pale stools
- Careful monitoring of blood glucose levels is important: hyperglycaemia may occur and need correcting
- Monitor for cardiac arrhythmias
- Monitor IVI sites for infection and inflammation
- Assess nutritional status (MUST): refer to dietician as patient recovers and begins to eat
- If jaundiced, assess discomfort caused by itching
- Assess ability and willingness to mobilise: assess risk of VTE
- Prior to discharge assess alcohol intake and advise to reduce/stop drinking: refer to counsellor
- Assess diet and smoking status and advise

## Primary care

### Nursing a patient with chronic pancreatitis

**HE&P**

- Explain that the pancreas has become permanently damaged by inflammation
- Advice will need to be given about medication for pain relief and lifestyle changes
- Lifestyle change advice should focus on avoiding alcohol consumption, smoking cessation: changing to a low fat diet (referral to counsellors/dieticians may be needed)
- Diabetes may be a complication of chronic pancreatitis: advise about recognising symptoms of diabetes and its management
- Pancreatic enzyme supplementation may be needed and this should be explained

Likely points of access to the healthcare system are general practice, emergency department, out-of-hours (OOH) service, and ambulance service

*Adult Nursing at a Glance*, First Edition. Andrée le May. © 2015 John Wiley & Sons, Ltd. Published 2015 by John Wiley & Sons, Ltd.
Companion website: www.ataglanceseries.com/nursing/adult

# Key facts

- Pancreatitis is inflammation of the pancreas. It can be acute or chronic.
- Most pancreatitis resolves spontaneously. Severe pancreatitis can be life threatening.
- Acute pancreatitis is, most commonly, caused by gallstones, or the over-consumption of alcohol. Rarer causes include trauma, drugs (e.g. oestrogen, corticosteroids), viral infection (e.g. mumps, coxsackie) and hyperlipidaemia. Sometimes there is no known cause (idiopathic).
- Pancreatitis is associated with auto-digestion of pancreatic tissue leading to oedema, bleeding and necrosis.
- Signs and symptoms depend on the severity of the inflammation. In mild or moderate pancreatitis there is constant upper abdominal pain of sudden onset – the pain may radiate through to the back; nausea and maybe vomiting, pyrexia and jaundice may be present. In severe pancreatitis pain will be severe, hypovolaemic shock, compromised respiration and kidney function may occur.
- Diagnosis is made by clinical examination, blood tests (amylase levels usually raised), ultrasound, CT scan.
- Mild/moderate pancreatitis is usually managed by IV fluids, nil by mouth, analgesia, recordings of vital signs for early detection of deterioration. Severe pancreatitis usually requires care in HDU/ICU with invasive monitoring. Surgery is only used to treat severe complications.
- Complications of acute pancreatitis include abscesses, intra-abdominal sepsis, necrosis of the transverse colon, respiratory (Type I) and renal failure, pancreatic haemorrhage and cardiac arrhythmias if electrolyte balance is disturbed. Secondary diabetes mellitus may occur.
- Exocrine and endocrine pancreatic insufficiency (causing diabetes and steatorrhoea) is associated with chronic pancreatitis.
- Chronic pancreatitis is usually caused by alcohol abuse leaving residual damage to the pancreas following acute pancreatitis.

# A and P

- The pancreas consists of a head, body and tail (above); these comprise exocrine and endocrine tissue.
- The endocrine tissue makes the hormones insulin and glucagon in the islets of Langerhans. These hormones control carbohydrate metabolism.
- The exocrine tissue makes pancreatic juice (water, mineral salts, the enzymes amylase and lipase, and the inactive enzyme precursors trypsinogen, chymotrypsinogen and procarboxypeptidase).

- Amylase is responsible for carbohydrate digestion.
- Lipase is responsible for fat digestion.
- Trypsinogen, chymotrypsinogen and procarboxypeptidase in their inactive form protect the pancreas from auto-digestion. Once released into the duodenum they are activated by enterokinase and become trypsin, chymotrypsin and carboxypeptidase: they metabolise proteins.
- Pancreatic juice travels to the duodenum via the pancreatic duct through the hepatopancreatic ampulla and then the common bile duct.
- The cells of the pancreatic duct secrete bicarbonate ions (pH of pancreatic juice = 8). This helps neutralise acidic chyme. Amylase and lipase work best at pH 6–8.
- Gallstones can move down the common bile duct and block the hepatopancreatic ampulla causing pancreatitis.
- Pancreatic juice secretion is regulated by secretin and cholecystokinin (CCK).

# Pancreatitis: essentials of best practice

Nursing care will depend on the severity of the pancreatitis but will always need to focus on:

✓ Accurate assessment and regular monitoring
✓ Symptom control and management

Pain, anxiety, nausea and vomiting are likely to be the patient's dominant problems (Section 1). Nurses should particularly monitor the patient for signs of hypovolaemic shock (due to excessive vomiting, bleeding), arrhythmias (Chapter 31), respiratory failure (Chapter 38) and alterations to blood glucose levels. Help with daily living activities will be needed for patients who are acutely ill.

If surgical intervention is required to alleviate complications, adherence to the principles of pre- and post-operative care (Section 1) is required.

If a patient has chronic pancreatitis, most of their care will be provided in primary care. In this situation practice nurses will largely be responsible for providing advice about

✓ Health education and promotion

---

**Patient information**

You will find very helpful patient-centred fact sheets at www. patient.co.uk/.

# 52 Nursing people with renal and urinary disorders

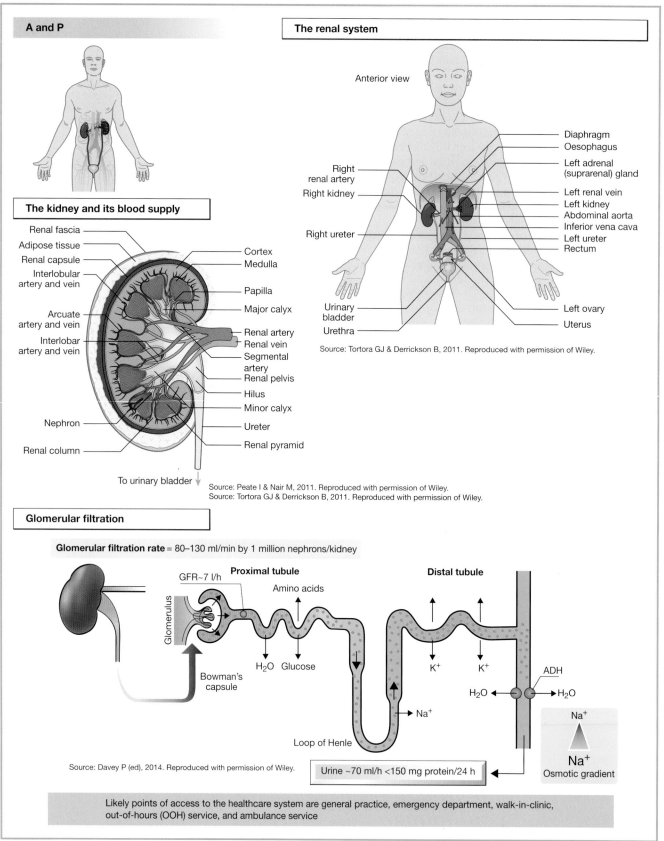

**A and P**

**The renal system**

Anterior view

Diaphragm
Oesophagus
Left adrenal (suprarenal) gland
Left renal vein
Left kidney
Abdominal aorta
Inferior vena cava
Left ureter
Rectum

Right renal artery
Right kidney

Right ureter

Urinary bladder
Urethra

Left ovary
Uterus

Source: Tortora GJ & Derrickson B, 2011. Reproduced with permission of Wiley.

**The kidney and its blood supply**

Renal fascia
Adipose tissue
Renal capsule
Interlobular artery and vein
Arcuate artery and vein
Interlobar artery and vein
Nephron
Renal column

Cortex
Medulla
Papilla
Major calyx
Renal artery
Renal vein
Segmental artery
Renal pelvis
Hilus
Minor calyx
Ureter
Renal pyramid

To urinary bladder

Source: Peate I & Nair M, 2011. Reproduced with permission of Wiley.
Source: Tortora GJ & Derrickson B, 2011. Reproduced with permission of Wiley.

**Glomerular filtration**

**Glomerular filtration rate** = 80–130 ml/min by 1 million nephrons/kidney

GFR~7 l/h

**Proximal tubule**

Amino acids

**Distal tubule**

Glomerulus

$H_2O$  Glucose

Bowman's capsule

$K^+$     $K^+$

ADH

$H_2O$ ← → $H_2O$

$Na^+$

Loop of Henle

$Na^+$

$Na^+$
Osmotic gradient

Urine ~70 ml/h <150 mg protein/24 h

Source: Davey P (ed), 2014. Reproduced with permission of Wiley.

Likely points of access to the healthcare system are general practice, emergency department, walk-in-clinic, out-of-hours (OOH) service, and ambulance service

*Adult Nursing at a Glance*, First Edition. Andrée le May. © 2015 John Wiley & Sons, Ltd. Published 2015 by John Wiley & Sons, Ltd.
Companion website: www.ataglanceseries.com/nursing/adult

# Key facts

- The renal and urinary system comprises two kidneys (the right is slightly lower than the left because of the position of the liver), two ureters, the urinary bladder and one urethra.
- This system is central to maintaining homeostasis.
- The kidneys regulate the body's fluid balance, electrolyte balance and the acid-base balance of the blood (renal acid-base control).
- People can live with only one kidney.
- Kidney transplantation saves lives.

# Common renal/urinary system disorders

- Glomerulonephritis
- Acute renal failure
- Chronic renal failure
- Urinary calculi
- Urinary tract infections.

Each is covered in the following pages. See Chapter 53 for common signs and symptoms associated with renal and urinary disorders.

# A and P

- The kidneys comprise three parts – the renal cortex, the renal medulla and the renal pelvis (above).
- The kidneys separate waste and excess water from blood and convert this filtrate into urine.
- Blood is brought to the kidneys by several arteries (above) for filtering. Once filtered, blood leaves the kidneys by the renal vein.
- Blood is filtered in the nephron. Each kidney consists of around 1 million nephrons.
- Each nephron is made up of a cup shaped Bowman's capsule holding a capillary network (glomerulus), a proximal convoluted tubule, a loop of Henle and a distal convoluted tubule. The distal convoluted tubule drains into collecting ducts which eventually drain the filtrate (urine) into the renal pelvis. The ureter takes urine from the renal pelvis to the urinary bladder.
- Urine formation involves three processes: filtration, selective reabsorption and secretion.
- Filtration occurs in the glomerulus (opposite).
- Blood is filtered through the glomeruli (glomerular filtration) into the Bowman's capsule. As a result of filtration the blood is separated into two parts – a filtrated blood product and the glomerular filtrate (water, waste products, salt, glucose and other chemicals). The filtrated blood product is taken from the glomerulus, via a capillary and venous network, to the renal vein and returned to the circulatory system. Capillaries also run along the course of the nephron allowing the exchange of water and solutes as the filtrate moves through to the collecting ducts.

- The glomeruli filter around 7 l of fluid/hour producing 50–100 ml of urine. Substances needed to maintain acid-base and fluid balance are selectively reabsorbed from the filtrate by osmosis, diffusion and active transportation as it passes from the glomeruli, via the proximal tubule, loop of Henle and distal tubule to the collecting ducts in the renal pelvis (above).
- Ions, creatinine, urea and some hormones are secreted into the renal tubules.
- Urine is stored in the bladder.
- Urine leaves the bladder via the urethra and is excreted.
- Urine comprises water (~96%) and solutes (~4%) from cellular metabolism: it is normally slightly acidic (pH 4.5–8).
- Antidiuretic hormone (ADH) regulates the amount of urine passed.
- The kidneys also have an endocrine function synthesising hormones.
- Renin and angiotensin regulate sodium and fluid retention and the expansion and contraction of blood vessels and have a role in BP control. Renin controls the glomerular blood flow and filtration rate.
- The kidneys produce erythropoietin which is carried via the blood to the bone marrow to stimulate red blood cell production. Dysfunction can cause anaemia.
- The kidneys produce calcitriol (maintains calcium and phosphate levels in the blood and bones) and synthesise vitamin D. Renal dysfunction can cause renal bone disease.

# Essentials of best practice

Disorders of the renal and urinary system can range from mild to severe. Nursing someone with any of these disorders may take place in the community, the GP Surgery, the ED or OOH service or in a hospital ward or specialist renal unit. The essentials of best practice required to care for common disorders are covered in the subsequent pages. In addition, Chapter 53 details assessment of the renal and urinary system, common signs and symptoms and emergencies.

## Patient information

There are several patient support groups and charities focusing on disorders of the renal and urinary systems. You can find most of them on the Self Help UK website www.self-help.org.uk.

You will also find very helpful patient-centred fact sheets at www.patient.co.uk/.

# 53 Signs, symptoms, assessment and emergencies

**Important assessments of the renal and urinary system** (based on Dougherty and Lister, 2011 and O'Brien, 2012)

Making a nursing assessment of a patient with a renal or urinary system disorder should focus on:
- Finding out about the history of the problem (see signs and symptoms below)
- Urinalysis – find more out about the properties of the patient's urine by observing and testing a fresh specimen of urine
  o Look at the urine for colour (e.g. orange may suggest obstructive jaundice: pink/red suggests blood*, green may suggest infection with pseudomonas*)
  o Look at the urine for clarity (cloudy may suggest infection*: sediment may suggest infection*)
  o Smell urine for unusual odours (fishy may suggest infection*: sweet smelling suggests ketones)
  o Urine dipstick analysis may confirm the presence (or absence) of, for example, glucose, blood, protein, ketones, bilirubin and also pH
  o Microscopy, culture and sensitivities – send for lab tests if* above
  o Measurement of BP
- Fluid balance: check for imbalance between input and output, reduced urine, no urine or excessive urine
- Monitor blood pressure: kidney damage can cause raised blood pressure
- Monitor other systems, for example heart rate and rhythms, respiratory rate, confusion
- Assess and monitor pain

**Some causes of acute urinary retention** (www.patient.co.uk)

| Men | Women | Men and women |
|---|---|---|
| Benign prostatic hypertrophy (BPH)<br>Meatal stenosis<br>Paraphimosis<br>Phimosis<br>Prostate cancer<br>Penile constricting bands<br>Balanitis<br>Prostatitis | Prolapse (urinary, cystocoele, rectocoele)<br>Pelvic mass (fibroid, malignancy, ovarian cyst)<br>Acute vulvovaginitis<br>Vaginal lichen planus<br>Post-partum complications | Bladder cancer<br>Calculi (stones)<br>Faecal impaction<br>Malignancies (GIT)<br>Urethral strictures<br>Foreign bodies<br>Bilharzia<br>Cystitis<br>Herpes simplex virus<br>Some drugs (e.g. opioids and anaesthetics)<br>Neurological problems e.g. multiple sclerosis, Parkinson's disease, nerve damage<br>Pelvic trauma<br>Post-operative complications (associated with pain, instrumentation, bed rest, bladder over-distension). |

*Adult Nursing at a Glance*, First Edition. Andrée le May. © 2015 John Wiley & Sons, Ltd. Published 2015 by John Wiley & Sons, Ltd.
Companion website: www.ataglanceseries.com/nursing/adult

## Common signs and symptoms
### Lower urinary tract infection
- Malaise (feeling under the weather)
- Pain/discomfort: including a burning sensation passing urine, loin pain, back pain, lower abdominal pain, suprapubic pain or tenderness
- Urinary frequency
- Passing small amounts of urine
- Smelly urine
- Cloudy urine
- Urgency sometimes coupled with incontinence
- Pyrexia
- Haematuria.

### Upper urinary tract infection
- Pain: back pain, side pain, groin pain
- Pyrexia and rigors
- Nausea and/or vomiting
- Diarrhoea
- Loss of appetite
- Tiredness.

Any urinary tract infection may be accompanied by:
- Anxiety
- Confusion in older people.

Blockage anywhere in the urinary tract (e.g. from renal stones) will cause severe pain, reduced amounts of urine and if left unresolved lead to renal failure (Chapter 57).

## Emergencies: renal and urinary system
### Acute urinary retention
- Recognising and responding to any sudden deterioration in a patient's condition is vital. The sudden inability to pass urine is acute urinary retention (AUR). The main causes are listed above.
- AUR is very painful and is treated by emergency catheterisation. See catheter care in Chapter 58.
- Once the immediate problem is solved management of the underlying cause becomes the priority. (Nursing care will vary depending on the cause.)
- Careful attention should be paid to urinary output once the catheter is removed.
- Monitoring temperature for signs of infection is also important following catheterisation.
- Complications include UTIs, renal failure and post-obstructive diuresis. Post-obstructive diuresis may lead to electrolyte imbalance with resultant risk of arrhythmias.

# Nursing people with glomerulonephritis

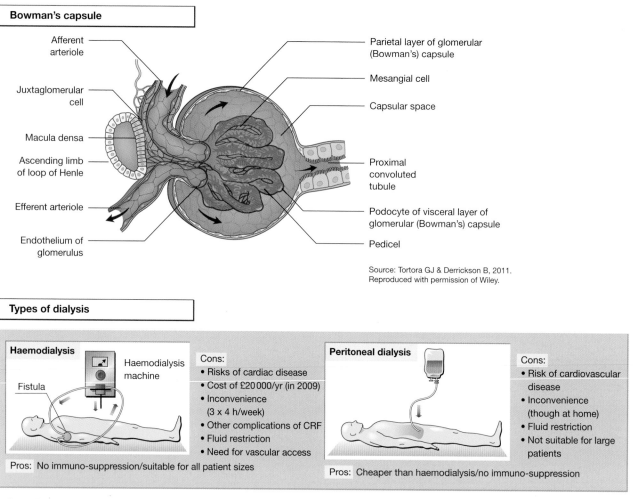

**Bowman's capsule**

- Afferent arteriole
- Juxtaglomerular cell
- Macula densa
- Ascending limb of loop of Henle
- Efferent arteriole
- Endothelium of glomerulus
- Parietal layer of glomerular (Bowman's) capsule
- Mesangial cell
- Capsular space
- Proximal convoluted tubule
- Podocyte of visceral layer of glomerular (Bowman's) capsule
- Pedicel

Source: Tortora GJ & Derrickson B, 2011.
Reproduced with permission of Wiley.

**Types of dialysis**

**Haemodialysis**

Fistula

Haemodialysis machine

Cons:
- Risks of cardiac disease
- Cost of £20 000/yr (in 2009)
- Inconvenience (3 x 4 h/week)
- Other complications of CRF
- Fluid restriction
- Need for vascular access

Pros: No immuno-suppression/suitable for all patient sizes

**Peritoneal dialysis**

Cons:
- Risk of cardiovascular disease
- Inconvenience (though at home)
- Fluid restriction
- Not suitable for large patients

Pros: Cheaper than haemodialysis/no immuno-suppression

Source: Davey P (ed), 2014. Reproduced with permission of Wiley.

Likely points of access to the healthcare system are general practice, emergency department, walk-in-clinic, and out-of-hours (OOH) service

# Key facts

- Glomerulonephritis (GN) means inflammation of the glomeruli.
- GN is characterised by the presence of protein, blood and casts (cylindrical structures formed in the nephrons) in urine.
- The normal amount of protein in urine is <150 mg/day. More protein than that suggests GN.
- GN accounts for renal failure in around one third of patients needing renal dialysis or renal transplant.
- GN affects both kidneys symmetrically.
- GN can be acute or chronic.
- Acute GN can underlie acute renal failure and nephrotic syndrome (proteinuria, oedema, hypoalbuminaemia) or present as haematuria and proteinuria and hypertension.
- Chronic GN can underlie chronic renal failure. In chronic renal failure kidneys may become small and fibrotic and there may be a history of proteinuria and haematuria.
- GN is also associated with systemic lupus erythematosus (SLE).
- Investigations used to diagnose GN include routine urinalysis and microscopy, 24 hour urine collection for protein excretion, serum creatinine and creatinine clearance, and renal ultrasound to establish the size of the kidneys. If the kidneys are normal in size biopsies may be taken.
- GN is usually classified into three types:
  - minimal change GN (treatment = corticosteroid therapy to produce remission);
  - membranous GN (requires drug therapy and has a mixed prognosis);
  - rapidly progressive GN (requires aggressive drug therapy).
- Raised blood pressure and raised cholesterol can result from GN. Aggressive drug therapy for both may slow the progress of the disease.
- Drugs that are toxic to the kidneys should be avoided (e.g. NSAIDs and acyclovir).

# Essentials of best practice

The nursing care of patients with glomerulonephritis will depend on the severity of the disease. There may be no treatment required, sometimes dietary changes are suggested (e.g. eating less salt to reduce the work of the kidneys), and treatment for hypertension (Chapter 28) can help. However, some people will require more active nursing care, either in the community or hospital, which focuses on:

✓ Accurate assessment and regular monitoring
✓ Communication with the healthcare team, patient and family
✓ Health education and promotion
✓ Discharge planning

Encouraging a patient to rest and minimise the work done by their kidneys and heart is important; however, convincing someone to rest and minimise exercise (and carry this on until they make as complete a recovery as possible) can be challenging. Fluid overload may be a problem so restrictions of fluid and sodium intake are needed: this will require careful explanation from the medical team and possibly the dietician. Contact with the dietician will also be needed for advice about reducing the amount of protein eaten to prevent uraemia and about reducing cholesterol. Patients should also be advised to contact their GP if they have any infections. Smoking can also make GN deteriorate so smoking cessation should be discussed and supported.

Some patients with severe GN will require dialysis which may take place at home or in hospital dialysis units (above).

## Patient information

There are several useful charities and support groups focusing on kidney disease:
The National Kidney Federation (NKF) www.kidney.org.uk/.
The British Kidney Patient Association www.britishkidney-pa.co.uk/.
The Scottish Kidney Federation www.scotskidneyfederation.org/.
You will find very helpful patient-centred fact sheets at www.patient.co.uk/.

# 55 Nursing people with acute renal failure

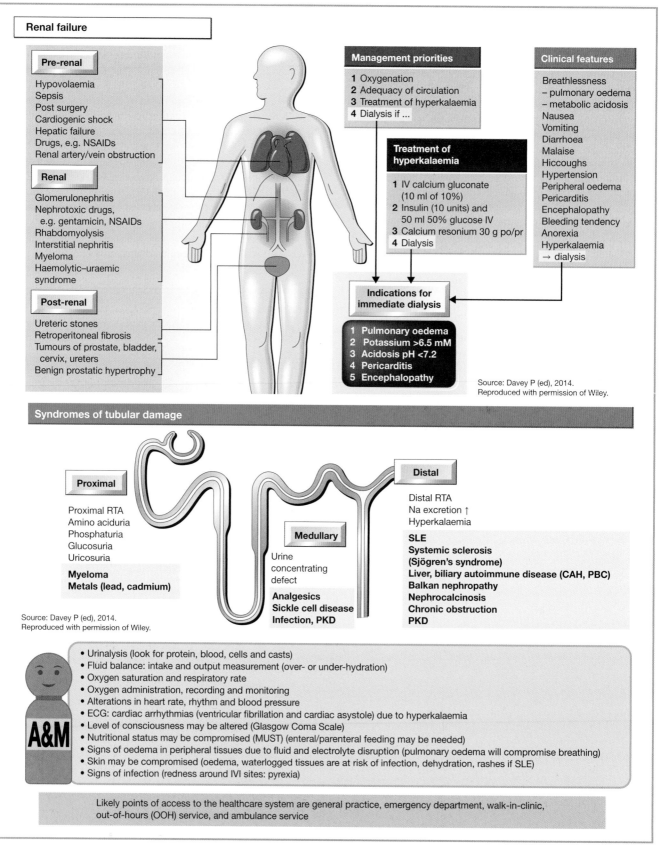

## Renal failure

### Pre-renal

Hypovolaemia
Sepsis
Post surgery
Cardiogenic shock
Hepatic failure
Drugs, e.g. NSAIDs
Renal artery/vein obstruction

### Renal

Glomerulonephritis
Nephrotoxic drugs,
  e.g. gentamicin, NSAIDs
Rhabdomyolysis
Interstitial nephritis
Myeloma
Haemolytic–uraemic
syndrome

### Post-renal

Ureteric stones
Retroperitoneal fibrosis
Tumours of prostate, bladder,
  cervix, ureters
Benign prostatic hypertrophy

### Management priorities

1 Oxygenation
2 Adequacy of circulation
3 Treatment of hyperkalaemia
4 Dialysis if ...

### Treatment of hyperkalaemia

1 IV calcium gluconate
   (10 ml of 10%)
2 Insulin (10 units) and
   50 ml 50% glucose IV
3 Calcium resonium 30 g po/pr
4 Dialysis

### Indications for immediate dialysis

1 **Pulmonary oedema**
2 **Potassium >6.5 mM**
3 **Acidosis pH <7.2**
4 **Pericarditis**
5 **Encephalopathy**

### Clinical features

Breathlessness
– pulmonary oedema
– metabolic acidosis
Nausea
Vomiting
Diarrhoea
Malaise
Hiccoughs
Hypertension
Peripheral oedema
Pericarditis
Encephalopathy
Bleeding tendency
Anorexia
Hyperkalaemia
→ dialysis

Source: Davey P (ed), 2014.
Reproduced with permission of Wiley.

## Syndromes of tubular damage

### Proximal

Proximal RTA
Amino aciduria
Phosphaturia
Glucosuria
Uricosuria

**Myeloma**
**Metals (lead, cadmium)**

### Medullary

Urine
concentrating
defect

**Analgesics**
**Sickle cell disease**
**Infection, PKD**

### Distal

Distal RTA
Na excretion ↑
Hyperkalaemia

**SLE**
**Systemic sclerosis**
**(Sjögren's syndrome)**
**Liver, biliary autoimmune disease (CAH, PBC)**
**Balkan nephropathy**
**Nephrocalcinosis**
**Chronic obstruction**
**PKD**

Source: Davey P (ed), 2014.
Reproduced with permission of Wiley.

**A&M**

• Urinalysis (look for protein, blood, cells and casts)
• Fluid balance: intake and output measurement (over- or under-hydration)
• Oxygen saturation and respiratory rate
• Oxygen administration, recording and monitoring
• Alterations in heart rate, rhythm and blood pressure
• ECG: cardiac arrhythmias (ventricular fibrillation and cardiac asystole) due to hyperkalaemia
• Level of consciousness may be altered (Glasgow Coma Scale)
• Nutritional status may be compromised (MUST) (enteral/parenteral feeding may be needed)
• Signs of oedema in peripheral tissues due to fluid and electrolyte disruption (pulmonary oedema will compromise breathing)
• Skin may be compromised (oedema, waterlogged tissues are at risk of infection, dehydration, rashes if SLE)
• Signs of infection (redness around IVI sites: pyrexia)

Likely points of access to the healthcare system are general practice, emergency department, walk-in-clinic, out-of-hours (OOH) service, and ambulance service

*Adult Nursing at a Glance*, First Edition. Andrée le May. © 2015 John Wiley & Sons, Ltd. Published 2015 by John Wiley & Sons, Ltd.
Companion website: www.ataglanceseries.com/nursing/adult

# Key facts

• Patients with acute renal failure will be seriously ill.

• Acute renal failure is a syndrome characterised by rapid decline (days – weeks) in glomerular filtration rate (GFR). This results in an accumulation of nitrogenous waste and problems regulating extracellular volume and electrolytes. Reduced (oliguria) or no urine (anuria) output may occur.

• Acute renal failure is also known as acute kidney injury (AKI).

• Acute renal failure results from a variety of causes (pre-renal, renal and post-renal) (opposite). Often it originates from outside the kidney.

• Pre-renal causes largely relate to hypo-perfusion of the kidneys. This mainly stems from other system failures, for example cardiovascular.

• Renal causes result from diseases affecting the kidney.

• Post-renal causes are associated with urinary tract obstructions.

• Patients with acute renal failure may present with a range of signs and symptoms (above).

• Treatment focuses on ensuring adequate oxygenation and circulation, management of the presenting symptoms and the underlying causes.

• Fluid overload may result in pulmonary oedema.

• Metabolic acidosis can occur. (In the healthy glomerulus carbonic acid is split forming bicarbonate and $H^+$ ions, bicarbonate is retained in the blood for circulation and the $H^+$ ions pass into the glomerular filtrate for excretion. If this doesn't happen $H^+$ ions are retained in the blood.)

• Dialysis (renal replacement therapy) may be required.

• Acute renal failure may be reversible (depending on the cause).

• Following the acute phase, when urine is characteristically reduced in quantity or absent, is a diuretic phase. During the diuretic phases the nephrons begin to function again but the tubules cannot concentrate urine so they produce large quantities (polyuria). This can be dehydrating and lead to electrolyte imbalance.

When this has resolved recovery and recuperation begin – sometimes taking many months.

• Acute renal failure, because it is often associated with other serious illnesses/problems (e.g. disruptions of the cardiovascular system and of fluid balance and acidosis) has a high mortality rate.

• Recovery can take a long time: accurate assessment and regular monitoring may be needed for several months.

# Essentials of best practice

Patients with acute renal failure will be nursed either in ITU/HDU or on a ward depending on the severity of their condition. The nursing care of patients with acute renal failure focuses largely on:

✓ Accurate assessment and regular monitoring

✓ Communication with the healthcare team, patient and family

Restoring and maintaining homeostasis is central to care. This will involve careful monitoring of fluid balance and skilled observation of the patient's condition for deterioration (or improvement) (above).

Haemodialysis may be necessary.

Acute renal failure can be very frightening for the patient and their family/carers so accurate, explanatory and empathic communication is essential.

## Patient information

There are several useful charities and support groups focusing on kidney disease:

The National Kidney Federation (NKF) www.kidney.org.uk/.

The British Kidney Patient Association www.britishkidney-pa. co.uk/.

The Scottish Kidney Federation www.scotskidneyfederation.org/.

You will find very helpful patient-centred fact sheets at www. patient.co.uk/.

# 56 Nursing people with chronic renal failure

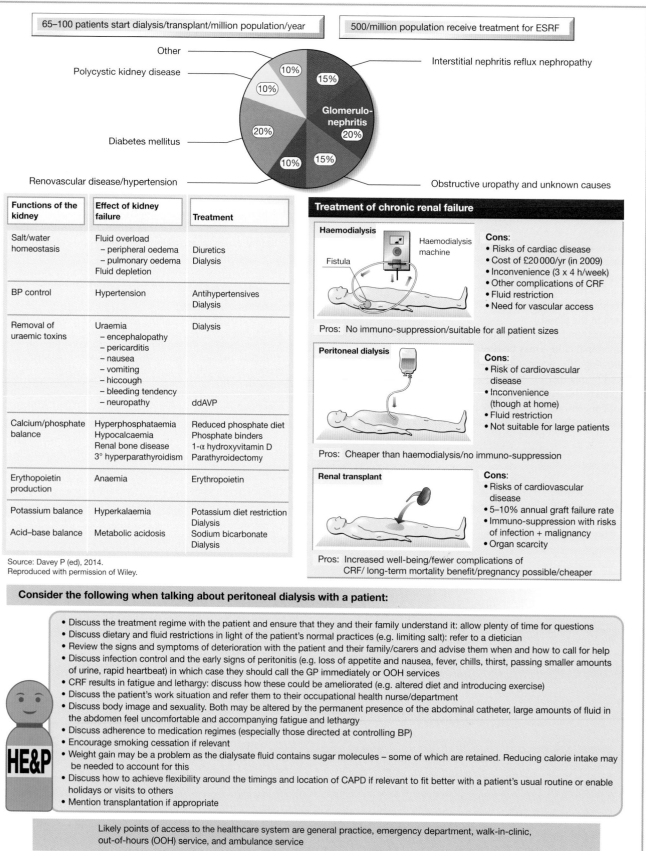

65–100 patients start dialysis/transplant/million population/year

500/million population receive treatment for ESRF

Other
Polycystic kidney disease
10%
10%
15% — Interstitial nephritis reflux nephropathy
Glomerulo-nephritis
20%
Diabetes mellitus — 20%
10%
15%
Renovascular disease/hypertension
Obstructive uropathy and unknown causes

| Functions of the kidney | Effect of kidney failure | Treatment |
|---|---|---|
| Salt/water homeostasis | Fluid overload<br>– peripheral oedema<br>– pulmonary oedema<br>Fluid depletion | Diuretics<br>Dialysis |
| BP control | Hypertension | Antihypertensives<br>Dialysis |
| Removal of uraemic toxins | Uraemia<br>– encephalopathy<br>– pericarditis<br>– nausea<br>– vomiting<br>– hiccough<br>– bleeding tendency<br>– neuropathy | Dialysis<br><br><br><br><br><br><br>ddAVP |
| Calcium/phosphate balance | Hyperphosphataemia<br>Hypocalcaemia<br>Renal bone disease<br>3° hyperparathyroidism | Reduced phosphate diet<br>Phosphate binders<br>1-α hydroxyvitamin D<br>Parathyroidectomy |
| Erythopoietin production | Anaemia | Erythropoietin |
| Potassium balance | Hyperkalaemia | Potassium diet restriction<br>Dialysis |
| Acid–base balance | Metabolic acidosis | Sodium bicarbonate<br>Dialysis |

Source: Davey P (ed), 2014.
Reproduced with permission of Wiley.

## Treatment of chronic renal failure

**Haemodialysis**
Fistula
Haemodialysis machine

Cons:
• Risks of cardiac disease
• Cost of £20 000/yr (in 2009)
• Inconvenience (3 x 4 h/week)
• Other complications of CRF
• Fluid restriction
• Need for vascular access

Pros: No immuno-suppression/suitable for all patient sizes

**Peritoneal dialysis**

Cons:
• Risk of cardiovascular disease
• Inconvenience (though at home)
• Fluid restriction
• Not suitable for large patients

Pros: Cheaper than haemodialysis/no immuno-suppression

**Renal transplant**

Cons:
• Risks of cardiovascular disease
• 5–10% annual graft failure rate
• Immuno-suppression with risks of infection + malignancy
• Organ scarcity

Pros: Increased well-being/fewer complications of CRF/ long-term mortality benefit/pregnancy possible/cheaper

## Consider the following when talking about peritoneal dialysis with a patient:

• Discuss the treatment regime with the patient and ensure that they and their family understand it: allow plenty of time for questions
• Discuss dietary and fluid restrictions in light of the patient's normal practices (e.g. limiting salt): refer to a dietician
• Review the signs and symptoms of deterioration with the patient and their family/carers and advise them when and how to call for help
• Discuss infection control and the early signs of peritonitis (e.g. loss of appetite and nausea, fever, chills, thirst, passing smaller amounts of urine, rapid heartbeat) in which case they should call the GP immediately or OOH services
• CRF results in fatigue and lethargy: discuss how these could be ameliorated (e.g. altered diet and introducing exercise)
• Discuss the patient's work situation and refer them to their occupational health nurse/department
• Discuss body image and sexuality. Both may be altered by the permanent presence of the abdominal catheter, large amounts of fluid in the abdomen feel uncomfortable and accompanying fatigue and lethargy
• Discuss adherence to medication regimes (especially those directed at controlling BP)
• Encourage smoking cessation if relevant
• Weight gain may be a problem as the dialysate fluid contains sugar molecules – some of which are retained. Reducing calorie intake may be needed to account for this
• Discuss how to achieve flexibility around the timings and location of CAPD if relevant to fit better with a patient's usual routine or enable holidays or visits to others
• Mention transplantation if appropriate

HE&P

Likely points of access to the healthcare system are general practice, emergency department, walk-in-clinic, out-of-hours (OOH) service, and ambulance service

*Adult Nursing at a Glance*, First Edition. Andrée le May. © 2015 John Wiley & Sons, Ltd. Published 2015 by John Wiley & Sons, Ltd.
Companion website: www.ataglanceseries.com/nursing/adult

# Key facts

- Chronic renal failure (CRF) is defined as a consistently, abnormally low glomerular filtration rate (GFR) for more than 3 months
- Chronic renal failure results from a variety of causes (opposite). CRF can have the same life threatening consequences as acute renal failure (Chapter 55).
- There is no cure for CRF.
- Chronic renal failure can progress to End Stage Renal Failure (ESRF) without transplantation.
- End of life care may need to be discussed and planned if transplantation is unlikely.
- Chronic renal failure means that the kidneys fail to function in a number of different ways (above).
- People with CRF may present with a range of signs and symptoms (above). CRF may have an insidious onset or present as a uraemic emergency.
- Investigations include renal ultrasound; biopsy; urinalysis for proteinuria, haematuria; serum creatinine clearance; blood tests for urea and creatinine levels, for example.
- Treatment focuses on managing the presenting symptoms (above), aggressive blood pressure control to reduce the speed of deterioration and renal replacement therapy (dialysis or transplantation).
- If possible patients should be prepared for dialysis (psychologically and physically) before their renal failure results in uraemia.
- There are two main dialysis options: haemodialysis and peritoneal dialysis (PD).
- Haemodialysis involves the diffusion of solutes and water from blood across a semi-permeable membrane held in a haemodialysis machine. Filtered blood is returned to the circulatory system.
- Haemodialysis requires vascular access. Creating an arteriovenous fistula is the preferred way of doing this however it can take 8–12 weeks for the fistula to mature before use (e.g. the vein walls thicken and dilate to enable repeated insertion of the needles required for dialysis). Before the fistula is ready for use, double lumen subclavian, jugular or femoral lines can be used.
- The fistula usually comprises a permanent anastomosis in the lower arm between the radial artery and the cephalic vein.
- The patient's arm with the fistula should not be used to take BP, nor be cannulated except for dialysis. Nor should tight strapping of any kind be applied to it since it will restrict blood flow through the fistula. Unconscious patients should not lie on the fistula arm.
- A synthetic graft may also be used if arterial disease is present. The site of the graft is usually the thigh or the forearm.
- Haemodialysis can result in cardiovascular instability.
- Peritoneal dialysis (PD) is an alternative to haemodialysis. There are two types: continuous ambulatory peritoneal dialysis (CAPD) and automated peritoneal dialysis (APD). Both use the peritoneal lining as the dialysis membrane. CAPD requires patients to instil around 2 litres of isotonic or hypertonic glucose solution four times a day into the peritoneal cavity through a permanent catheter placed through the abdominal wall. Once instilled, the fluid is left in place for several (~6) hours and then, containing excess fluid, solutes and waste products, it is drained out. This needs to be done four times a day. Alternatively, the catheter is connected to a machine which does this overnight (APD).
- PD means patients can be more independent of healthcare services once they are proficient in the technique.
- Dehydration, constipation and peritonitis are risks associated with PD.
- Dialysis requires patients to keep to strict dietary and fluid restrictions.
- Renal transplantation is often the most effective treatment option but is limited by the availability of suitable kidneys.

# Essentials of best practice

Patients with CRF are likely to be cared for in a variety of locations by different members of the multi-disciplinary team. Many nurses (e.g. community nurses, practice nurses, ward, HDU or ITU nurses, specialist renal nurses, specialist palliative care nurses and consultant nurses) will be involved in a person's care as their condition progresses. Practice nurses, as well as their role in maintaining the general health of people with CRF in the community, may have been involved in the initial stages of care if chronic kidney disease (CKD) was identified routinely by the GP, or in conjunction with the management of other diseases.

The nursing care of patients with chronic renal failure, depends largely on the stage of their disease and their treatment plan. Restoring and maintaining homeostasis is however, central to care, as is helping the patient and family achieve the best quality of life possible within the constraints of CRF and its treatment.

For those with ESRF end of life care will be a central component of care (Section 1). For those at other stages of CRF care will focus largely on:

✓ Accurate assessment and regular monitoring
✓ Communication with the healthcare team, patient and family
✓ Health education and promotion

Chronic renal failure and the need for dialysis can be very frightening for the patient and their family/carers so accurate, explanatory and empathic communication is essential. Self-management of CAPD at home relies on careful teaching and confidence building (above). Raising the possibility of kidney donation by relatives might be appropriate.

---

## Patient information

There are several useful charities and support groups focusing on kidney disease:
The National Kidney Federation (NKF) www.kidney.org.uk/.
The British Kidney Patient Association www.britishkidney-pa.co.uk/.
The Scottish Kidney Federation www.scotskidneyfederation.org/
You will find very helpful patient-centred fact sheets at www.patient.co.uk/.

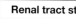

# 57 Nursing people with urinary calculi

## Renal tract stones

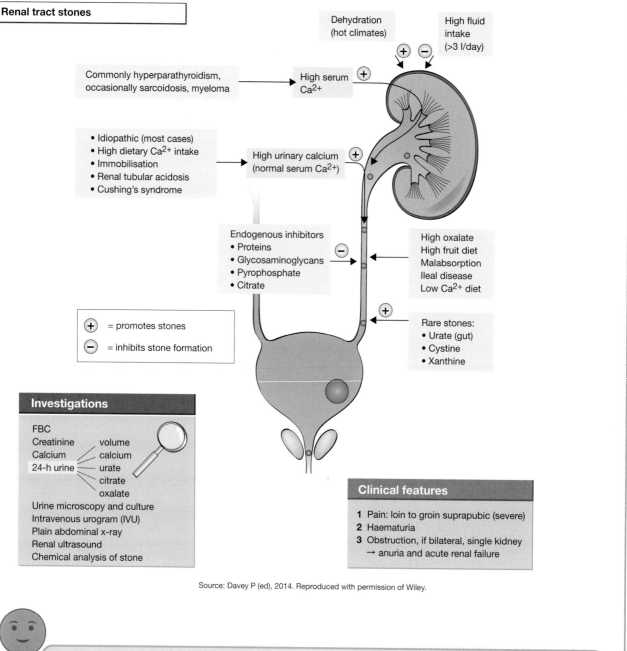

Dehydration (hot climates)

High fluid intake (>3 l/day)

Commonly hyperparathyroidism, occasionally sarcoidosis, myeloma → High serum $Ca^{2+}$

- Idiopathic (most cases)
- High dietary $Ca^{2+}$ intake
- Immobilisation
- Renal tubular acidosis
- Cushing's syndrome

→ High urinary calcium (normal serum $Ca^{2+}$)

Endogenous inhibitors
- Proteins
- Glycosaminoglycans
- Pyrophosphate
- Citrate

High oxalate
High fruit diet
Malabsorption
Ileal disease
Low $Ca^{2+}$ diet

Rare stones:
- Urate (gut)
- Cystine
- Xanthine

(+) = promotes stones
(−) = inhibits stone formation

### Investigations

FBC
Creatinine — volume
Calcium — calcium
24-h urine — urate
— citrate
— oxalate
Urine microscopy and culture
Intravenous urogram (IVU)
Plain abdominal x-ray
Renal ultrasound
Chemical analysis of stone

### Clinical features

1 Pain: loin to groin suprapubic (severe)
2 Haematuria
3 Obstruction, if bilateral, single kidney
→ anuria and acute renal failure

Source: Davey P (ed), 2014. Reproduced with permission of Wiley.

**HE&P**

Advise a patient prior to discharge from hospital to:
- Drink ~3 litres fluid/day unless advised otherwise
- Contact their GP if kidney pain worsens, passing urine becomes painful, urine becomes blood stained or diminishes in amount
- If the stone was made up of calcium oxalate, dietary changes may prevent recurrence: reduce fruit and vegetables containing oxalate (e.g. beetroot, rhubarb, parsley, almonds, peanuts, cashew nuts, leeks) and chocolate
- Do not reduce the amount of calcium that you consume unless you are specifically advised to by your GP
- Your GP might want to review your usual medications if any might have caused your kidney stones

Likely points of access to the healthcare system are general practice, emergency department, walk-in-clinic, out-of-hours (OOH) service, and ambulance service

# Key facts

- Urinary calculi (stones) are solid concentrations of solutes in the urinary tract formed when they precipitate from the urine.
- Most calculi contain calcium oxylate.
- More men than women get urinary calculi.
- Most calculi are idiopathic (above).
- Calculi present with haematuria and often very severe, sharp pain in the loin (acute renal colic) as the stones are moved along the ureter by peristalsis, suprapubic pain, dysuria, UTIs and urinary tract obstruction.
- Acute or chronic renal failure can result from obstruction or consequent infection.
- Investigations may include imaging of the calculi, blood tests for renal function, urinalysis, microscopy, culture and sensitivities to check for infection.
- Immediate management focuses on pain control: renal colic is extremely painful. Control of nausea with anti-emetics. Increased fluid intake is recommended (~3 litres/day unless advised otherwise). Fluid balance needs regular assessment as diminishing urinary output or anuria suggests blockage to both kidneys: this is a medical emergency.
- Around 80% of calculi pass spontaneously without complication.
- Most calculi are managed without surgery by extracorporeal shock wave lithotripsy (ESWL), percutaneous nephrostomy, ureteroscopy and lithotripsy which reduces the stones to smaller particles, or extraction of the calculi.
- Open surgery is rare – ureterolithotomy or nephrolithotomy.

# Essentials of best practice

The nursing care of patients with obstruction of the urinary tract due to calculi focuses largely on pain control (Section 1) and careful observations for deterioration. Fluid balance is important in identifying early signs of diminishing urine output. Nursing care will therefore focus on:

✓ Accurate assessment and regular monitoring
✓ Communication with the healthcare team, patient and family
✓ Symptom control and management
✓ Health education and promotion
✓ Discharge planning

If surgery is needed, the principles of pre- and post-operative care in Section 1 should be adhered to.

## Patient information

There are several useful charities and support groups focusing on kidney disease:

The National Kidney Federation (NKF) www.kidney.org.uk/.

The British Kidney Patient Association www.britishkidney-pa.co.uk/.

The Scottish Kidney Federation www.scotskidneyfederation.org/.

You will find very helpful patient-centred fact sheets at www.patient.co.uk/.

# 58 Nursing people with urinary tract infections

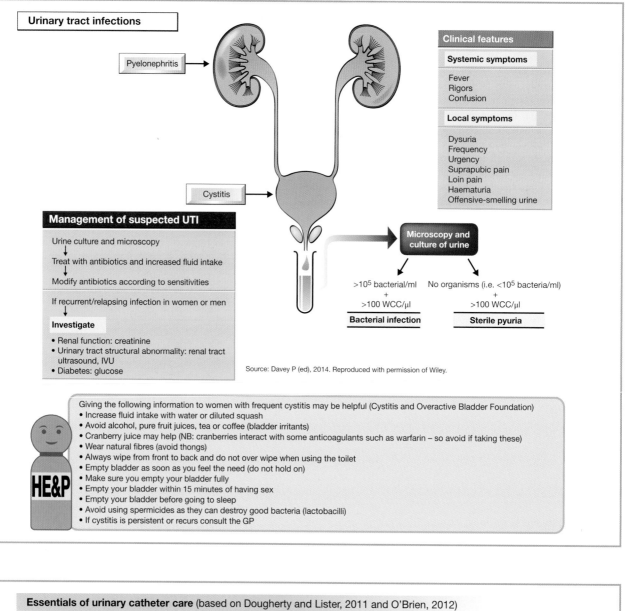

**Urinary tract infections**

Pyelonephritis

Cystitis

**Clinical features**

**Systemic symptoms**

Fever
Rigors
Confusion

**Local symptoms**

Dysuria
Frequency
Urgency
Suprapubic pain
Loin pain
Haematuria
Offensive-smelling urine

**Management of suspected UTI**

Urine culture and microscopy

Treat with antibiotics and increased fluid intake

Modify antibiotics according to sensitivities

If recurrent/relapsing infection in women or men

**Investigate**

• Renal function: creatinine
• Urinary tract structural abnormality: renal tract ultrasound, IVU
• Diabetes: glucose

**Microscopy and culture of urine**

>10⁵ bacterial/ml
+
>100 WCC/μl

**Bacterial infection**

No organisms (i.e. <10⁵ bacteria/ml)
+
>100 WCC/μl

**Sterile pyuria**

Source: Davey P (ed), 2014. Reproduced with permission of Wiley.

**HE&P**

Giving the following information to women with frequent cystitis may be helpful (Cystitis and Overactive Bladder Foundation)
• Increase fluid intake with water or diluted squash
• Avoid alcohol, pure fruit juices, tea or coffee (bladder irritants)
• Cranberry juice may help (NB: cranberries interact with some anticoagulants such as warfarin – so avoid if taking these)
• Wear natural fibres (avoid thongs)
• Always wipe from front to back and do not over wipe when using the toilet
• Empty bladder as soon as you feel the need (do not hold on)
• Make sure you empty your bladder fully
• Empty your bladder within 15 minutes of having sex
• Empty your bladder before going to sleep
• Avoid using spermicides as they can destroy good bacteria (lactobacilli)
• If cystitis is persistent or recurs consult the GP

**Essentials of urinary catheter care** (based on Dougherty and Lister, 2011 and O'Brien, 2012)

• Urinary catheterisation is the **aseptic** insertion of a specifically designed tube into the bladder, to drain urine, instil medication or allow the removal of debris and blood clots. Catheters can be inserted via the urethra or suprapubically
• Catheterisation should be used cautiously due to the risks of infection, altered body image, disturbed mobility and discomfort
• The best catheter is selected for each patient (consider e.g. size, length, material, for short-term or long-term use)
• Once inserted the catheter is attached to a drainage bag that suits the needs of the patient
• Continual care of the urinary drainage system (the catheter and the bag or a catheter and catheter valve) is needed to minimise infection and retain patency
• The bag should be emptied regularly (explain what you're doing, gather equipment, wash hands and put on gloves, swab clean outlet valve, open, collect urine in sterile jug, close valve, swab clean again, measure and record urine, wash hands)
• Bags should be changed when the catheter is changed or when the bag leaks or in line with manufacturer's instructions
• Valves are useful for some people: they allow intermittent emptying of the bladder through release of the valve. Valves need changing in line with manufacturer's instructions
• Cleaning the urethral meatus should be done as part of routine washing with soap and water
• Catheters need changing in line with the manufacturer's instruction or the patient's therapeutic needs
• Removal of a catheter should be done aseptically following the local policy/guidelines

Likely points of access to the healthcare system are general practice, emergency department, walk-in-clinic, out-of-hours (OOH) service, and ambulance service

*Adult Nursing at a Glance*, First Edition. Andrée le May. © 2015 John Wiley & Sons, Ltd. Published 2015 by John Wiley & Sons, Ltd.
Companion website: www.ataglanceseries.com/nursing/adult

# Key facts

- Urinary tract infections (UTI) are very common.
- UTIs are more common in women which may be because women have a shorter urethra than men and most UTIs occur because bowel flora are introduced into the bladder via the urethra.
- UTIs are commonly attributed to sexual intercourse, incomplete emptying of the bladder (e.g. neurogenic bladder in multiple sclerosis, spinal cord injury), urinary calculi, diabetes mellitus, structural abnormalities of the urinary tract and urethral catheters.
- Symptoms include fever, pain, frequency, urgency and smelly urine (above).
- Confusion often accompanies UTIs in older people – it may even be the only clue to these UTIs.
- If symptoms are in the bladder the inflammation caused by infection is called cystitis. Cystitis may be acute or chronic.
- Inflammation caused by infection of the pelvis of the kidney is called pyelonephritis.
- Investigations include urinalysis with a dip stick for nitrites (suggesting gram-negative bacteria), protein, blood, and leukocytes (inflammatory response); microscopy, culture and sensitivities of a clean catch of urine; renal tract imaging to look for underlying causes, for example structural abnormalities.
- Treatment is with antibiotics. Usually oral therapy is sufficient, however acute pyelonephritis may require IV antibiotics.
- Persistent pyelonephritis may result in renal failure requiring dialysis.
- Increased fluid intake (~3 litres/day) is recommended to flush the kidneys, prevent urinary stasis in the bladder and decrease bacterial replication.

# Essentials of best practice

The care of patients with urinary tract infections is largely focused on the GP, with treatment with oral antibiotics being the first course of action. In the main, people with urinary tract infections require no specific nursing care. Sometimes, however, urinary tract infections require more active management with intravenous antibiotics and this may require a short stay in hospital. If this is the case, nursing care should focus on:

✓ Accurate assessment and regular monitoring
✓ Communication with the healthcare team, patient and family
✓ Health education and promotion
✓ Symptom control and management
✓ Discharge planning

Urinary tract infections (and dehydration) may be the cause of some older people being admitted to hospital for investigations of confusion and deterioration of their general health.

Seeing the practice nurse or family planning nurse for contraception may prompt, mainly women, to discuss urinary tract infections. Advice about preventing these should be given (above).

## Patient information

There are several useful charities and support groups focusing on urinary tract infections:
The Cystitis and Overactive Bladder Foundation www.cobfoundation.org.
You will find very helpful patient-centred fact sheets at www.patient.co.uk/.

# 59 Nursing people with blood/lymph disorders

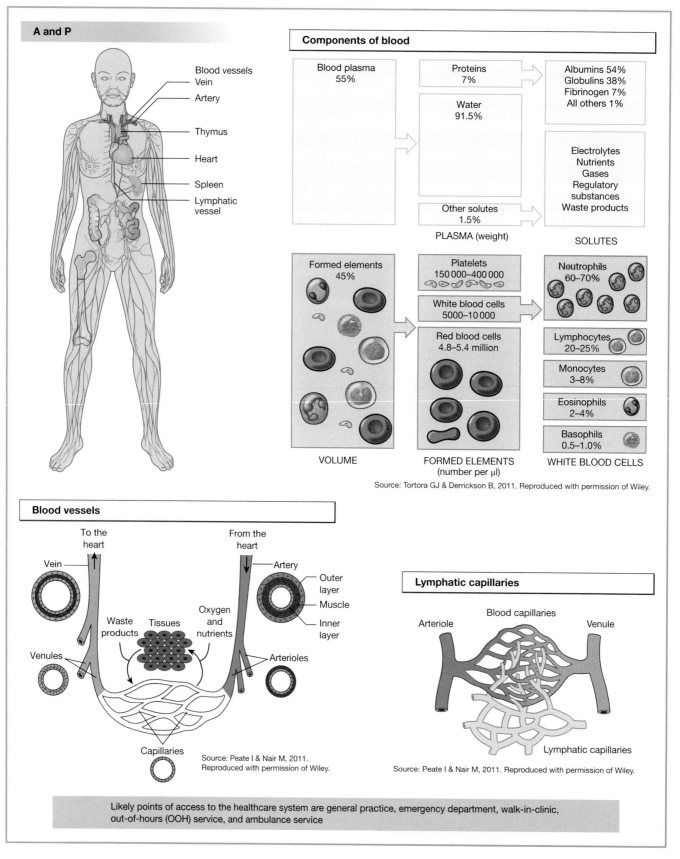

**A and P**

Blood vessels
Vein
Artery
Thymus
Heart
Spleen
Lymphatic vessel

**Components of blood**

Blood plasma 55%

Proteins 7%

Water 91.5%

Other solutes 1.5%

PLASMA (weight)

Albumins 54%
Globulins 38%
Fibrinogen 7%
All others 1%

Electrolytes
Nutrients
Gases
Regulatory substances
Waste products

SOLUTES

Formed elements 45%

Platelets 150 000–400 000

White blood cells 5000–10 000

Red blood cells 4.8–5.4 million

Neutrophils 60–70%

Lymphocytes 20–25%

Monocytes 3–8%

Eosinophils 2–4%

Basophils 0.5–1.0%

VOLUME

FORMED ELEMENTS (number per µl)

WHITE BLOOD CELLS

Source: Tortora GJ & Derrickson B, 2011. Reproduced with permission of Wiley.

**Blood vessels**

To the heart
Vein
From the heart
Artery
Outer layer
Muscle
Inner layer
Waste products
Tissues
Oxygen and nutrients
Venules
Arterioles
Capillaries

Source: Peate I & Nair M, 2011.
Reproduced with permission of Wiley.

**Lymphatic capillaries**

Blood capillaries
Arteriole
Venule
Lymphatic capillaries

Source: Peate I & Nair M, 2011. Reproduced with permission of Wiley.

Likely points of access to the healthcare system are general practice, emergency department, walk-in-clinic, out-of-hours (OOH) service, and ambulance service

*Adult Nursing at a Glance*, First Edition. Andrée le May. © 2015 John Wiley & Sons, Ltd. Published 2015 by John Wiley & Sons, Ltd.
Companion website: www.ataglanceseries.com/nursing/adult

# Key facts

- The circulatory system is essential in the movement of nutrients, oxygen and hormones to the body's cells, the disposal of waste from cellular metabolism and the body's ability to protect itself from infection.
- The circulatory system includes two interlinked systems: one associated with the circulation of blood and the other with the circulation of lymph.
- Blood is transported around the body in a network of blood vessels leading to and from the heart. This network is made up of veins, venules, capillaries, arterioles and arteries.
- The average adult person has ~5 litres of blood circulating in their body.
- 55% of blood is made up of fluid (plasma): the remaining 45% comprises 'formed elements' – red blood cells, white blood cells and platelets.
- The lymphatic system is made up of lymph vessels, lymph nodes, the spleen and the thymus gland. The lymph vessels drain into two ducts – the left lymphatic and the thoracic ducts: these ducts drain into the subclavian veins.
- The lymphatic system primarily helps destroy pathogens, filters waste, removes dead cells and toxins from cells and interstitial spaces: it also transports some nutrients, oxygen and hormones.
- Lymph, a clear fluid, is transported in the lymphatic system.
- This entire circulatory system is important in homeostasis.

# Common circulatory system disorders

- Anaemias
- Neutropenia
- Leukaemias
- Lymphomas
- Platelet disorders
- Clotting disorders.

Each is covered in the following pages. See Chapter 60 for common signs and symptoms associated with disorders of the blood and lymphatic systems.

# A and P

- Blood is made up of plasma (55%) and red blood cells, white blood cells and platelets (the remaining 45%). Plasma is the fluid content and the rest is the formed content of blood.
- Plasma is pale yellow and made up of ~90% water and ~10% solutes (mainly proteins with ~1% inorganic salts).
- Plasma proteins, synthesised in the liver, constitute three groups: albumin, fibrinogen and globulins.
- Albumin maintains plasma osmotic pressure. Fibrinogen is central to blood clotting. Alpha and beta globulins transport lipids and fat-soluble vitamins. Gamma globulins are immunoglobulins and important in immunity.
- Plasma's osmolality is usually between 285–295 mOsmol/kg. Keeping this within normal range is important for blood cell survival (e.g. if osmolality is too high red blood cells shrivel (crenate) and die: if it is too low they rupture (haemolysis) and die).

- IV replacement fluids need to be close to plasma osmolality.
- Red blood cells, white blood cells and platelets are produced in the bone marrow from undifferentiated stem cells. As the stem cell divides and matures it becomes either a red blood cell, or a white blood cell or a platelet.
- Red blood cells (erythrocytes) are biconcave discs. There are ~4–5.5 million red blood cells/cubic mm of blood. Mature red blood cells do not have a nucleus and organelles – this increases their potential for carrying haemoglobin, which in turn increases the amount of oxygen they can transport. Red blood cells also transport $CO_2$ from the cells to the lungs as carbaminohaemoglobin; they also enable the conversion of $CO_2$ to carbonic acid (and then bicarbonate and hydrogen ions) through the enzyme carbonic anhydrase. Red blood cells have a life span of around 120 days. Erythropoietin, a hormone produced by the kidneys, controls the production of red blood cells. They are broken down in the spleen by macrophages.
- White blood cells (leucocytes) have nuclei, can move out of the blood vessels into tissues and play an important role in immunity and inflammation. There are around 25 000/cubic mm of blood. An increase in number is called leucocytosis and a decrease leucopenia. There are two types of leucocytes – granulocytes (neutrophils, eosinophils, basophils) and agranulocytes (monocytes and lymphocytes). Lymphocytes are transported in lymph to lymph nodes and the spleen.
- Platelets are very small blood cells central to preventing blood loss. They form platelet plugs to seal blood vessels and also release blood clotting components. Increased platelets can cause unwanted blood clots and too few, unwanted bleeding.
- Blood is carried from the heart in arteries to the capillaries (the microcirculatory system) where most of the exchange of nutrients, electrolytes, water, gases and waste occurs through the capillaries' thin walls, then back to the heart in veins. (NB: arteries usually carry oxygenated blood and veins deoxygenated blood, with the exception of the pulmonary artery and vein where this is the other way round.)
- Lymph circulates through the lymphatic system.

# Essentials of best practice

Disorders of the circulatory system can range from mild to severe. Nursing someone with any of these disorders may take place in the community, the GP surgery, the ED or OOH service or in a hospital ward or specialist haematology or oncology unit. The essentials of best practice required to care for common disorders are covered in the subsequent pages. In addition Chapter 60 details assessment of these systems, common signs and symptoms and emergencies.

## Patient information

There are several patient support groups and charities focusing on disorders of the blood and lymph systems. You can find most of them on the Self Help UK website www.self-help.org.uk.
You will also find very helpful patient-centred fact sheets at www.patient.co.uk/.

# 60 Signs, symptoms, assessment and emergencies

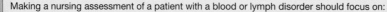

### Important assessments of the blood and lymphatic systems

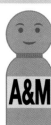

**A&M** Making a nursing assessment of a patient with a blood or lymph disorder should focus on:
- Finding out about the history of the problem (see signs and symptoms below)
- Monitoring other systems, for example respiratory rate and confusion as well as heart rate and rhythms
- Assessing and monitoring pain

### Medical management of pulmonary embolism

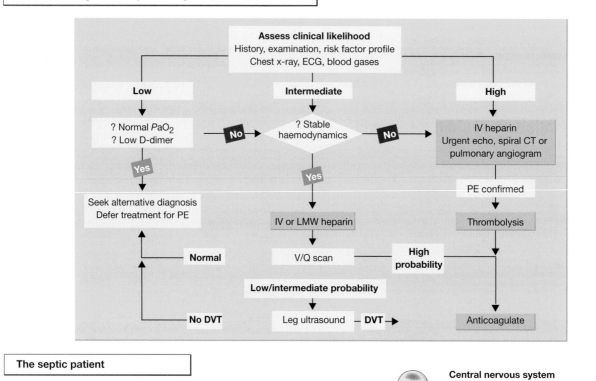

### The septic patient

**Consequences of infection**
- Petechial rash in meningococcal disease
- Embolic lesions in endocarditis, *Staphylococcus* or *Candida* infections
- Poor peripheral perfusion or evidence of gangrene in some severe systemic infections (e.g. meningococcal)

**Retina**
**Fungal emboli**
- Disseminated candidaemia

**Skin**
**Evidence of source of sepsis**
- IV line site infections
- Needle tracks
- Leg ulcers or pressure sores
- Boils or cellulitis

**Central nervous system**
**Meningeal irritation**
- Meningitis
- Sudden change in consciousness or focal neurological signs
- Cerebral abscess

**Heart**
New murmurs
- Endocarditis

**Rectum**
**Rectal abscess**
- Enterobacteraciae

**Genital tract**
**Tampon**
- Toxic shock syndrome

Source: Davey P (ed), 2014. Reproduced with permission of Wiley.

*Adult Nursing at a Glance*, First Edition. Andrée le May. © 2015 John Wiley & Sons, Ltd. Published 2015 by John Wiley & Sons, Ltd.
Companion website: www.ataglanceseries.com/nursing/adult

**People at risk of deep vein thrombosis should be advised what to look for:** (www.patient.co.uk)

**HE&P**

- Pain/tenderness in the calf
- Calf swelling
- Redness and warmth in the calf

Also give advice about avoiding long periods of immobility (e.g. bed rest, sitting in one position, and/or plane, train, car and coach journeys)

Regularly walking around or exercising the legs is important

Being overweight can increase the risk of developing a DVT so advice about weight reduction might also be appropriate

Smoking cessation should also be advised if appropriate

It is important to emphasise that seeking medical advice is critical if a person suspects a DVT since part of the DVT may break off, travel to the lung and cause a clot (PE) which could be fatal

Likely points of access to the healthcare system are general practice, walk-in-clinic, out-of-hours (OOH) service, emergency department, and ambulance service

# Common signs and symptoms
## Blood circulatory system

Tiredness
Breathlessness
Feeling faint
Chest pain if an underlying heart problem
Pain/discomfort
Bruising/purpura
Swelling
Rash
Skin feels hot
Redness of area on skin
Malaise (feeling under the weather)
Pallor
Pyrexia if infection
Unintentional weight loss.

## Lymphatic system

Oedema
Swollen lymph nodes
Malaise
Sweats
Unintentional weight loss.

# Emergencies: circulatory system
## Pulmonary embolism

- Pulmonary embolism (PE) is a blockage in the pulmonary arterial system.
- Emboli can result from a blood clot emanating from a DVT (in the leg or pelvis) or fat from a fractured long bone or orthopaedic surgery, or amniotic fluid or air (e.g. from bronchial trauma) or a small piece of tumour.
- PE is a medical emergency (opposite).
- Symptoms and signs can be varied and may include:
  - breathlessness;
  - cough;
  - haemoptysis (coughing up blood);
  - pleuritic pain;
  - dizziness and fainting;
  - hypoxia (confusion, agitation);
  - circulatory collapse (hypotension, tachycardia and hypoxia).

- Treatment will include oxygen administration, heparin initially – which will be changed to warfarin following diagnosis: thrombolysis if appropriate.
- Risk factors include: bed rest, immobility, surgery, lower limb problems (fracture, thrombophlebitis), malignancy, previous venous thromboembolism (VTE) (either a DVT or PE), hypertension, chronic dialysis, obesity, COPD.
- PE can present without many warning signs so being constantly alert to the possibility of PE is very important (above).
- Nursing care: if you are the first to notice the deterioration of a patient's condition should focus on getting immediate help and staying with the patient.
- Subsequent care will depend on the prescribed treatment but will always involve accurate, frequent observations of vital signs and reporting these appropriately.
- Clear explanation is essential to patients and their families/carers after PE. Advice about reducing risks (e.g. avoiding immobility) and adhering to prescribed anticoagulant medication (and its monitoring) is important.
- PE is a frightening experience for all concerned so appropriate information will help to reassure the patient.

## Sepsis

- Sepsis is an infection with a systemic response – raised or lowered temperature (>38°C or <36°C), increased respiratory rate (>20 breaths/minute), tachycardia (>90 beats/minute) and a raised or lowered white blood cells count.
- Recognising and responding to these signs is vital in preventing a rapid deterioration in a patient's condition with the possibility of progression to septic shock.
- Sepsis can occur for many reasons (e.g. bacterial or fungal infections, poor resistance/increased susceptibility to infection, a response to surgery or a wound infection, a result of infection from invasive procedures, e.g. IV infusions, urinary catheters).
- Septic shock is sepsis with organ dysfunction and hypotension despite adequate fluid resuscitation. It may manifest in, for example, acute confused state, coma, adult respiratory distress syndrome (ARDS), circulatory failure, acute renal failure or haemostatic failure.
- Care focuses on treating the cause and presenting signs and symptoms and evaluating organ function for deterioration (or improvement). Nursing care will be in direct response to medical intervention (e.g. administration of antibiotics, management of IVIs) and monitoring vital signs.
- Accurate, frequent monitoring and reporting of vital signs is critical.

# 61 Nursing people with anaemias

## Anaemia classification

| Microcytic | Normochromic | Macrocytic | |
|---|---|---|---|
| • Fe deficiency<br>• Thalassaemia<br><br>MCV <80 fl | • Chronic disease<br>• Acute bleed<br>• Mixed B$_{12}$, Fe deficiency<br><br>MCV 80–95 fl | • Folate/B$_{12}$ deficiency<br>• Low T$_4$<br>• Haemolytic anaemias<br>• Myelodysplasia<br>MCV > 100 fl | Red cell |

Source: Davey P (ed), 2014. Reproduced with permission of Wiley.

## Defining the main types of anaemia (www.patient.co.uk)

| | |
|---|---|
| **Iron deficiency anaemia** | Iron deficiency anaemia is the most common cause of anaemia in the UK. Iron deficiency may occur because of blood loss (e.g. through menstruation, GIT bleeding), an iron deficient diet, pregnancy, poor absorption of iron (e.g. coeliac disease) or hook worm infection. |
| **Thalassaemia** | Thalassaemia is a genetic condition that affects the alpha or beta chains of haemoglobin. Consequently there is insufficient normal haemoglobin and the red blood cells break down easily. Thalassaemia is associated with being of Mediterranean or Asian origin. |
| **Aplastic anaemia** | Aplastic anaemia is a disorder of the bone marrow resulting in a deficiency of all blood cells. |
| **Pernicious anaemia** | In pernicious anaemia vitamin B$_{12}$ cannot be absorbed. Antibodies are formed against intrinsic factor or against the cells in the stomach that make intrinsic factor, this stops intrinsic factor from attaching to vitamin B$_{12}$ and prevents its absorption. |
| **Haemolytic anaemias** | A group of anaemias (e.g. sickle cell disease, thalassaemia) where red blood cell life is shortened. |

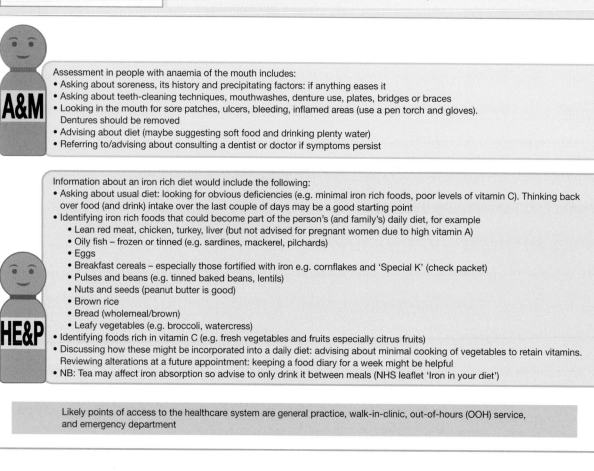

**A&M**

Assessment in people with anaemia of the mouth includes:
- Asking about soreness, its history and precipitating factors: if anything eases it
- Asking about teeth-cleaning techniques, mouthwashes, denture use, plates, bridges or braces
- Looking in the mouth for sore patches, ulcers, bleeding, inflamed areas (use a pen torch and gloves). Dentures should be removed
- Advising about diet (maybe suggesting soft food and drinking plenty water)
- Referring to/advising about consulting a dentist or doctor if symptoms persist

**HE&P**

Information about an iron rich diet would include the following:
- Asking about usual diet: looking for obvious deficiencies (e.g. minimal iron rich foods, poor levels of vitamin C). Thinking back over food (and drink) intake over the last couple of days may be a good starting point
- Identifying iron rich foods that could become part of the person's (and family's) daily diet, for example
  - Lean red meat, chicken, turkey, liver (but not advised for pregnant women due to high vitamin A)
  - Oily fish – frozen or tinned (e.g. sardines, mackerel, pilchards)
  - Eggs
  - Breakfast cereals – especially those fortified with iron e.g. cornflakes and 'Special K' (check packet)
  - Pulses and beans (e.g. tinned baked beans, lentils)
  - Nuts and seeds (peanut butter is good)
  - Brown rice
  - Bread (wholemeal/brown)
  - Leafy vegetables (e.g. broccoli, watercress)
- Identifying foods rich in vitamin C (e.g. fresh vegetables and fruits especially citrus fruits)
- Discussing how these might be incorporated into a daily diet: advising about minimal cooking of vegetables to retain vitamins. Reviewing alterations at a future appointment: keeping a food diary for a week might be helpful
- NB: Tea may affect iron absorption so advise to only drink it between meals (NHS leaflet 'Iron in your diet')

Likely points of access to the healthcare system are general practice, walk-in-clinic, out-of-hours (OOH) service, and emergency department

*Adult Nursing at a Glance*, First Edition. Andrée le May. © 2015 John Wiley & Sons, Ltd. Published 2015 by John Wiley & Sons, Ltd.
Companion website: www.ataglanceseries.com/nursing/adult

# Key facts

- Anaemia occurs when haemoglobin is reduced by more than two standard deviations from the mean for that person. Anaemia occurs because there are insufficient/poorly functioning red blood cells (RBC) or there is a reduction in haemoglobin (Hb) in each RBC.
- Reduced haemoglobin means that RBC carry less oxygen.
- Haemoglobin levels normally vary between individuals. Women tend to have lower levels than men.
- WHO (2011) defined anaemia as less than 12 g/dl Hb for non-pregnant women; less than 11 g/dl Hb for pregnant women and less than 13 g/dl Hb for men.
- Anaemias are caused by different illnesses/deficiencies (above).
- Nutritional deficiencies can cause anaemia. Iron deficiency is the most common cause of anaemia in the world. (Folate, vitamin $B_{12}$ and vitamin A deficiencies are also important.)
- Anaemias are usually classified according the RBC size (opposite): microcytic/hypochromic anaemia (small red blood cells with less haemoglobin than normal); normochromic/normocytic (normal haemoglobin, normal sized red blood cells); macrocytic (red blood cells are larger than normal).
- Symptoms and signs of anaemia depend on underlying pathologies but may include:
  - tiredness;
  - peripheral oedema, for example swollen feet;
  - breathlessness;
  - feeling faint;
  - angina if underlying heart problems;
  - pallor may be seen in conjunctiva;
  - spoon shaped nails in long-standing anaemia.
- Diagnosis is made by examination, history and blood tests (e.g. full blood count, haemoglobin concentration, haematocrit (or packed cell volume – PCV), blood film). For some people, bone marrow examination and other specific tests will also be done.
- Treatment is of the underlying disease. It may include hospitalisation or be carried out in primary care. Options include:
  - iron supplements (and dietary advice);
  - blood transfusion;
  - recombinant erythropoietin;
  - vitamin supplements/replacements.

# Essentials of best practice

The nursing care of people with anaemia will depend on the severity of their disease and its underlying pathology. For some people no treatment will be required except for advice about dietary changes (e.g. eating food rich in iron and also ensuring an adequate intake of vitamin C (vitamin C may help the body to absorb iron) and protein), for others iron or vitamin $B_{12}$ supplements may be prescribed: in severe cases some people will need blood transfusions.

Hypoxia related to anaemia may cause tiredness, breathlessness and associated anxiety. Advice should be given about how to alleviate each of these, for example making sure that rest is planned into daily routines may help to control tiredness and help with breathlessness, sitting upright also may help reduce feelings of breathlessness (see Chapter 36). Some people may also report sore mouths, which will affect their appetite, and an oral assessment (opposite) should be carried out if this is the case. Smoking can also impact on anaemia so smoking cessation should be discussed and supported.

Whilst for the majority of people nursing care is likely to be provided by practice nurses and community nurses some people will require more active nursing care in hospital. Hospitalisation is likely to be associated with, for instance, severe blood loss or when someone is diagnosed with aplastic anaemia or requires transfusions for haemolytic anaemias. In these instances care will largely focus on:

✓ Accurate assessment and regular monitoring (e.g. transfusions, sickle cell crises)
✓ Communication with the healthcare team, patient and family
✓ Symptom control and management (e.g. tiredness and breathlessness)
✓ Health education and promotion (e.g. about diet, alleviating symptoms associated with their condition)
✓ Risk assessment and management (e.g. VTE and pressure ulcers due to immobility)
✓ Discharge planning

Help may be needed, in or out of hospital, with activities of daily living if the patient is very tired or breathless.

Some people may also need advice about supplementary benefits to enable them to make significant changes to their diet or sickness benefits if they cannot work, and referral to a social worker or Citizen's Advice Bureau may be helpful.

## Patient information

There are several useful charities and support groups focusing on anaemia:
The Aplastic Anaemia Trust www.theaat.org.uk.
The United Kingdom Thalassemia Society www.ukts.org.
The Pernicious Anaemia Society www.pernicious-anaemia-society.org.
You will find very helpful patient-centred fact sheets at www.patient.co.uk.

# 62 Nursing people with neutropenia

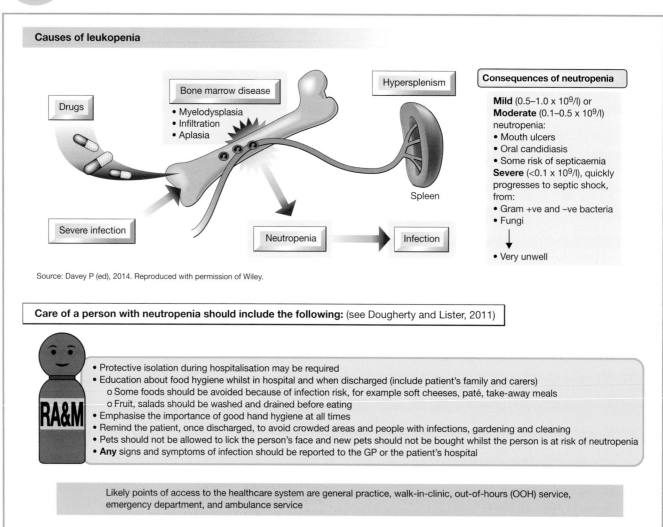

## Causes of leukopenia

Drugs

Bone marrow disease
• Myelodysplasia
• Infiltration
• Aplasia

Hypersplenism

Spleen

Severe infection

Neutropenia → Infection

### Consequences of neutropenia

**Mild** (0.5–1.0 x $10^9$/l) or **Moderate** (0.1–0.5 x $10^9$/l) neutropenia:
• Mouth ulcers
• Oral candidiasis
• Some risk of septicaemia
**Severe** (<0.1 x $10^9$/l), quickly progresses to septic shock, from:
• Gram +ve and –ve bacteria
• Fungi
  ↓
• Very unwell

Source: Davey P (ed), 2014. Reproduced with permission of Wiley.

---

**Care of a person with neutropenia should include the following:** (see Dougherty and Lister, 2011)

• Protective isolation during hospitalisation may be required
• Education about food hygiene whilst in hospital and when discharged (include patient's family and carers)
  o Some foods should be avoided because of infection risk, for example soft cheeses, paté, take-away meals
  o Fruit, salads should be washed and drained before eating
• Emphasise the importance of good hand hygiene at all times
• Remind the patient, once discharged, to avoid crowded areas and people with infections, gardening and cleaning
• Pets should not be allowed to lick the person's face and new pets should not be bought whilst the person is at risk of neutropenia
• **Any** signs and symptoms of infection should be reported to the GP or the patient's hospital

Likely points of access to the healthcare system are general practice, walk-in-clinic, out-of-hours (OOH) service, emergency department, and ambulance service

# Key facts

• White blood cells (leucocytes) are made in the bone marrow. There are two types of leucocytes: granulocytes (neutrophils, eosinophils, basophils) and agranulocytes (monocytes and lymphocytes).

• White blood cells' (WBC) main functions are associated with infection control and inflammatory responses. Any reduction or damage to them can have lethal consequences.

• Leukopenia occurs when the number of effective WBC is reduced: this can be associated with bone marrow diseases (e.g. leukaemias), certain cytotoxic anticancer drugs and severe infections (below).

# Neutropenia

• Neutropenia is a reduction in circulating neutrophils. Neutrophils fight infection especially those caused by bacteria and fungi. A low level puts people at risk of infection.

• Neutropenia can be congenital, associated with particular ethnic origins (e.g. people of African descent), acquired due to ineffective/decreased neutrophil production (e.g. in aplastic anaemia, chemotherapy, radiotherapy, alcohol abuse, human immunodeficiency virus (HIV), bone marrow infiltration with cancer), accelerated neutrophil turnover in blood (e.g. malaria, acute bacterial infections), an autoimmune reaction or due to thyroid dysfunction.

• Mild neutropenia may result in no symptoms but some people have mouth ulcers and oral thrush: mild/moderate neutropenia has some risk of septicaemia: severe neutropenia is linked to septic shock and may be fatal. In mild cases treatment, with monitoring, may be carried out in primary care.

• Symptoms and signs of neutropenia depend on the underlying cause and severity of the neutropenia: they may include pyrexia, obvious signs of inflammation/infection, for example around IVI line sites, signs of infection related to specific parts of the body, for example pneumonia, or rashes. These early signs of infection are important to record and report – for example a temperature of 37.5 °C or more in cancer-linked neutropenia may be the first sign of a person developing febrile neutropenia – which can rapidly progress to sepsis.

• The Multinational Association for Supportive Care in Cancer (MASCC) has produced a risk assessment tool for use with people with cancer who are at risk of developing febrile neutropenia.

• In people with febrile neutropenia early treatment (within 30 minutes of being alerted) is critical to their survival – neutropenic sepsis is a medical emergency.

• In febrile neutropenia rapid treatment of the underlying cause and prevention of shock are key to survival: this necessitates hospitalisation.

• NICE guidance is available for the treatment of neutropenic sepsis in patients with cancer.

# Essentials of best practice

The nursing care of people with neutropenia will depend on its severity and the underlying pathology. For some people, no treatment will be required except for advice about early signs and symptoms of infection to be alert to and seek immediate medical advice about. Some patients undergoing chemotherapy which might induce neutropenia are advised to seek early advice if their temperature is elevated, they feel unwell, have a sore throat, pain urinating, coughs/breathlessness or have redness/swelling around an infusion site. Written instructions about what to look out for and who to contact are important for patients and their families and carers to have and adhere to. Some patients may be offered prophylactic treatment with antibiotics or granulocyte colony-stimulating factor (G-CSF) which stimulates bone marrow to produce blood cells.

In instances of febrile neutropenia (which can quickly progress to septic neutropenia), nursing care will be in hospital and will largely focus on:

✓ Accurate assessment and regular monitoring
✓ Communication with the healthcare team, patient and family
✓ Risk assessment and management

## Patient information

There are several useful charities and support groups focusing on neutropenia and leukaemia:
Macmillan Cancer Support www.macmillan.org.uk.
Cancer Research UK www.cancerresearchuk.org.
You will find very helpful patient-centred fact sheets at www.patient.co.uk.

# 63 Nursing people with leukaemia

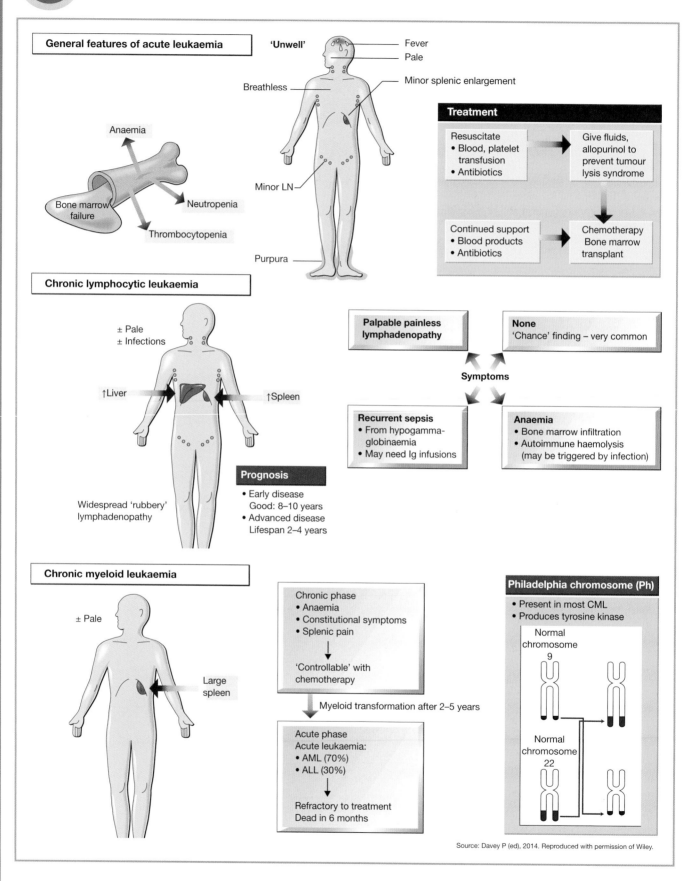

**General features of acute leukaemia**

'Unwell'
Fever
Pale
Minor splenic enlargement
Breathless
Minor LN
Purpura

Anaemia
Bone marrow failure
Neutropenia
Thrombocytopenia

**Treatment**

Resuscitate
- Blood, platelet transfusion
- Antibiotics

Give fluids, allopurinol to prevent tumour lysis syndrome

Continued support
- Blood products
- Antibiotics

Chemotherapy
Bone marrow transplant

**Chronic lymphocytic leukaemia**

± Pale
± Infections

↑Liver
↑Spleen

Widespread 'rubbery' lymphadenopathy

**Prognosis**
- Early disease
  Good: 8–10 years
- Advanced disease
  Lifespan 2–4 years

**Palpable painless lymphadenopathy**

**None**
'Chance' finding – very common

**Symptoms**

**Recurrent sepsis**
- From hypogamma-globinaemia
- May need Ig infusions

**Anaemia**
- Bone marrow infiltration
- Autoimmune haemolysis (may be triggered by infection)

**Chronic myeloid leukaemia**

± Pale

Large spleen

Chronic phase
- Anaemia
- Constitutional symptoms
- Splenic pain

'Controllable' with chemotherapy

Myeloid transformation after 2–5 years

Acute phase
Acute leukaemia:
- AML (70%)
- ALL (30%)

Refractory to treatment
Dead in 6 months

**Philadelphia chromosome (Ph)**
- Present in most CML
- Produces tyrosine kinase

Normal chromosome 9

Normal chromosome 22

Source: Davey P (ed), 2014. Reproduced with permission of Wiley.

*Adult Nursing at a Glance*, First Edition. Andrée le May. © 2015 John Wiley & Sons, Ltd. Published 2015 by John Wiley & Sons, Ltd.
Companion website: www.ataglanceseries.com/nursing/adult

**Giving advice about the early signs of neutropenia will include reminding a patient and their family/carers to seek immediate medical advice if:**

**HE&P**

- Their temperature is elevated
- They feel unwell
- Have a sore throat or pain urinating or a cough/breathlessness
- Have redness/swelling around an infusion site

Written instructions about what to look out for and who to contact should be given alongside verbal advice.

Likely points of access to the healthcare system are general practice, walk-in-clinic, out-of-hours (OOH) service, emergency department, and ambulance service

## Key facts

- Leukaemia is cancer of the blood or bone marrow.
- Leukaemia can be acute or chronic (opposite).
- Leukaemias are named after the stem cell line that is affected (e.g. in Acute Myeloid Leukaemia (AML) the myeloid line is affected, in Chronic Lymphocytic Leukaemia (CLL) it is the lymphoid line). The affected white blood cells (blasts) are immature and proliferate taking over the space in the bone marrow preventing other blood cells (e.g. red blood cells and platelets) from developing.
- The main types of leukaemia affecting adults in the UK are AML and CLL.
- Although rare in the UK, AML is the most common acute leukaemia in adults. AML is associated with increasing age and peaks at around 70 years of age.
- Chronic Lymphocytic Leukaemia (CLL) and Chronic Myeloid Leukaemia (CML) are chronic leukaemias. The incidence of CLL increases with age, CLL is more common in men. CML is rare and usually occurs in middle age.
- Acute leukaemia, without treatment, can progress very quickly resulting in death within a few months. Chronic leukaemia tends to develop slowly.

## Acute Myeloid Leukaemia

- The cause of AML may be associated with chromosomal anomalies or be linked to past chemotherapy, radiation, smoking and benzene exposure as well as other chronic blood disorders such as aplastic anaemia, paroxysmal nocturnal haemoglobinuria (rare and linked with anaemia, red blood cells are destroyed in the blood stream, urine contains iron and may be red/black in the morning).
- Signs and symptoms of AML are associated with anaemia, leucopenia, and thrombocytopenia (low platelet count). These manifest as tiredness, breathlessness, infections (fever and malaise), bleeding (and bruising), weight loss and anorexia, and sweats.
- Diagnosis is through examination, history and blood tests together with bone marrow aspiration.
- Treatment will depend on the severity of the presenting symptoms – some people can be very ill and vulnerable to infection. Blood transfusion to correct anaemia, antibiotics to counteract infection and platelets or fresh frozen plasma to prevent bleeding may be required. Allopurinol may be given to lower uric acid levels. Nursing care will revolve around the management of these regimens and reassuring the patient and their family and carers.
- After a person's condition has been stabilised, treatment with chemotherapy will start. During this time nursing care will focus on observing for and minimising the side-effects of chemotherapy (e.g. nausea and vomiting, a sore mouth, and chemotherapy induced neutropenia – see Chapter 62). Treatment can continue for some months.
- Stem cell transplantation may be a treatment option.

## Chronic Lymphocytic Leukaemia

- CLL is characterised by large numbers of abnormal lymphocytes which spill into the blood stream.
- CLL is a chronic, mainly incurable, condition.
- In CLL B lymphocytes are functionally immature.
- CLL may progress slowly and many people with CLL are diagnosed by chance through a routine blood test.
- For those with signs and symptoms these include: fever, weight loss, night sweats, infections, anaemia (tiredness and breathlessness) and thrombocytopenia (bruising: purpura).
- Diagnosis is made through examination, history and blood tests (e.g. full blood count and blood film).
- Treatment focuses on symptoms and may be carried out in primary care, as an outpatient or if need be as an in-patient.
- Nursing care is largely about providing psychological support, educating patients and their family/carers about drug regimens and side-effects, dealing with tiredness and breathlessness and when to seek help (e.g. infections).
- Some younger patients may have stem cell transplants.

## Essentials of best practice

The nursing care of people with leukaemia will depend on its severity and the underlying pathology. For some people, no treatment will be required except for advice about early signs and symptoms of infection to be alert to and seek immediate medical advice about. Some patients undergoing chemotherapy will need care focused on relieving the side-effects they are experiencing at the time and advice about recognising the early signs of neutropenia. Written instructions about what to look out for and whom to contact are important for patients and their families and carers to have and adhere to.
Nursing care will include:

✓ Accurate assessment and regular monitoring
✓ Communication with the healthcare team, patient and family
✓ Symptom control and management
✓ Risk assessment and management
✓ Health education and promotion
✓ Discharge planning

### Patient information

There are several charities and support groups focusing on leukaemia:
Macmillan Cancer Support www.macmillan.org.uk.
Cancer Research UK www.cancerresearchuk.org.
The Leukaemia Cancer Society www.leukaemiasociety.org.
You will find very helpful patient-centred fact sheets at www.patient.co.uk.

# 64 Nursing people with platelet/coagulation disorders

## Blood clotting factors (Peate and Nair: 383)

| Factor | Common name |
|--------|-------------|
| I | Fibrinogen |
| II | Prothrombin |
| V | Proaccelerin, labile factor |
| VII | Proconvertin |
| VIII | Antihaemophilic factor A |
| IX | Antihaemophilic factor B |
| X | Thrombokinase, Stuart–Power factor |
| XI | Antihaemophilic factor C |
| XII | Hagerman factor |
| XIII | Fibrin stabilising factor |

Source: Peate I & Nair M, 2011. Reproduced with permission of Wiley.

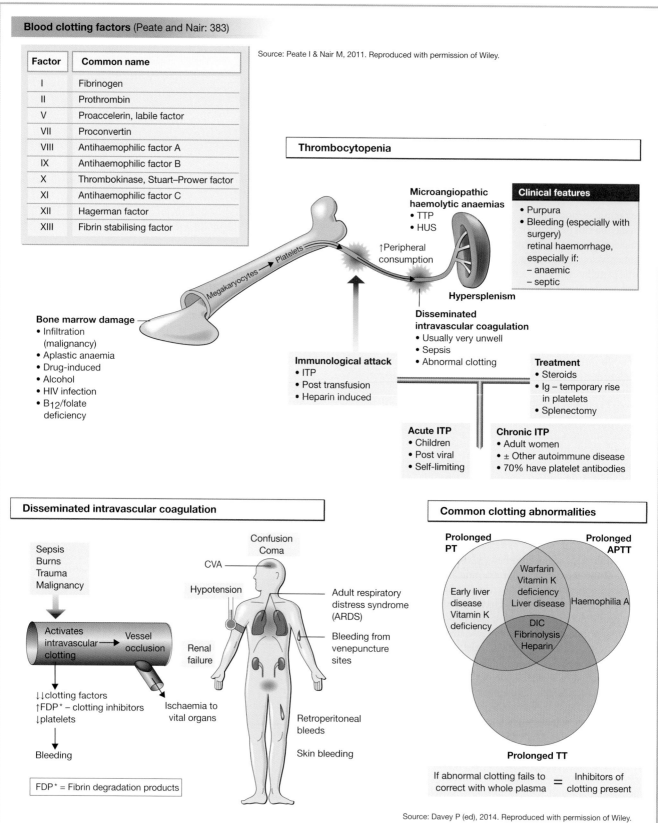

### Thrombocytopenia

**Microangiopathic haemolytic anaemias**
- TTP
- HUS

↑Peripheral consumption

**Hypersplenism**

**Clinical features**
- Purpura
- Bleeding (especially with surgery) retinal haemorrhage, especially if:
  – anaemic
  – septic

Megakaryocytes → Platelets

**Bone marrow damage**
- Infiltration (malignancy)
- Aplastic anaemia
- Drug-induced
- Alcohol
- HIV infection
- B$_{12}$/folate deficiency

**Immunological attack**
- ITP
- Post transfusion
- Heparin induced

**Disseminated intravascular coagulation**
- Usually very unwell
- Sepsis
- Abnormal clotting

**Treatment**
- Steroids
- Ig – temporary rise in platelets
- Splenectomy

**Acute ITP**
- Children
- Post viral
- Self-limiting

**Chronic ITP**
- Adult women
- ± Other autoimmune disease
- 70% have platelet antibodies

### Disseminated intravascular coagulation

Sepsis
Burns
Trauma
Malignancy

Activates intravascular clotting → Vessel occlusion

↓↓clotting factors
↑FDP* – clotting inhibitors
↓platelets

Bleeding

FDP* = Fibrin degradation products

Confusion
Coma

CVA

Hypotension

Renal failure

Adult respiratory distress syndrome (ARDS)

Bleeding from venepuncture sites

Ischaemia to vital organs

Retroperitoneal bleeds

Skin bleeding

### Common clotting abnormalities

**Prolonged PT**

**Prolonged APTT**

Warfarin
Vitamin K deficiency
Liver disease

Early liver disease
Vitamin K deficiency

Haemophilia A

DIC
Fibrinolysis
Heparin

**Prolonged TT**

If abnormal clotting fails to correct with whole plasma = Inhibitors of clotting present

Source: Davey P (ed), 2014. Reproduced with permission of Wiley.

*Adult Nursing at a Glance*, First Edition. Andrée le May. © 2015 John Wiley & Sons, Ltd. Published 2015 by John Wiley & Sons, Ltd.
Companion website: www.ataglanceseries.com/nursing/adult

# Key facts

- Platelets are very small blood cells (thrombocytes) produced in the bone marrow.
- They have no nucleus and live for around 5–9 days. Dead platelets are removed by macrophages in the spleen and liver.
- A platelet's surface contains proteins that allow it to adhere to other proteins (e.g. collagen).
- Platelets are important in clotting and preventing blood loss – they therefore are central to maintaining haemostasis.
- Disorders of platelets are linked to excessive bleeding (low numbers) or thrombosis (high numbers) resulting in VTE, strokes and myocardial infarctions.

# Haemostasis A and P

Haemostasis is a series of steps that stop bleeding and prevent blood loss. Haemostasis helps to maintain the body's homeostasis. Haemostasis comprises three phases:

1 Local vasoconstriction
2 Platelet aggregation
3 Coagulation.

Platelets have a role in all three. In step 1 platelets release thromboxanes promoting vasoconstriction. In step 2 platelets stick to the exposed collagen in damaged blood vessels via von Willebrand's factor (VWF). Platelets release substances to attract other platelets to the site; they stick together and form a platelet plug. The platelets aggregate to each other by cross-linking with fibrinogen. These plugs prevent blood loss from the vessel. If damage to the blood vessel is too extensive for vasoconstriction and the platelet plug to control blood loss blood clotting (coagulation) takes place. Coagulation (step 3) needs certain clotting factors (opposite) synthesised in the liver/acquired from the diet. Platelets release thromboplastinogenase which combines with antihaemophilic factor to convert thromboplastinogen into thromboplastin – this is the start of a cascade of conversions which eventually results in fibrin and clot formation. Coagulation inhibitors are activated to restrict clot formation to the damaged site. Once healing, fibrinolysis occurs restoring the patency of the vessel. Find out more on the coagulation cascade at www.youtube.com/watch?v=xNZEERMSeyM.

# Thrombocytopenia

- Thrombocytopenia is a reduction in the number of platelets. This may be because too few platelets are produced or too many platelets are destroyed.
- Under-production is usually linked to aplastic anaemia, bone marrow damage due to, for example, leukaemia, lymphoma, vitamin B$_{12}$ or folate deficiency, HIV infection. Excess destruction can be linked to viral or bacterial infection, liver disease, disseminated intravascular coagulation (DIC), connective tissue disease (e.g. systemic lupus erythematosus), hypersplenism (above).
- Thrombocytopenia presents as purpura, petechiae, mucosal bleeding, nose bleeds or heavy periods.
- There are several different types of thrombocytopenia (e.g. immune thrombocytopenic purpura (ITP), thrombotic thrombocytopenic purpura (TTP), haemolytic uraemic syndrome (HUS), bone marrow infiltration, post-transfusion purpura) (above).

- Treatment depends on the type of thrombocytopenia and may range from steroids to transfusions, to IV immunoglobulin. Nursing care will centre on the management of these regimens, protecting patients from injury because of the likelihood of bleeding and bruising, monitoring the patient for signs of bleeding (e.g. in urine or stools: cerebral bleeds may be signalled by headaches) and reassuring the patient and their family/carers.
- Patients with disseminated intravascular coagulation will be extremely ill and need specialist care in intensive care units.

# Thrombocytosis

- Thrombocytosis is an increase in platelets. This can occur in myeloproliferative disease, for example essential thrombocythaemia, or be secondary to anaemia or inflammation.
- The risk associated with thrombocytosis largely lies in the risk of thrombosis development (see Chapter 60).
- Prophylaxis against thrombosis should be given as well as advice about identifying signs and symptoms of a Deep Vein Thrombosis (DVT)/Pulmonary Embolus (PE).

# Coagulation disorders

- Disorders of coagulation affect clotting factors.
- These disorders are categorised through routine coagulation tests – activated partial thromboplastin time (APTT), prothrombin time (PT) and thrombin time (TT) (above).
- Coagulation disorders can be inherited (e.g. haemophilia A, haemophilia B and von Willebrand's disease) or acquired (e.g. DIC, liver disease and vitamin K deficiency).
- Treatment will depend on the underlying pathology.

# Essentials of best practice

The nursing care of people with platelet or clotting disorders will depend on the severity of the disease. For some people. no treatment will be required except for advice about things to avoid (e.g. contact sports, aspirin preparations, needle stick injury or cuts) and carrying clear medic alerts to draw attention to their illness. Others will require replacement of clotting factors, prophylaxis if they have a risk of thrombosis and some patients may be very ill (e.g. with DIC or liver disease) and require specialist hospitalised care. Nursing care of anyone in hospital will focus on:

✓ Accurate assessment and regular monitoring
✓ Communication with the healthcare team, patient and family
✓ Symptom control and management
✓ Risk assessment and management
✓ Discharge planning

---

**Patient information**

There are several charities and support groups, for example:
The Haemophilia Society www.haemophilia.org.uk.
The ITP Support Association www.itpsupport.org.uk.
You will find very helpful patient-centred fact sheets at www.patient.co.uk.

**65** # Nursing people with lymphomas

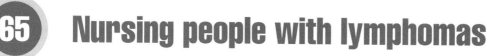

---

**Active monitoring (watchful waiting) for people with low grade non-Hodgkin's lymphoma will include:**

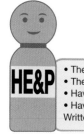

- Regular visits to either the GP or haematologist as an outpatient (this may include blood tests, x-rays and CT scans)
- Discussing with the patient and their family/carers what could suggest progression of their lymphoma and necessitate the commencement of treatment. Any of these should be immediately reported to the GP/ haematologist:
  - o Presentation of new symptoms, for example night sweats, fevers and/or weight loss
  - o New enlarged lymph nodes not associated with infection
  - o Pain in other parts of the body

People who are in the 'watch and wait' group may be anxious about their disease management and lack confidence in recognising its progression – information about symptoms and what to do if they occur is important. Offering support and opportunities to discuss their lymphoma outside the scheduled appointment times may also be helpful. Specialist cancer nurses as well as practice nurses should be able to do this

(Sometimes watchful waiting is called active monitoring as this is more acceptable to patients)

---

**Giving advice about the early signs of neutropenia will include reminding a patient and their family/carers to seek immediate medical advice if:**

- Their temperature is elevated
- They feel unwell
- Have a sore throat or pain urinating or a cough/breathlessness
- Have redness/swelling around an infusion site

Written instructions about what to look out for and who to contact should be given alongside verbal advice

---

Likely points of access to the healthcare system are general practice, walk-in-clinic, out-of-hours (OOH) service, emergency department, and ambulance service

*Adult Nursing at a Glance*, First Edition. Andrée le May. © 2015 John Wiley & Sons, Ltd. Published 2015 by John Wiley & Sons, Ltd.
Companion website: www.ataglanceseries.com/nursing/adult

# Key facts

- Lymphomas are cancers of cells in the lymphatic system.
- There are two main types of lymphoma: Hodgkin's lymphoma and non-Hodgkin's lymphoma.

# Hodgkin's lymphoma

- Hodgkin's lymphoma is rare, usually affecting younger adults aged between 20–30 and older people after 70.
- Hodgkin's lymphoma affects B lymphocytes. These lymphocytes collect in lymph nodes which then get bigger and form malignant tumours. These abnormal cells can travel to other parts of the lymphatic system so people may develop several cancerous lymph nodes and an enlarged spleen.
- Symptoms include:
  - persistent swollen lymph nodes without infection;
  - night sweats;
  - fever;
  - weight loss;
  - tiredness;
  - anorexia;
  - anaemia;
  - itching;
  - general malaise;
  - symptoms associated with increased tumour size (e.g. cough or breathlessness if tumour is in the chest).
- Diagnosis is by biopsy of a swollen lymph node. Staging occurs after confirmation of the diagnosis and usually includes CT and MRI scans, blood tests and a bone marrow biopsy.
- Treatment depends on staging but will usually include chemotherapy and radiotherapy. During this time, nursing care will focus on observing for and minimising the side-effects of chemotherapy (e.g. nausea and vomiting, a sore mouth, and chemotherapy induced neutropenia – see Chapter 62).
- Prognosis is usually good.

# Non-Hodgkin's lymphoma

- Non-Hodgkin's lymphoma is a cancer affecting lymphocytes.
- There are several types of non-Hodgkin's lymphoma that are fast growing (high grade) and slow growing (low grade).
- The cancerous lymphocytes gather in lymph nodes and form tumours: they also travel within and outside the lymphatic system to other lymph nodes, the spleen and via the blood system to other parts of the body where they form lymphoma tumours.
- Non-Hodgkin's lymphoma is a relatively common cancer mainly found in people over 60 years of age. Men are more commonly affected than women.
- Signs and symptoms are similar to Hodgkin's lymphoma plus pain from lymphomas that have grown outside the lymphatic system.

- Diagnosis is by biopsy and grading. CT and MRI scans, blood tests and bone marrow biopsy are used in staging the lymphoma.
- High-grade lymphomas grow more quickly and are more aggressive than low-grade tumours.
- Treatment will depend on grade and staging. Low-grade slow-growing tumours may not require immediate treatment but careful monitoring (above). Other more virulent lymphomas will require treatment with chemotherapy, monoclonal antibodies or radiotherapy. Stem cell transplants are sometimes used.
- Some non-Hodgkin's lymphomas can be cured or controlled.
- Nursing care is largely about delivering, and monitoring responses to chemotherapy and radiotherapy, alleviating side-effects of these treatments, providing psychological support, educating patients and their family/carers about drug regimens, dealing with tiredness and advising about when to seek help (e.g. infections).

# Essentials of best practice

The nursing care of people with lymphomas will depend on the severity of the disease and the presenting symptoms. For some people, no treatment will be required except active monitoring, for others hospitalisation and aggressive chemotherapy will be needed. If active monitoring is the case the patient and their family/carers need to be aware of changes that should be reported to their doctor. Some patients undergoing chemotherapy will need nursing care focused on relieving the symptoms they are experiencing, possibly help with daily living activities and advice about recognising the early signs of neutropenia (above). Written instructions about what to look out for and who to contact are important for patients and their families and carers to have and adhere to.

Nursing care will include:
- ✓ Accurate assessment and regular monitoring
- ✓ Communication with the healthcare team, patient and family
- ✓ Symptom control and management
- ✓ Risk assessment and management
- ✓ Health education and promotion
- ✓ Discharge planning

## Patient information

There are several charities and support groups focusing on lymphoma:
Macmillan Cancer Support www.macmillan.org.uk.
Cancer Research UK www.cancerresearchuk.org.
The Lymphoma Association www.lymphomas.org.uk.
You will find very helpful patient-centred fact sheets at www.patient.co.uk.

# 66 Nursing people with endocrine disorders

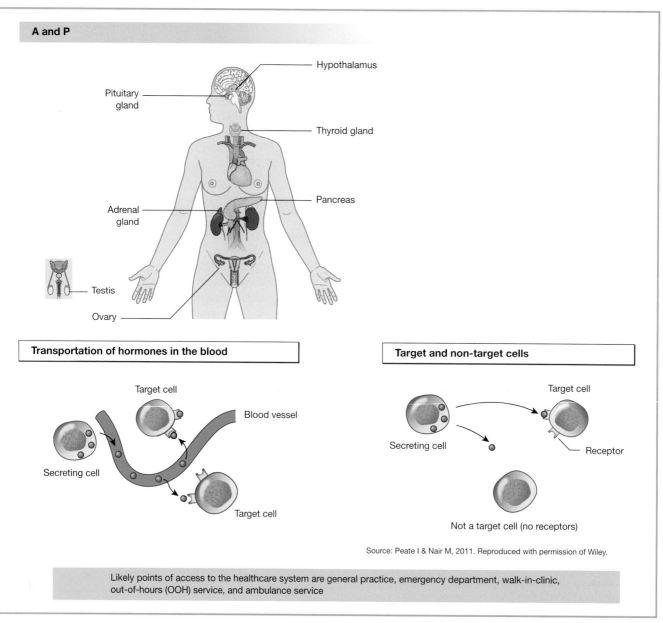

**A and P**

Hypothalamus

Pituitary gland

Thyroid gland

Pancreas

Adrenal gland

Testis

Ovary

**Transportation of hormones in the blood**

Target cell

Blood vessel

Secreting cell

Target cell

**Target and non-target cells**

Target cell

Secreting cell

Receptor

Not a target cell (no receptors)

Source: Peate I & Nair M, 2011. Reproduced with permission of Wiley.

Likely points of access to the healthcare system are general practice, emergency department, walk-in-clinic, out-of-hours (OOH) service, and ambulance service

*Adult Nursing at a Glance*, First Edition. Andrée le May. © 2015 John Wiley & Sons, Ltd. Published 2015 by John Wiley & Sons, Ltd.
Companion website: www.ataglanceseries.com/nursing/adult

# Key facts

- The endocrine system contributes to, for example, maintaining homeostasis, coordinating the body's storage and use of carbohydrates, proteins and fats for energy, regulating growth, metabolism, ions (e.g. sodium, potassium and calcium) and reproduction and responding to external stimuli (e.g. temperature, stress).
- The endocrine system does this by producing hormones.
- The endocrine system comprises three parts:
  1 endocrine glands (organs whose sole function is to produce hormones – pituitary, thyroid, parathyroid and adrenal glands);
  2 organs that produce large amounts of hormones but have other functions (hypothalamus and pancreas);
  3 hormone-producing cells in organs that have many other functions other than producing hormones (e.g. stomach, small intestines, ovaries, testes).
- Each part of the endocrine system is served by a rich blood supply enabling hormones to be easily transported around the body.
- The endocrine system's influence extends throughout the body so failure in any part of it can have significant consequences for a person's health.

# Endocrine system disorders

Include:
- Diabetes mellitus
- Hypo/hyperthyroidism
- Adrenal disease
- Diabetes insipidus
- Acromegaly
- Prolactin hypersecretion
- Hyper/hypocalcaemia
- Hypogonadism.

These are covered in the following pages. The endocrine system's influence is immense, meaning that a coherent list of common signs and symptoms, assessments and emergencies cannot feasibly be produced.

# A and P

- Hormones are chemical messengers which have a variety of effects throughout the body. They are manufactured in the various glands and organs of the endocrine system (above).

- Hormones are released in response to internal or external stimuli and their production is usually controlled by negative feedback mechanisms.
- These stimuli are known as *humoral* (a response to changing levels of ions and nutrients in blood, e.g. the parathyroid hormone is produced in response to falling calcium ions); *neural* (a response to stimulation by the nervous system, e.g. the hypothalamus which controls many of the pituitary activities or increased sympathetic nervous system activity, which stimulates the adrenal glands to release adrenalin and noradrenaline); *hormonal* (a response to hormones released by other organs, e.g. the release of thyroid stimulating hormone from the anterior pituitary gland stimulates the thyroid gland to release thyroxine).
- Hormones are secreted by one cell (secreting cell) and impact on another which has a receptor for that particular hormone (target cell) (above).
- Once they have carried out their work, hormones are destroyed in the target cell, the liver and/or the kidneys. They (or usually the breakdown products) are excreted in urine and faeces.
- Nurses are most likely to provide care for people with diabetes (Chapter 68) either in hospital or the community. They may also occasionally care for people with some of the other endocrine disorders summarised in Chapter 67.

# Essentials of best practice

Disorders of the endocrine system can range from mild to severe. Nursing someone with any of these disorders may take place in the community, the GP surgery, the ED or OOH service or in a hospital ward or specialist unit. The essentials of best practice required to care for common disorders are covered in the subsequent pages.

## Patient information

There are several patient support groups and charities focusing on disorders of the endocrine system. You can find most of them on the Self Help UK website www.self-help.org.uk.
You will also find very helpful patient-centred fact sheets at www.patient.co.uk/.

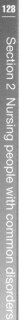

# 67 Summary of disorders of the endocrine system

**Table 67a** Functions of the endocrine system.

| Hormones controlled by the hypothalamus/pituitary | | | Non-hypothalamus/pituitary control | | |
|---|---|---|---|---|---|
| **Hypothalamus**<br>controls releasing and inhibiting factors of hormones that are produced by the anterior lobe of the pituitary gland. It also releases two hormones directly into the posterior lobe of the pituitary | **Pituitary**<br>**anterior lobe** produces hormones in response to stimulation or inhibition by substances released by the hypothalamus. They work on a number of target glands/organs | **Thyroid** | **Adrenal glands: adrenal medulla** secretes catecholamines (adrenaline, noradrenaline and dopamine)<br>**adrenal cortex** secretes corticosteroids | **Parathyroid glands** (posterior lobes of thyroid) secrete parathyroid hormone (PTH) which controls plasma calcium levels. PTH largely acts on kidney and intestine to absorb calcium | **Pancreas**<br>islets of Langerhans cells secrete various hormones.<br>Alpha – glucagon<br>Beta – insulin<br>Delta – somatostatin |
| Growth hormone releasing factor | Growth hormone (GH)<br>Stimulates growth of body cells | | | | |
| Growth hormone release inhibiting factor | (GH inhibited) | | | | |
| Thyroid releasing hormone (TRH) | Thyroid stimulating hormone (TSH)<br>Stimulates release of thyroid hormone (NB iodine needed) | Thyroid hormone (2 forms); thyroxine ($T_4$) and triiodothyronine ($T_3$)<br>Affect basal metabolic rate. Increase $O_2$ consumption by cells. Increase production of body heat. | | | |
| Corticotrophin releasing hormone (CRH) | Adrenocorticotrophic hormone (ACTH)<br>Stimulates release of corticosteroids | | Corticosteroids (mineralocorticoids – affects concentration of electrolytes in blood e.g. aldosterone<br>glucocorticoids – mainly influence cell metabolism, suppress immune system and inflammatory response, help repair damaged cells<br>gonadocorticoids – adrenal sex hormones – androgens and oestrogens) | | |
| Prolactin releasing hormone | Prolactin<br>Stimulates milk production in **mammary glands**. Also stimulates corpus luteum in **ovary** to produce progesterone | | | | |
| Prolactin inhibiting hormone | (Prolactin inhibited) | | | | |
| Gonadotrophin releasing hormone | Gonadotrophin<br>Follicle stimulating hormone<br>Early maturation of ovarian follicles and oestrogen secretion<br>Sperm production in **testes**<br>Luteinising hormone<br>Final maturation of ovarian follicles and oestrogen secretion: testosterone secretion<br>**Pituitary posterior lobe**<br>Oxytocin<br>Uterine contraction, 'let down' reflex in breast feeding<br>Antidiuretic hormone (ADH)<br>Increases water retention by kidneys | | | | |

*Adult Nursing at a Glance*, First Edition. Andrée le May. © 2015 John Wiley & Sons, Ltd. Published 2015 by John Wiley & Sons, Ltd.
Companion website: www.ataglanceseries.com/nursing/adult

**Table 67b** Common problems linked to imbalances in hormones in adults.

| Hormone | Clinical consequences | Medical management (depending on cause) | Essentials of nursing care |
|---|---|---|---|
| Growth hormone | Acromegaly: raised GH in adulthood due to benign pituitary tumour. Signs and symptoms include enlarged hands, feet, jaw, nose, tongue, protruding jaw; tiredness; joint pain; deep voice; oily skin. | Suppress GH/surgery/pituitary radiotherapy. | Reassurance and explanation of changes to body image. Education about medication regimens. Pre- and post-operative care if needed. |
| Thyroxine | Hyperthyroidism: excess thyroxine causing e.g. irritability, mood swings, heat intolerance, sweating, tachycardia, palpitations. Hypothyroidism: reduced thyroxine due to disease of the thyroid or pituitary causing e.g. intolerance of cold, weight gain, depression, cloudy thinking and lethargy. | Hyperthyroidism: decrease thyroid hormone synthesis (antithyroid drugs, surgery, radio-iodine). Hypothyroidism: increase and titrate $T_4$ or $T_3$. | Education about medication regimens. Explanation of any side-effects. Pre- and post-operative care if needed. In hypothyroidism improvement may take weeks as medication is titrated. |
| Glucocorticoids | Cushing's disease: excess glucocorticoids (commonly associated with over prescription of synthetic corticosteroids). It is important that nurses recognise the signs and symptoms: diabetes mellitus, infections, weight gain, moon-shaped face, skin thinning, bruising, poor wound healing. Hunch-shape to back from vertebral collapse. | Reduce cortisol levels. Drugs to lower cortisol levels, surgery. Ongoing follow up. | Managing symptoms is the central component of nursing care alongside education and reassurance. |
| Corticosteroids | Addison's disease is when the adrenal cortex is destroyed and there is no cortisol secretion. It is likely to be an autoimmune disease, or caused by medication, TB, HIV. Signs and symptoms include skin discoloration, postural hypotension, weight loss, nausea, abdominal pain, fatigue. More seriously patients can develop an Addisonian crisis which can be fatal if untreated – here the absence of cortisol results in severe shock. Signs and symptoms include severe abdominal, leg or lower back pain, vomiting and diarrhoea, dehydration, hypotension, hypoglycaemia, altered consciousness. | Long-term replacement of glucocorticoids and mineralocorticoids. In Addisonian crisis rapid intra-venous intervention to restore steroid, sodium and glucose balance is needed. Once stabilised, oral replacement of hormones. | Education about medications and when to take extra steroids if infections or are stressed. Advise family/carers too. Emphasise the importance of seeking advice and also wearing a medic alert disc and carrying a steroid card. Diligent monitoring of a patient's condition during and following Addisonian crisis is necessary. Careful attention to fluid balance and IVI sites. NB: Elevated temperature (indicative of infection) and altered blood pressure (report hypotension). |
| Parathyroid hormone (PTH) | Hypercalcaemia: raised plasma calcium. Usually linked to raised PTH or malignancy. Hypocalcaemia: reduced PTH. | Acute hypercalcaemia is a medical emergency (initial rapid rehydration lowers calcium). Maybe steroid therapy. Surgery. Hypocalcaemia requires replacement of calcium and vitamin D supplements. | People with acute hypercalcaemia are likely to be very ill and require attentive nursing care until their condition stabilises. Care will involve help with activities of daily living, 24-hour urine collection for calcium analysis. Be attentive for tetany. Pre- and post-operative care if needed. For people with hypocalcaemia education regarding medication and exposure to sunlight. |
| Antidiuretic hormone | Diabetes insipidus: passing large amounts (over 3 litres in 24 hours) of dilute urine. | Restricted fluids: ADH replacement. | Accurate recording of fluid balance. Education about fluid intake and medications. |
| Prolactin | Hyperprolactinaemia: abnormal or inappropriate milk production in men or women and amenorrhoea. Infertility. Erectile dysfunction. Reduced libido. | Inhibition of prolactin/surgery/pituitary radiotherapy. | Education about medication regimens. Explanation of any side-effects. Pre- and post-operative care if needed. |
| Oestrogen/ testosterone | Hypogonadism. | Hormone replacement. | Education about medication regimens. |
| Insulin | Diabetes Mellitus | **See Chapter 68.** | **See Chapter 68.** |

# 68 Nursing people with diabetes mellitus

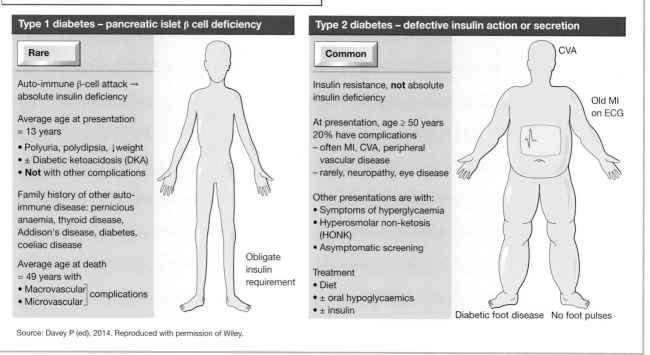

Type 1 and Type 2 diabetes

**Type 1 diabetes – pancreatic islet β cell deficiency**

Rare

Auto-immune β-cell attack → absolute insulin deficiency

Average age at presentation = 13 years
• Polyuria, polydipsia, ↓weight
• ± Diabetic ketoacidosis (DKA)
• **Not** with other complications

Family history of other auto-immune disease: pernicious anaemia, thyroid disease, Addison's disease, diabetes, coeliac disease

Average age at death = 49 years with
• Macrovascular ⎤ complications
• Microvascular ⎦

Obligate insulin requirement

**Type 2 diabetes – defective insulin action or secretion**

Common

Insulin resistance, **not** absolute insulin deficiency

At presentation, age ≥ 50 years
20% have complications
– often MI, CVA, peripheral vascular disease
– rarely, neuropathy, eye disease

Other presentations are with:
• Symptoms of hyperglycaemia
• Hyperosmolar non-ketosis (HONK)
• Asymptomatic screening

Treatment
• Diet
• ± oral hypoglycaemics
• ± insulin

CVA

Old MI on ECG

Diabetic foot disease    No foot pulses

Source: Davey P (ed), 2014. Reproduced with permission of Wiley.

## Key facts

• Diabetes mellitus is a disease characterised by raised blood glucose levels. In people with diabetes a random test for blood glucose will show an elevated blood glucose level of >11.1 mmol/l.
• Diabetes mellitus can take two forms – Type 1 diabetes (a relatively rare condition) and Type 2 diabetes (becoming increasingly common).
• Type 1 diabetes is associated with a total lack of/deficiency in insulin because of pancreatic islet β cell deficiency. This may have an autoimmune origin.
• Type 2 diabetes is associated with insulin resistance rather than deficiency. In this type of diabetes the body's cells become resistant to the effects of insulin and require more to keep blood glucose levels within normal limits. Type 2 diabetes is usually linked to being overweight.
• Type 1 diabetes usually presents in people aged below 30 whereas Type 2 diabetes presents usually in people aged around 50 or over.
• Type 2 diabetes is common in South Asian and African Caribbean people.
• Some pregnant women can get gestational diabetes and require specialist care. They may have a risk of developing Type 2 diabetes later.
• Treatment is with injected insulin replacement in people with Type 1 diabetes and with diet, lifestyle changes and oral drugs to reduce hyperglycaemia in people with Type 2 diabetes.
• Diagnosis and monitoring of people with Type 2 diabetes involves testing the blood for blood glucose level and for HbA1c (glycated haemoglobin) – a measure of average blood glucose over a few weeks or months. Urinalysis will also show glucose.

• Symptoms of diabetes include: increased thirst, increased urine output, tiredness and weight loss.
• Diabetes is linked to long-term complications (below).
• Nurses will care for people with either type of diabetes mellitus: there are differences in the care associated with each type of diabetes.

## A and P

The pancreas consists of a head, body and tail (Chapter 51) and has both exocrine and endocrine functions. Exocrine tissue secretes digestive enzymes into the small intestine. The endocrine cells of the pancreas are scattered through the exocrine tissue clustered together as islets of Langerhans. Each islet has three types of cells (alpha, beta and delta) which secrete various hormones.
• Alpha – glucagon
• Beta (β) – insulin
• Delta – somatostatin.
Insulin and glucagon affect blood glucose levels and the metabolism of proteins and lipids: they work in partnership to maintain blood glucose within normal limits.

When food is digested glucose passes through the intestine wall into the blood stream, in response to this insulin is released from the β cells of the islets of Langerhans to maintain blood glucose levels within normal limits. Insulin does this by enabling body cells (e.g. in muscle, adipose tissue) to take up glucose for energy and the liver to store glucose as glycogen for release at another time. When blood glucose levels drop so does insulin.

*Adult Nursing at a Glance*, First Edition. Andrée le May. © 2015 John Wiley & Sons, Ltd. Published 2015 by John Wiley & Sons, Ltd.
Companion website: www.ataglanceseries.com/nursing/adult

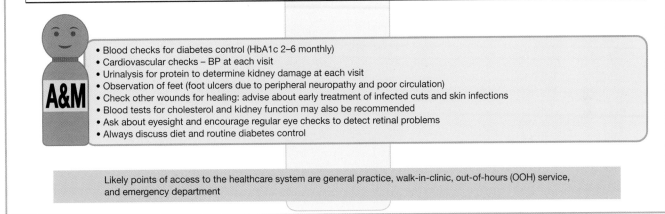

**Primary care**

You will need to discuss the following with a person newly diagnosed with Type 2 diabetes:

- How you can work together. Motivating a person to take control of the management of their diabetes is a very important aspect of treatment since much relies of accurate self-monitoring, being motivated to stick to dietary restrictions, medications and exercise regimens
- Keeping blood glucose within agreed limits
  - o Discussion of lifestyle changes including, for example, losing weight if overweight or waist measurement exceeds 31.5 inches (women)/37 inches (men), exercising regularly (20 minutes of brisk walking or equivalent for 5 days a week), drawing attention to foods and drinks that may increase blood glucose levels or elevate lipids (referral to a dietician may be useful)
  - o Discussion of medication regimens. Discussion if taking glucose lowering drugs about the signs and symptoms of hypoglycaemia and what to do (sugary drink/starchy snack)
  - o Discussion of self-monitoring of blood glucose (SMBG)
  - o Discussion of regular HbA1c monitoring (2–6 monthly) and review appointments
  - o Discussion of long-term complications and how to avoid these together with the need for regular monitoring, for example cardiovascular system monitoring, eye checks (elevated blood glucose levels can damage blood vessels), foot care
  - o Advice on alcohol intake and smoking cessation if necessary
  - o Advice about pneumonia and flu immunisations (infections can alter blood glucose levels)

**HE&P**

**Primary care**

A person with Type 2 diabetes will require regular checks of their health over their remaining lifetime. These will include:

- Blood checks for diabetes control (HbA1c 2–6 monthly)
- Cardiovascular checks – BP at each visit
- Urinalysis for protein to determine kidney damage at each visit
- Observation of feet (foot ulcers due to peripheral neuropathy and poor circulation)
- Check other wounds for healing: advise about early treatment of infected cuts and skin infections
- Blood tests for cholesterol and kidney function may also be recommended
- Ask about eyesight and encourage regular eye checks to detect retinal problems
- Always discuss diet and routine diabetes control

**A&M**

Likely points of access to the healthcare system are general practice, walk-in-clinic, out-of-hours (OOH) service, and emergency department

Glucagon is secreted when blood glucose levels fall prompting the liver to convert glycogen to glucose, fat and proteins are also converted to glucose and hypoglycaemia is averted. Glucagon is inhibited by insulin.

Somatostatin inhibits insulin and glucagon release in the pancreas.

In diabetes, glucagon raises blood glucose levels too much either because there is no insulin to inhibit it or the body has become resistant to the effects of insulin.

## Essentials of best practice

The nursing care of people with diabetes will depend on the type of diabetes they have.

For people with Type 1 diabetes, regular injections of insulin, careful attention to diet and close self-monitoring of blood glucose levels will enable them to maintain blood glucose levels within normal limits. People are usually diagnosed with Type 1 diabetes in childhood or adolescence and so by the time adulthood is reached they are skilled at controlling their diabetes effectively. However, extra stresses placed on the body by, for example, infection, trauma, surgery, inadequate attention to diet or failure to use insulin correctly may necessitate a re-appraisal of their condition and intervention by specialist diabetes nurses or practice nurses. Difficulties may also occur for people if they develop dementia or other age-related illnesses. Some people may develop diabetic ketoacidosis (DKA) as a result of severe hyperglycaemia and be admitted to hospital: they will require close monitoring of vital signs and level of consciousness, rehydration, electrolyte balance restoration and insulin therapy. Any underlying infection will also need treating which may necessitate the administration of antibiotics or other medications.

Ongoing monitoring of people with Type 1 diabetes is likely to be undertaken by practice nurses who will also be alert to possible long term problems associated with diabetes (above).

For the majority of people with Type 2 diabetes their nursing care will be provided by practice nurses and community nurses. This care will focus initially around:
- ✓ Accurate assessment and regular monitoring
- ✓ Communication with the healthcare team, patient and family
- ✓ Health education and promotion

People with diabetes should also be advised to have regular eye checks, cardiovascular checks, flu and pneumonia vaccinations and visit a podiatrist regularly.

**Patient information**

Diabetes UK has useful information and support groups: www.diabetes.org.uk.
Other self-help groups can be found at SelfHelpUK www.self-help.org.uk.
You will find very helpful patient-centred fact sheets at www.patient.co.uk.

# 69 Nursing people with immune disorders

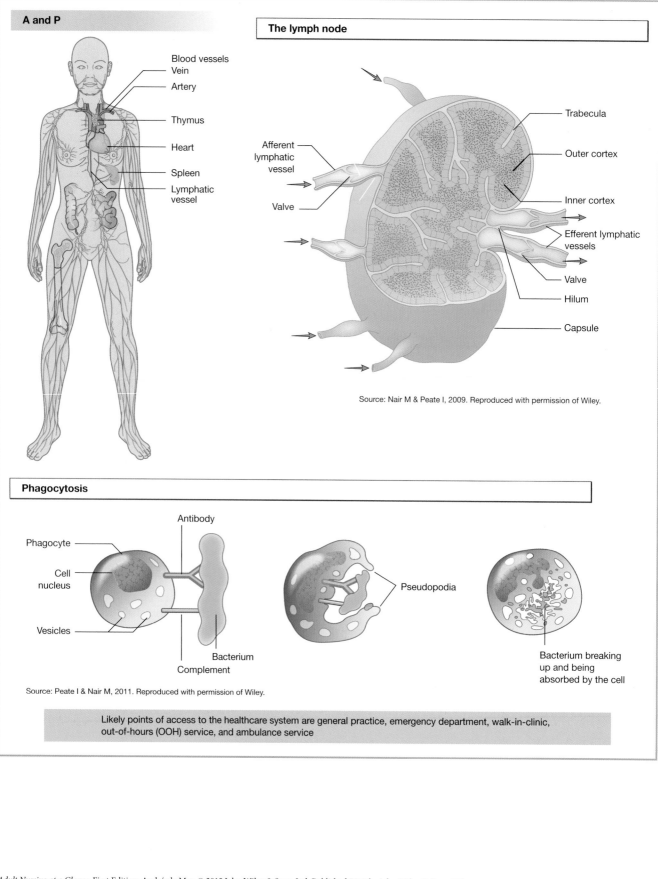

**A and P**

- Blood vessels
  - Vein
  - Artery
- Thymus
- Heart
- Spleen
- Lymphatic vessel

**The lymph node**

- Afferent lymphatic vessel
- Valve
- Trabecula
- Outer cortex
- Inner cortex
- Efferent lymphatic vessels
- Valve
- Hilum
- Capsule

Source: Nair M & Peate I, 2009. Reproduced with permission of Wiley.

**Phagocytosis**

- Phagocyte
- Cell nucleus
- Vesicles
- Antibody
- Bacterium
- Complement
- Pseudopodia
- Bacterium breaking up and being absorbed by the cell

Source: Peate I & Nair M, 2011. Reproduced with permission of Wiley.

Likely points of access to the healthcare system are general practice, emergency department, walk-in-clinic, out-of-hours (OOH) service, and ambulance service

# Key facts

• The body's defence mechanisms against infection and disease are numerous: they include barriers such as the skin (Chapter 72), cilia in the nose/bronchi, eyelashes, various organ's bactericidal secretions, for example lysozyme in tears and hydrochloric acid in the stomach, platelets' ability to plug blood vessels and contribute to clotting and wound healing and the work of the immune system.

• The immune system is a complicated system comprising the blood and lymphatic systems (Chapter 59), organs (the spleen, the thymus), mucosa-associated lymphoid tissue (e.g. in the gastro-intestinal tract, lungs, genito-urinary tract) and lymph nodes (below).

• Whilst the immune system's main role is protecting the body from disease it can over-perform (hypersensitivity) for example in anaphylactic shock, under-perform (immunodeficiency) or malfunction causing autoimmune diseases in which the body's immune system attacks its own cells (e.g. rheumatoid arthritis).

• Innate immunity is the immunity a person has by birth.

• Adaptive immunity is the immunity acquired either naturally through having an illness and producing antibodies or artificially through vaccination.

• The immune system's influence extends throughout the body so failure in any part of it can have significant consequences for a person's health.

# Immune system disorders

• Hypersensitivity and allergic reactions
• Autoimmune disorders
• Immunodeficiency.

These are covered in the following pages. A list of common signs and symptoms and emergencies associated with disorders of the immune system is provided in Chapter 70.

# A and P

Once the physical barriers associated with the body's defences have been penetrated, the immune system activates other defence mechanisms. The first set of mechanisms limit the spread of invading pathogens through inflammation and phagocytosis. The second set of mechanisms is cell-mediated and/or antibody-mediated (humoral) immunity and involves B and T lymphocytes.

• Inflammation is an immediate, non-specific protective reaction to injury that includes histamine release from mast cells, vasodilation, leakage of plasma proteins and white blood cells from nearby capillaries, phagocytosis and clotting.

• White blood cells (leucocytes) are a central component of the immune system. There are two types of leucocytes – granulocytes (neutrophils, eosinophils, basophils) and agranulocytes (monocytes and lymphocytes).

• Granulocytes (neutrophils, eosinophils and basophils) and monocytes destroy pathogens by phagocytosis (engulfing and ingesting) (above).

• Lymphocytes move between the blood and lymph systems.

• Lymphocytes are important to immunity in a number of different ways. There are two overarching types: T lymphocytes and B lymphocytes.

• T lymphocytes originate in red bone marrow but migrate to and mature in the thymus. These lymphocytes learn to differentiate between cells that are part of a person's body (self cells) and cells that are not (non-self cells) for example bacteria or transplanted cells or viruses. T lymphocytes are antigen specific and destroy non-self cells in a process called cell-mediated immunity.

• Certain T lymphocytes (T-helper and T-suppressor) are believed to control the immune system. The immune response is stimulated by T-helper cells (e.g. they help B lymphocytes change into antibody producing cells) and T-suppressor cells prevent over stimulation of the system.

• Cytotoxic T lymphocytes work independently against cells infected with viruses or mutated to cancer cells.

• T lymphocytes remember antigens – this helps the immune system work more quickly.

• B lymphocytes come from bone marrow and once mature are differentiated into plasma cells that secrete antibodies (immunoglobulins) and memory cells.

• Antibodies lock onto and inactivate pathogens.

• Memory cells remember the antigen and are ready to activate antibodies specific to that antigen at its next invasion. This process is called antibody-mediated (humoral) immunity.

• Antibody-mediated response is known as primary or secondary. The primary response occurs when the immune system first encounters an antigen and produces a specific antibody (it can take up to 2 weeks): subsequent encounters result in much quicker antibody production (the secondary response) because of the help of memory cells.

• Lymphocytes and antibodies proliferate in the spleen. The spleen filters dead blood cells and pathogens ready for phagocytosis.

• The lymph nodes (opposite) also provide a place for lymphocyte and antibody proliferation, filter dead/damaged blood cells, pathogens and cancer cells from the lymph ready for phagocytosis.

• Mucosa-associated lymphatic tissue detects pathogens entering the body.

# Essentials of best practice

Disorders of the immune system can range from mild to severe. Nursing someone with any of these disorders may take place in the community, the GP surgery, the ED or in a hospital ward or specialist unit (see later).

## Patient information

There are several patient support groups and charities focusing on disorders of the immune system or autoimmune diseases. You can find most of them on the Self Help UK website http://www.self-help.org.uk.
You will also find very helpful patient-centred fact sheets at www.patient.co.uk/.

# 70 Signs, symptoms and emergencies

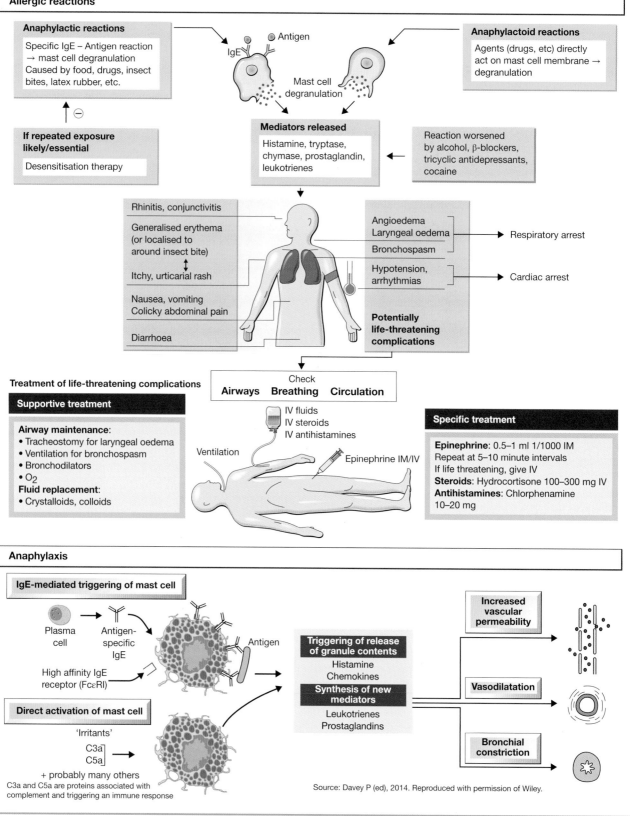

## Allergic reactions

### Anaphylactic reactions

Specific IgE – Antigen reaction → mast cell degranulation
Caused by food, drugs, insect bites, latex rubber, etc.

### Anaphylactoid reactions

Agents (drugs, etc) directly act on mast cell membrane → degranulation

Antigen
IgE
Mast cell degranulation

### If repeated exposure likely/essential

Desensitisation therapy

### Mediators released

Histamine, tryptase, chymase, prostaglandin, leukotrienes

Reaction worsened by alcohol, β-blockers, tricyclic antidepressants, cocaine

Rhinitis, conjunctivitis

Generalised erythema (or localised to around insect bite)

Itchy, urticarial rash

Nausea, vomiting
Colicky abdominal pain

Diarrhoea

Angioedema
Laryngeal oedema → Respiratory arrest

Bronchospasm

Hypotension, arrhythmias → Cardiac arrest

**Potentially life-threatening complications**

### Treatment of life-threatening complications

Check
**Airways Breathing Circulation**

#### Supportive treatment

**Airway maintenance:**
• Tracheostomy for laryngeal oedema
• Ventilation for bronchospasm
• Bronchodilators
• $O_2$
**Fluid replacement:**
• Crystalloids, colloids

IV fluids
IV steroids
IV antihistamines

Ventilation

Epinephrine IM/IV

#### Specific treatment

**Epinephrine**: 0.5–1 ml 1/1000 IM
Repeat at 5–10 minute intervals
If life threatening, give IV
**Steroids**: Hydrocortisone 100–300 mg IV
**Antihistamines**: Chlorphenamine 10–20 mg

## Anaphylaxis

### IgE-mediated triggering of mast cell

Plasma cell

Antigen-specific IgE

High affinity IgE receptor (FcεRI)

Antigen

### Direct activation of mast cell

'Irritants'
C3a
C5a

+ probably many others
C3a and C5a are proteins associated with complement and triggering an immune response

**Triggering of release of granule contents**
Histamine
Chemokines
**Synthesis of new mediators**
Leukotrienes
Prostaglandins

**Increased vascular permeability**

**Vasodilatation**

**Bronchial constriction**

Source: Davey P (ed), 2014. Reproduced with permission of Wiley.

*Adult Nursing at a Glance*, First Edition. Andrée le May. © 2015 John Wiley & Sons, Ltd. Published 2015 by John Wiley & Sons, Ltd.
Companion website: www.ataglanceseries.com/nursing/adult

# Signs and symptoms
## Immunodeficiency

- Increased susceptibility to infection.
- Infections in unusual locations.
- In antibody deficiency disorders: recurrent bacterial infections.
- Deficiencies in complement may present with glomerulonephritis or systemic lupus erythematosus.

**Hypersensitivity** to certain substances can result in allergic reactions (opposite) or anaphylactic shock.

The following signs and symptoms are associated with allergies. Inhalant allergies (e.g. house-dust mites, pollens, animal fur):

- Sneezing, blocked and runny nose
- Itchy eyes, red eyes, weepy eyes
- Headache
- Sinus pain
- Asthma.

Food allergies:

- Eczema in children – rarely in adults.
- Oral allergy syndrome – swelling of lips and tongue (usually associated with peaches, nectarines, almonds, apples).

The following signs and symptoms may occur in people with anaphylaxis (rapid onset usually).

- Urticaria or erythema
- Generalised pruritus
- Angioedema (deep tissue swelling)
- Bronchospasm
- Laryngeal oedema
- Airway obstruction
- Nausea, vomiting
- Cardiac arrhythmias
- Hypotension
- Cardiorespiratory arrest.

# Emergencies: immune system
## Anaphylactic shock

- Anaphylaxis is a medical emergency (above) to which a rapid response is required. Nurses might encounter people having anaphylactic reactions in any setting ranging from the GP practice to the ED.
- If you are the first person to be with someone having an anaphylactic reaction, call for help, check the person's condition and continue to monitor Airway, Breathing and Circulation and act accordingly until help arrives.
- Try to find out the cause of the reaction (if known) and if they have an auto-inject pen if they've used it (if not, help administer a dose).
- Patients who have had anaphylactic shock will need to be observed closely for a number of hours post-recovery.
- Further investigations to find out the cause of the reaction will be needed following recovery, and subsequent advice/education given about managing future encounters with the antigen (e.g. avoiding particular foods, medicines; the use of adrenalin (epinephrine) pre-filled auto-inject pens; carrying medic alert cards/bracelets; family education about immediate care).

The nursing care required by people with allergies is usually associated with health education and promotion and risk assessment and management – it is largely carried out in primary care.

## Patient information

Information about allergies can be obtained from Allergy UK. www.allergyuk.org.

# 71 Nursing people with immunodeficiency and auto-immune diseases

## Some examples of secondary immunodeficiency

| Cause | Aspect of immune system affected | Consequences |
|---|---|---|
| Asplenia | Humoral | Overwhelming sepsis (*Pneumococcus, Meningococcus, Haemophilus, Staphylococcus, Capnocytophaga* [dog bites]); severe malaria and babesiosis |
| Diabetes | Humoral and phagocytic systems | Bacterial infections, candidiasis, abscesses |
| Renal failure (uraemia) | Humoral and cellular | Bacterial and viral infections (hepatitis B) |
| HIV infection | Cellular | Opportunist infections: CMV, *Toxoplasma*, herpes viruses, *Pneumocystis*, *Candida* |
| Lymphoma, myeloma | Cellular and humoral | Viral, bacterial and fungal infections |
| Plasmapheresis | Humoral | Bacterial infections |
| Irradiation | Cellular and humoral | Bacterial, viral, fungal, opportunist infections |
| Chemotherapy, immunosuppressive drugs | Cellular, humoral, phagocytic system | Any type; secondary malignancy due to viruses (EBV, papilloma viruses) |
| Corticosteroids | Cellular, phagocytic system | Viral infections, opportunist infections (*Pneumocystis*) |

Source: Davey P (ed), 2014. Reproduced with permission of Wiley.

## Common AIDS-defining illnesses

Oesophageal candidiasis
*Pneumocystis carinii* pneumonia
Tuberculosis
KS
CMV retinitis
Lymphoma

Cerebral toxoplasmosis
Progressive or disseminated herpes simplex
Recurrent herpes zoster
Recurrent bacterial pneumonia

Likely points of access to the healthcare system are general practice, out-of-hours (OOH) service, emergency department, and ambulance service

*Adult Nursing at a Glance*, First Edition. Andrée le May. © 2015 John Wiley & Sons, Ltd. Published 2015 by John Wiley & Sons, Ltd.
Companion website: www.ataglanceseries.com/nursing/adult

# Key facts

- Immunodeficiency means that the immune system is deficient in some way. We can categorise these deficiencies largely into primary and secondary immunodeficiencies and auto-immune diseases.
- People should be investigated for immunodeficiencies if they have increased susceptibility to infection. This may manifest as serious infections needing intravenous antibiotics or infections in unusual places (e.g. abscesses in the liver or brain) or infections from unusual pathogens.
- There are different types of immunodeficiencies but the most common are usually secondary to other diseases/illnesses or treatments (above). Nursing care will need to focus on the primary disease (e.g. diabetes and its control) as well as the secondary conditions (e.g. poor wound healing and repeated infections).
- Primary immunodeficiency is rare (and usually diagnosed in childhood): it may result in deficiencies associated with, for example, antibodies, phagocytes, complement proteins, lymphocytes.
- Symptoms and signs of immunodeficiency will depend on the underlying causes.
- Treatment for immunodeficiency focuses on the underlying disease. This may include hospitalisation or be carried out in primary care. Nurses may have a variety of roles ranging from health education and promotion to care of a severely immunocompromised patient in ITU.
- Nursing a person who is immunocompromised may require protective isolation.
- Auto-immune diseases occur because the immune system starts to attack the body's own cells. There are several auto-immune diseases (e.g. Addison's disease (Chapter 67), multiple sclerosis (Chapter 85) and rheumatoid arthritis (Chapter 78)). The nursing care required by people with auto-immune diseases varies and is focused on the signs and symptoms of each condition.

# HIV infection and AIDS

- Human Immunodeficiency Virus (HIV) is a retrovirus that infects T-helper cells compromising their surface protein CD4 and macrophages. Gradually the immune system becomes seriously affected and susceptible to many different types of infections and rarely cancers (e.g. non-Hodgkin's lymphoma or Kaposi's sarcoma (KS)).
- The blood-borne virus can be transmitted in a variety of ways (e.g. through sexual intercourse, contaminated blood products, needle stick injuries or intravenous drug abuse and through maternal–child transmission).
- HIV tends to be asymptomatic after initial infection and this period without signs and symptoms can last for several years. During this time the virus can still be highly infectious.

- HIV may then progress to being symptomatic but is only classified as Acquired Immunodeficiency Syndrome (AIDS) when the person has what is termed as an AIDS-defining illness (above).
- Diagnosis of HIV is made by detection of anti-HIV antibodies.
- Treatment of HIV is usually through combinations of drugs, for example Highly Active Anti-Retroviral Therapy (HAART) and treatment of opportunistic infections. Better treatment over the last few years has resulted in HIV being a much less severe disease than first anticipated and many people having good health with HIV.
- People living with AIDS may have many debilitating problems, some of which nurses can help with, for example breathlessness due to pneumonia or Kaposi's sarcoma and fever. Symptom control and management are very important.
- Some people with AIDS will be severely ill (e.g. with cerebral infections or AIDS-related dementia) or reaching the end of their lives: they will require appropriate care.
- People with HIV/AIDS will usually be linked to a specialist nurse who will advise them about the progress of their illness and how to maintain their health.
- Health education about the spread of HIV/AIDS is an essential element of minimising the transmission of the virus. Advising about safe sex through condom use, safer IV drug use by never sharing needles and always safely disposing of them and always using reputable tattoo parlours is important.

# Essentials of best practice

The nursing care of people with immunodeficiency will depend on the severity of their disease and its underlying pathology. For some people, treatment will focus on the presenting problem, for example poor wound healing, recurrent infections, pain or limited mobility (rheumatoid arthritis) whilst for others expert advice about their disease course and expectations will be needed. For people with HIV, advice about adhering to drug regimens, knowing the warning signs of deterioration, seeking advice about infections early and the need for protected sexual activity will be the mainstays of health education and promotion.

## Patient information

There are several charities and support groups focusing on immunodeficiency:

The Terrence Higgins Trust provides information and support for people with HIV/AIDS and their families and carers. www.tht. org.uk.

Addison's Disease Self Help Group www.addisons.org.uk.

You will find very helpful patient-centred fact sheets at www. patient.co.uk.

# 72 Nursing people with skin disorders

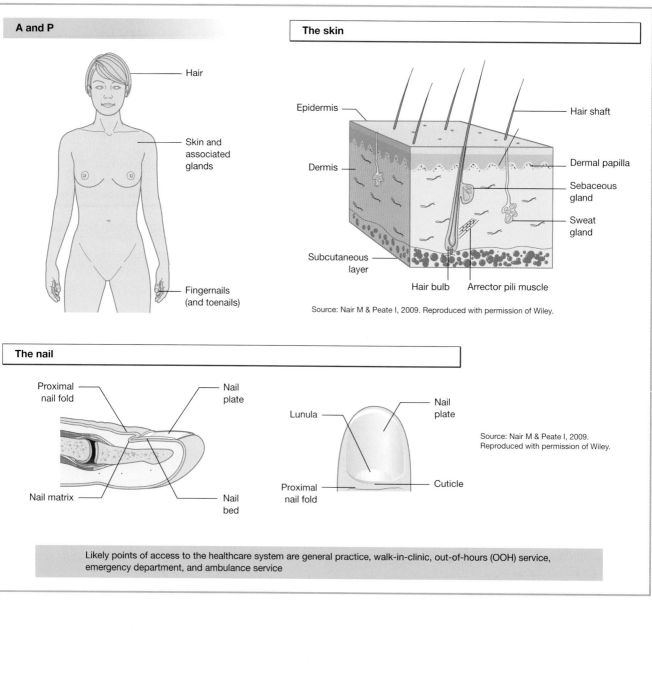

## A and P

- Hair
- Skin and associated glands
- Fingernails (and toenails)

## The skin

- Epidermis
- Dermis
- Subcutaneous layer
- Hair shaft
- Dermal papilla
- Sebaceous gland
- Sweat gland
- Hair bulb
- Arrector pili muscle

Source: Nair M & Peate I, 2009. Reproduced with permission of Wiley.

## The nail

- Proximal nail fold
- Nail plate
- Nail matrix
- Nail bed

- Lunula
- Nail plate
- Proximal nail fold
- Cuticle

Source: Nair M & Peate I, 2009. Reproduced with permission of Wiley.

Likely points of access to the healthcare system are general practice, walk-in-clinic, out-of-hours (OOH) service, emergency department, and ambulance service

*Adult Nursing at a Glance*, First Edition. Andrée le May. © 2015 John Wiley & Sons, Ltd. Published 2015 by John Wiley & Sons, Ltd.
Companion website: www.ataglanceseries.com/nursing/adult

# Key facts

- The skin is critical to survival, health and wellbeing.
- The skin is a waterproof barrier against the external environment, a primary means of defence against injury and infection and essential in maintaining homeostasis (e.g. temperature control).
- The skin comprises an epidermis and dermis (above).
- The nails, hair and exocrine skin glands (sweat, sebaceous and apocrine) are also usually categorised as accessory skin structures (above).
- The skin has several functions including:
  - protection, for example defence mechanism against injury or infection; against dehydration; against harmful UV light;
  - sensation, for example touch, pain, irritations, it senses changes in external environments (heat, cold);
  - thermoregulation so that body temperature stays within survivable limits;
  - excretion, for example of waste in sweat contributes to the body's ability to discard toxins;
  - absorption of therapeutic substances and toxins, oxygen, carbon dioxide;
  - Vitamin D synthesis requires the skin to absorb UV rays from the sun to activate a precursor molecule for calcitriol.
- Observing the skin can tell healthcare professionals a lot about a person's general health and specific illness (Chapter 73).
- Damage to the skin can have physical and psychological consequences. Skin, hair and nails are important in making up our body image.

# Common skin disorders

- Rashes and blistering disorders
- Eczema
- Psoriasis.

Each is covered in the following pages. See Chapter 73 for common signs and symptoms associated with disorders of the skin.

The skin is also an indicator of the health of other parts of the body (for example colour: cyanosis may indicate respiratory or cardiovascular disease, yellowness may indicate jaundice; turgor may indicate hydration or dehydration; oedema may indicate cardiovascular problems; swelling, heat and redness may indicate infection; itchiness may indicate liver problems or malignancy).

# A and P

- The epidermis of the skin is the thinner top layer that we can see. It is comprised of several types of cells (keratinocytes, melanocytes, Langerhans cells and Merkel cells). Keratinocytes produce a tough fibrous protein (keratin) which protects against pathogens, chemicals and heat. Keratinocytes produce a waterproofing substance. Melanocytes produce melanin, the pigment that gives skin its colour and protects it from damage by sunlight. Langerhans cells regulate immune reactions in the skin. Merkel cells are associated with tactile sensation.
- The dermis lies below the epidermis. It is comprised of connective tissue containing collagen and elastin and holds blood vessels, hair follicles, sebaceous glands, sweat glands, nerves, lymph vessels and smooth muscles.
- Hair inhibits heat loss and protects the scalp and eyes (eyelashes and eyebrows). When erector pili muscles contract, hair stands on end (goose-bumps) trapping an insulting layer of air between the hairs. Sebaceous glands are linked to hair follicles and secrete sebum which contributes to waterproofing the skin. Sebum is also slightly acidic and bactericidal.
- Nails are tightly packed hardened dead epidermal cells that form a protective covering for the fingers and toes.

# Essentials of best practice

Disorders of the skin can range from mild to severe. Nursing someone with any of these disorders may take place in the community, the GP surgery, the ED or OOH service or in a hospital ward or specialist dermatology unit. The essentials of best practice required to care for common disorders are covered in the subsequent pages. In addition, Chapter 73 details assessment of the skin, and common signs and symptoms.

---

**Patient information**

There are several patient support groups and charities focusing on disorders of the skin. You can find most of them on the Self Help UK website http://www.self-help.org.uk.

You will also find very helpful patient-centred fact sheets at www.patient.co.uk/.

# 73 Signs, symptoms and assessment

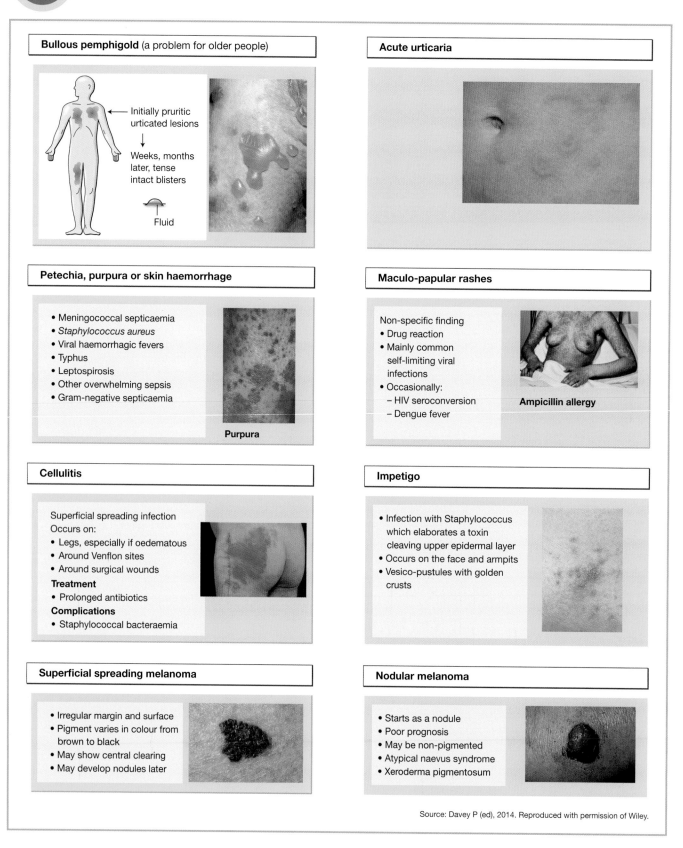

**Bullous pemphigold** (a problem for older people)

Initially pruritic urticated lesions

Weeks, months later, tense intact blisters

Fluid

**Petechia, purpura or skin haemorrhage**

- Meningococcal septicaemia
- *Staphylococcus aureus*
- Viral haemorrhagic fevers
- Typhus
- Leptospirosis
- Other overwhelming sepsis
- Gram-negative septicaemia

**Purpura**

**Cellulitis**

Superficial spreading infection
Occurs on:
- Legs, especially if oedematous
- Around Venflon sites
- Around surgical wounds

**Treatment**
- Prolonged antibiotics

**Complications**
- Staphylococcal bacteraemia

**Superficial spreading melanoma**

- Irregular margin and surface
- Pigment varies in colour from brown to black
- May show central clearing
- May develop nodules later

**Acute urticaria**

**Maculo-papular rashes**

Non-specific finding
- Drug reaction
- Mainly common self-limiting viral infections
- Occasionally:
  – HIV seroconversion
  – Dengue fever

**Ampicillin allergy**

**Impetigo**

- Infection with Staphylococcus which elaborates a toxin cleaving upper epidermal layer
- Occurs on the face and armpits
- Vesico-pustules with golden crusts

**Nodular melanoma**

- Starts as a nodule
- Poor prognosis
- May be non-pigmented
- Atypical naevus syndrome
- Xeroderma pigmentosum

Source: Davey P (ed), 2014. Reproduced with permission of Wiley.

*Adult Nursing at a Glance*, First Edition. Andrée le May. © 2015 John Wiley & Sons, Ltd. Published 2015 by John Wiley & Sons, Ltd.
Companion website: www.ataglanceseries.com/nursing/adult

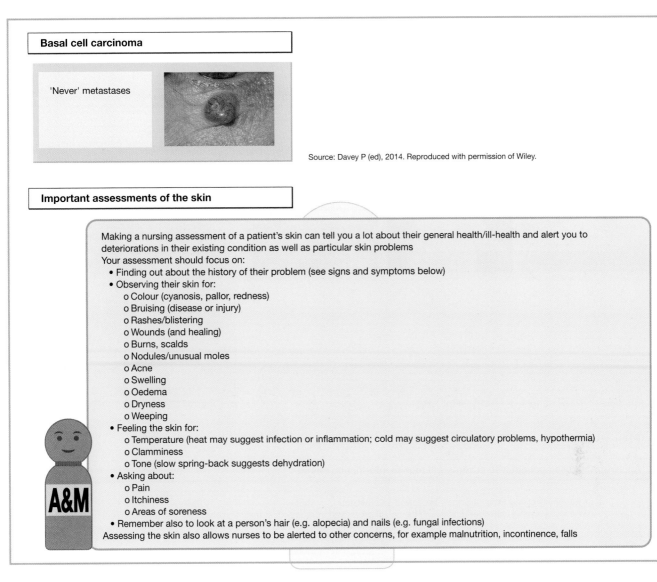

**Basal cell carcinoma**

'Never' metastases

Source: Davey P (ed), 2014. Reproduced with permission of Wiley.

**Important assessments of the skin**

Making a nursing assessment of a patient's skin can tell you a lot about their general health/ill-health and alert you to deteriorations in their existing condition as well as particular skin problems

Your assessment should focus on:
- Finding out about the history of their problem (see signs and symptoms below)
- Observing their skin for:
  - Colour (cyanosis, pallor, redness)
  - Bruising (disease or injury)
  - Rashes/blistering
  - Wounds (and healing)
  - Burns, scalds
  - Nodules/unusual moles
  - Acne
  - Swelling
  - Oedema
  - Dryness
  - Weeping
- Feeling the skin for:
  - Temperature (heat may suggest infection or inflammation; cold may suggest circulatory problems, hypothermia)
  - Clamminess
  - Tone (slow spring-back suggests dehydration)
- Asking about:
  - Pain
  - Itchiness
  - Areas of soreness
- Remember also to look at a person's hair (e.g. alopecia) and nails (e.g. fungal infections)

Assessing the skin also allows nurses to be alerted to other concerns, for example malnutrition, incontinence, falls

A&M

# Common signs and symptoms

Rash/blistering

Eruptions (e.g. boils, abscesses)

Dryness

Papery appearance (topical steroid use)

Skin feels hot (cold)

Redness of area on skin

Infection (e.g. cellulitis)

Scaly patches

Bleeding from moles

Itchiness

Weeping areas

Pain/discomfort

Bruising

Swelling

Pallor

Cyanosis

Wounds (which may be infected)

Burns/scalds

Oedema

Malaise (feeling under the weather)

Pyrexia if infection.

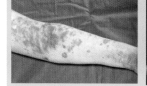

# 74 Nursing people with eczema or psoriasis

## Eczema/dermatitis: symptoms and signs

**Symptoms**
Itchy, ill-defined red patches

**Acute signs**
Erythema, oedema, vesicles, serum exudates

**Chronic signs**
• Lichenification
• Scaling

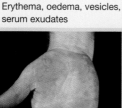

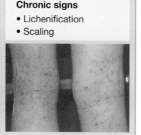

## Psoriasis

• 3% of population affected
• Lesions can occur anywhere, but often predominantly on extensor surfaces and scalp
• 5% develop arthritis
• Occasionally causes erythroderma and generalised pustular psoriasis
• Acute guttate attack may be provoked by group A streptococcal sore throat

Distribution

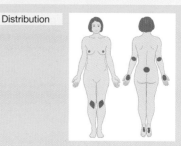

Source: Davey P (ed), 2014. Reproduced with permission of Wiley.

## Primary care

### A newly diagnosed patient with eczema will require information about:

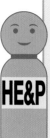

• Eczema (National Eczema Society has lots of information)
• Keeping eczema under control through the use of prescribed moisturisers to minimise dry, scaly skin (e.g. emollient bath oils/shower gels, emollient creams/lotions/ointments). Emollients (non-cosmetic moisturisers) should be applied gently and lightly, avoiding rubbing that may damage the skin, every day (usually more than once a day). This routine should continue even if no eczema is visible to stop flare-ups
• Using soap substitutes because soap dries the skin
• Applying topical corticosteroid treatments, as prescribed, may be necessary if emollient use doesn't work
• (If eczema gets worse after using emollients or topical corticosteroid creams see the doctor (it may be an allergy to the cream))
• Taking oral anti-histamines as prescribed
• Avoiding perfumed soaps, shampoos, shower gels, cosmetics
• Regularly bathing or showering will keep the skin clean and prevent infection
• Isolating and avoiding triggers (e.g. some food stuffs, animal fur, certain cosmetic preparations, stress)

## Ward care

### A person with severe erythrodermic psoriasis and skin failure will require close monitoring of:

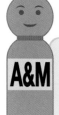

• Thermoregulation (warmth, management of pyrexia and rigors)
• Loss of fluid through the skin (oral fluids): fluid balance (input and output)
• Nutritional intake (loss of protein – refer to dietician)
• Pain (analgesics)
• Condition for deterioration (e.g. infection: level of consciousness: cardiac function – heart rate, respiratory rate, BP)
**Report any deterioration (skin or other system) immediately**

Likely points of access to the healthcare system are general practice, walk-in-clinic, and out-of-hours (OOH) service

*Adult Nursing at a Glance*, First Edition. Andrée le May. © 2015 John Wiley & Sons, Ltd. Published 2015 by John Wiley & Sons, Ltd.
Companion website: www.ataglanceseries.com/nursing/adult

# Key facts

- Eczema is an inflammation of the skin. Its severity can range from mild to severe.
- Eczema typically presents with reddened, itchy, scaly patches which may be on the face or in the body's flexures.
- Scratching typically may cause infections.
- Eczema tends to flare up from time to time, sometimes in response to known triggers.
- Eczema cannot be cured but patients can manage it very successfully through the use of emollients, atopic corticosteroid treatments, oral antihistamines and avoiding triggers (above).
- Eczema is usually managed in the community so practice nurses are likely to have a large part to play in health education and promotion and symptom control and management. Specialist dermatological nurses will also be involved – although their involvement may be associated more with severe eczema. Occupational health nurses will be involved in care if eczema is work related (either through contact with irritants or as a result of work-related stress).
- Contact dermatitis may also be work related (although not always) and should be considered before a diagnosis of eczema is confirmed. Isolating and avoiding triggers are critical parts of its management.
- Severe eczema can result in the need for hospitalisation especially if skin failure occurs (below and above).
- Psoriasis presents with inflamed, reddened, silver scaled lesions usually on extensor surfaces of the body (e.g. knees, elbows).
- Psoriasis can be mild or severe. There are several types.
- Guttate psoriasis is linked to a sore throat and small patches of psoriasis occur over the body. It can last from a few weeks to a few months then often disappears.
- Generalised pustular and erythrodermic psoriasis can be a very serious condition resulting in skin failure and requiring hospitalisation (below).
- Skin failure can lead to failure of thermoregulation, fluid loss, and infection.
- Some people with psoriasis may have psoriatic arthritis which results in painful and swollen joints.

- Psoriasis may be exacerbated by stress, infections, smoking, some medications (e.g. antimalarials), sunlight, hormonal changes (puberty and menopause), and alcohol.
- Treatment for psoriasis includes keeping the skin moisturised, vitamin D-based treatments, corticosteroids (above).
- Some people with severe psoriasis may be treated with phototherapy with UV B light.

# Essentials of best practice

The nursing care of people with any skin condition will depend on the severity of their disease and its underlying pathology. For some people, no treatment will be required except for advice about keeping their skin moisturised or using appropriate topical applications.

Whilst for the majority of people nursing care is likely to be provided by practice nurses, some people will require more intensive nursing care in hospital. Hospitalisation is likely to be associated with, for instance, severe infection or skin failure. In these instances care will largely focus on:

✓ Accurate assessment and regular monitoring (e.g. if there is skin failure)
✓ Communication with the healthcare team, patient and family
✓ Symptom control and management (e.g. itching, pyrexia, tiredness)
✓ Health education and promotion (e.g. alleviating symptoms associated with their condition and avoiding triggers)
✓ Discharge planning

Help may be needed in, or out of hospital with activities of daily living if the patient is debilitated.

## Patient information

There are several useful charities and support groups focusing on eczema and psoriasis:
The National Eczema Society www.eczema.org.
The Psoriasis Association www.psoriasis-association.org.uk.
You will find very helpful patient-centred fact sheets at www.patient.co.uk.

# 75 Nursing people with musculoskeletal disorders

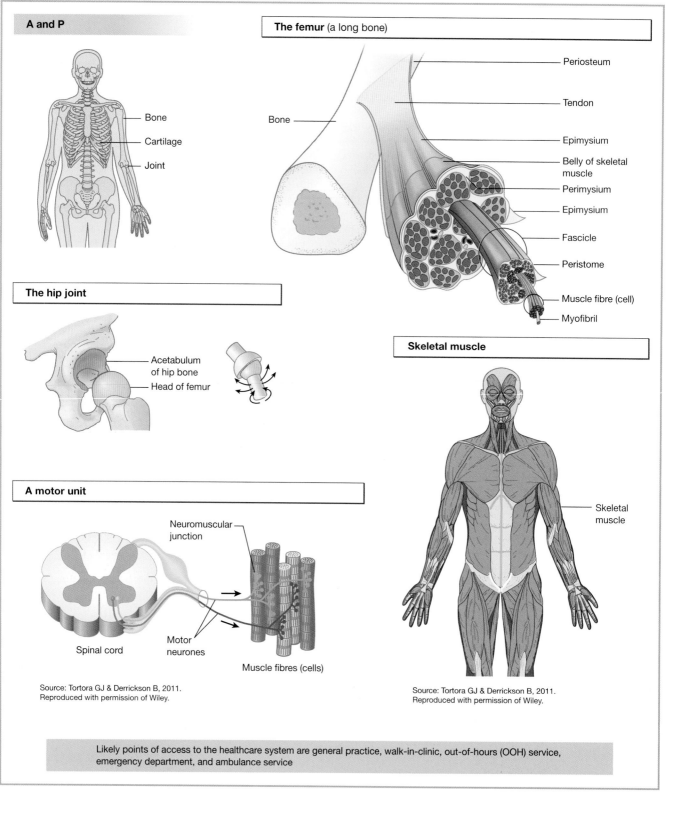

**A and P**

- Bone
- Cartilage
- Joint

**The femur** (a long bone)

- Bone
- Periosteum
- Tendon
- Epimysium
- Belly of skeletal muscle
- Perimysium
- Epimysium
- Fascicle
- Peristome
- Muscle fibre (cell)
- Myofibril

**The hip joint**

- Acetabulum of hip bone
- Head of femur

**Skeletal muscle**

- Skeletal muscle

**A motor unit**

- Neuromuscular junction
- Spinal cord
- Motor neurones
- Muscle fibres (cells)

Source: Tortora GJ & Derrickson B, 2011.
Reproduced with permission of Wiley.

Source: Tortora GJ & Derrickson B, 2011.
Reproduced with permission of Wiley.

Likely points of access to the healthcare system are general practice, walk-in-clinic, out-of-hours (OOH) service, emergency department, and ambulance service

*Adult Nursing at a Glance*, First Edition. Andrée le May. © 2015 John Wiley & Sons, Ltd. Published 2015 by John Wiley & Sons, Ltd.
Companion website: www.ataglanceseries.com/nursing/adult

# Key facts

- The musculoskeletal system comprises a complex structure of bones, ligaments, tendons, joints and skeletal muscles which give the body structure and strength protecting internal organs and tissues from damage and works alongside the nervous system enabling us to move.
- The skeleton comprises an axial skeleton and an appendicular skeleton. The axial skeleton consists of the skull, the vertebral column, the ribs and the sternum. The appendicular skeleton comprises the pectoral and pelvic girdles and the bones of the upper and lower limbs.
- Bone continues to be renewed and repaired throughout life (bone remodelling). Abnormalities in this process can result in either heavy and thick bone formation or formation of bones that are weak and easily broken.
- Most bones store and release minerals (e.g. calcium, magnesium and phosphorous).
- Red bone marrow is involved in the manufacture of blood cells and yellow bone marrow in the storage of lipids.
- Joints are where two bones meet and articulate.
- Skeletal muscles are responsible for movement, maintaining posture and stabilising joints.
- Skeletal muscles contract and relax causing bone movement under the control of the nervous system.
- Muscles also produce heat which contributes to maintaining the body's temperature.
- Damage to the musculoskeletal system can have physical, social and psychological consequences. Our posture, ability to move, physique and shape are all important in making up our body image.
- Observing somebody's movement can tell healthcare professionals a lot about a person's general health *and* specific illnesses/disorders.

# Common musculoskeletal disorders

- Fractures
- Osteoporosis
- Osteomyelitis
- Osteoarthritis
- Rheumatoid arthritis
- Myopathies
- Strains.

Each is covered in the following pages. See Chapter 76 for common signs and symptoms associated with disorders of the musculoskeletal systems.

# A and P

## Bones

- The skeleton is made up of a mix of long (e.g. humerus, femur, tibia), short (e.g. carpals and metacarpals), flat (e.g. ribs, sternum), irregular (e.g. ossicles of the ear – malleus, stapes and incus) and sesamoid (patella and hyoid) bones.
- Bones are living organs made up of different cells including osteocytes which are mature bone cells and vessels. Bones develop pre-natally from cartilage and continue to regenerate throughout life. Bone formation is called ossification.
- Bone strength comes from their protein matrix and mineral deposits. Deficiencies in either can cause problems.
- Bones have their own blood supply which takes nutrients and oxygen to the bone and waste from it.
- Haversian and Volkmann's canals form passages for blood vessels, lymph vessels and nerves to pass through.

## Joints

- Joints can be categorised as fibrous (e.g. radioulnar joints: these allow little movement), cartilaginous (e.g. symphysis pubis: little movement) and synovial (movable, synovial fluid filled, cartilage lined joints of e.g. the knee, elbow and hip).
- Ligaments are fibrous connective tissues holding bones together in a joint: ligaments also hold fibrous joints together.

## Skeletal muscles

- Skeletal muscles are made up of muscle cells (fibres), blood vessels, connective and nervous tissues. Skeletal muscle fibres are bunched together into fascicles and surrounded by connective tissue (above).
- Skeletal muscles have three types of muscle fibres (slow oxidative, fast oxidative-glycolytic and fast glycolytic) enabling muscles to work in various ways.
- Skeletal muscles are stimulated to contract by the release of acetylcholine (ACh) at the neuromuscular junction (opposite). Relaxation occurs when ACh is broken down by acetylcholinesterase (AChE).
- Muscle fibres get energy to contract from adenosine triphosphate (ATP). This process usually uses oxygen (aerobic) but in strenuous exercise muscles get extra energy through anaerobic respiration (without oxygen) too.
- Lactic acid and diminished oxygen are byproducts of anaerobic respiration resulting in muscle pain and weakness.
- Tendons attach muscle to bone and allow movement of joints to occur.

# Essentials of best practice

Disorders of the musculoskeletal system can range from mild to severe. Nursing someone with any of these disorders may take place in the community, the GP surgery, the ED or in a hospital ward or specialist unit. The essentials of best practice required to care for common disorders are covered in the subsequent pages. In addition, Chapter 76 details assessment of this system as well as common signs and symptoms.

---

## Patient information

There are several patient support groups and charities focusing on disorders of the musculoskeletal system. You can find most of them on the Self Help UK website http://www.self-help.org.uk. You will also find very helpful patient-centred fact sheets at www.patient.co.uk/.

# 76 Signs, symptoms and assessment

## Important assessments of the musculoskeletal system

Making a nursing assessment of a patient's musculoskeletal system can tell you a lot about their general health/ill-health and alert you to deteriorations in their existing condition as well as particular system problems. (NB: In major trauma remember ABCDE.)

Your assessment should focus on:

- Finding out about the history of their problem (see signs and symptoms below)
- Observing for:
  - o Unsteadiness
  - o Coordination
  - o Tremor
  - o Inability to weight bear
  - o Incomplete ranges of movements
  - o Abnormal appearance of limbs
  - o Abnormal rigidity or floppiness
  - o Uneven or stooped stature
  - o Muscle wasting
  - o Protrusions through skin (e.g. fractures)
  - o Bleeding (estimate blood loss)
  - o Swellings
  - o Bruising
  - o Misshapen joints (bony swellings)
  - o Contractures
  - o Pain
  - o A person holding a limb for support may suggest injury
- Feeling the skin for:
  - o Temperature (heat may suggest infection or inflammation e.g. of joints; cold may suggest hypothermia – this may be important as a consequence e.g. of exposure to the environment following trauma/fractures)
  - o Clamminess may suggest pain/shock
- Asking about:
  - o Pain
  - o Joint stiffness
  - o Areas of soreness
  - o Areas of weakness
  - o Trauma (which may or may not be accidental)
  - o Mobility aides
  - o Prostheses
  - o Restricted movement (this may be important in hospital to ensure that the appropriate care is planned – for example help with mobility and also exercises if movement is curtailed by bed-rest/illness)

Assessing the musculoskeletal system also allows nurses to be alerted to other concerns such as malnutrition, incontinence, falls. Discussing your assessment with other members of the multi-disciplinary team (especially physiotherapists and occupational therapists) is important

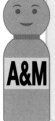

# Common signs and symptoms

- Unsteadiness
- Problems with coordination
- Tremor
- Falls
- Uneven or stooped stature
- Dorsal kyphosis (dowager's hump)
- Tibial bowing (rickets)
- Loss of function and inability to weight bear
- Incomplete ranges of movements
- Protrusions through skin in fractures and bleeding
- Bruising

- Muscle wasting
- Limb weakness
- Swellings/redness/heat, for example around joints
- Misshapen joints
- Contractures
- Pain/aching
- Malaise (feeling under the weather)
- Pyrexia if infection
- Cognitive impairment may be a feature of Parkinson's disease
- Altered consciousness following head injury
- REMEMBER: Trauma may also present problems with Airway, Breathing and Circulation.

# 77 Nursing people with disorders of bones

**The stages of broken bone repair** (Peate, 2011: 235)

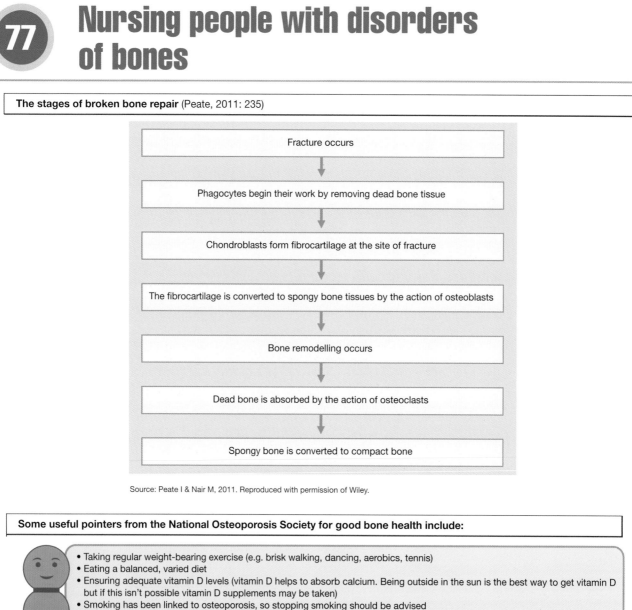

Source: Peate I & Nair M, 2011. Reproduced with permission of Wiley.

**Some useful pointers from the National Osteoporosis Society for good bone health include:**

- Taking regular weight-bearing exercise (e.g. brisk walking, dancing, aerobics, tennis)
- Eating a balanced, varied diet
- Ensuring adequate vitamin D levels (vitamin D helps to absorb calcium. Being outside in the sun is the best way to get vitamin D but if this isn't possible vitamin D supplements may be taken)
- Smoking has been linked to osteoporosis, so stopping smoking should be advised
- Not drinking too much alcohol – this reduces the chance of being unsteady and also the damage caused by alcohol to the skeleton
- Taking care not to trip or fall (be aware of hazards both in and out of the home). Some older people may wear hip protectors
- Seeking advice from the GP/pharmacist about the optimum levels of dietary supplements to take
- Keeping a check on underlying health problems that might affect balance and steadiness (e.g. hypertension, dizziness)

**HE&P**

Likely points of access to the healthcare system are general practice, walk-in-clinic, out-of-hours (OOH) service, emergency department, and ambulance service

# Key facts

- Nurses frequently provide care for people with fractures and osteoporosis and more rarely osteomyelitis.
- Fractures are a common reason for ED attendance and hospitalisation.
- Fractures occur when abnormal force is exerted on a normal bone or moderate force on a diseased bone (e.g. one with metastases or osteoporosis).
- Fractures can be
  - simple (clean breaks with no protrusion through the skin);
  - compound (breaks through the skin);
  - complicated (another structure involved e.g. nerve, blood vessel);
  - comminuted (more than two fragments of bone);
  - greenstick (incomplete);
  - pathological (bone weakened by disease).
- Fracture repair takes place in a number of stages (above).
- Fracture repair may be complicated by blood loss, infection, fat embolism following fracture/cutting of long bones, VTE, compartment syndrome (bleeding/swelling within a tightly enclosed space e.g. a bundle of tightly confined muscle fibres: acute signs and symptoms include intense pain, pins and needles/tingling/burning sensations on skin, paralysis, pallor and lack of pulse), poor union of bones or arthritis.
- Compartment syndrome is an emergency.
- Osteoporosis is common: it is found most commonly in older women but also in men.
- In women, osteoporosis is associated with oestrogen withdrawal (e.g. following menopause – especially if early menopause, late menarche or if women have had a long history of oligomenorrhoea (athletes, women who have/had anorexia nervosa)). Other risk factors include smoking, excessive alcohol consumption, steroid use, a sedentary lifestyle or a positive family history.
- Osteoporosis may be secondary to another disease such as thyrotoxicosis, Cushing's disease or cirrhosis of the liver.
- Treatment for osteoporosis will include lifestyle advice (opposite) and supplements of calcium and vitamin D. Hormonal therapy may be considered.
- Practice nurses and other public health nurses should emphasise the importance of preventing osteoporosis through continued health education and promotion of good bone health (below).
- Other bone diseases may result from deficiencies in the parathyroid glands and the kidneys (renal bone disease).
- Osteomyelitis is an infection of the bone. It may result from an open (compound) fracture or from spread via the circulatory system. Osteomyelitis is rare in adults: when it occurs it may be linked to an infection with staphylococcus, infections related to diabetes and diabetic foot infections, spinal TB, hospital acquired septicaemia from IVI lines.

# Essentials of best practice: fractures

The nursing care required by someone with a fracture will depend on its severity, type, location and their associated condition. Length of stay in hospital may depend on the level of support available to help with activities of daily living.

Nurses will work with people with fractures in the ED, in the community (e.g. immediately following a fall or after discharge from hospital) and in hospital wards and specialist orthopaedic units.

A person with a fracture will require immediate pain relief, reassurance and explanation about investigations (x-rays) and treatment (e.g. methods of reduction and immobilisation: their likely length of stay, whether or not they will have a plaster cast). They will need help with their usual activities of daily living and maintaining dignity whether they are in hospital or at home.

Fracture repair may necessitate general anaesthesia, so the principles of pre- and post-operative care should be adhered to: some reductions will require special post-operative care to maintain the reduced bone's position (e.g. through the use of traction or external fixation).

Observations following reduction should focus on colour, warmth, sensation and movement of the limb.

Following reduction explanation about the procedure and recovery of function will be needed – this should include, for those being discharged home quickly, advice about cast/frame care, wound care, mobility (e.g. how to use crutches), exercises, eating a balanced diet. A contact number for advice should also be given.

For people staying longer in hospital, physiotherapy and occupational therapy support will be available and a personalised rehabilitation plan designed which spans their stay in hospital and their return home. Some people (e.g. older women following repair of a fractured neck of femur) will need advice about and treatment for osteoporosis.

Care will largely focus on:

✓ Accurate assessment and regular monitoring (e.g. pre- and post-operative care (see Section 1), for signs and symptoms of compartment syndrome, haemorrhage, shock, VTEs, fat emboli (following fracture or surgery involving long bones), infection

✓ Communication with the healthcare team, patient and family

✓ Symptom control and management (e.g. pain relief, immobility, rehabilitation regimen)

✓ Health education and promotion (e.g. about levels of activity, pain relief and maintaining good bone health (above))

✓ Risk assessment and management (e.g. pressure ulcer risk, VTE risk)

✓ Discharge planning (post-discharge medication and advice about signs and symptoms of complications, e.g. infections: advice about mobilisation)

## Patient information

There are several useful charities and support groups focusing on bone disorders:
The National Osteoporosis Society provides information about osteoporosis www.nos.org.uk.
You will find very helpful patient-centred fact sheets at www.patient.co.uk.

# 78 Nursing people with joint disorders

## Common types of arthropathy

| Type of arthropathy | Common signs and symptoms | Treatment | Aspects of nursing care |
|---|---|---|---|
| **Osteoarthritis** | Joint pain (insidious onset with usually slow progression to severe) aggravated by activity and relieved by rest<br>Joint stiffness ('gelling' after inactivity)<br>Bony swellings especially in the hands (Heberden's nodes & Bouchard's nodes)<br>Reduced range of movement in affected joints | Pain relief tailored to needs (this may include injections of corticosteroids into joints)<br>Maintaining function and symptom management<br>Physiotherapy and occupational therapy – exercises and also adaptations for daily living<br>Weight loss, if overweight, may reduce pain if lower limb joints affected<br>Surgical replacement of joints (e.g. knee, hip) | Discussion of pain management and monitoring its success<br>Advice about weight loss and healthy eating if necessary<br>Pre- and post-operative care if joint replacement surgery<br>Working closely with the multi-disciplinary team |
| **Gout and pseudogout** | **Gout**<br>Joint pain, usually in one joint (monoarthritis) (often the big toe). Swelling, tenderness and redness of surrounding tissues<br>Acute gout may progress to chronic gout exacerbated by exercise, excessive alcohol, diet high in purines<br>Uric acid crystals can form tophi on fingers, ear cartilage (below)<br>(Renal colic if kidney stones)<br>**Pseudogout**<br>Monoarthritis | **Gout and pseudogout**<br>Pain relief with non-steroidal anti-inflammatory drugs<br>Steroids injected into the joint<br><br>**Gout**<br>Uric acid lowering medication<br>Lifestyle/dietary modification | Advice about lifestyle/dietary alterations (see below) and pain relief<br>Discussing effectiveness of uric-acid lowering medications in gout |
| **Rheumatoid arthritis** | Joint swelling, pain, stiffness and tenderness<br>Smaller joints of hands, feet and wrists tend to be affected first with subsequent involvement of larger joints<br>Tenosynovitis | Tailored rehabilitation and pain relief to minimise symptoms and improve prognosis<br>Multi-disciplinary involvement (physiotherapy for e.g. exercise and local symptomatic treatment; occupational therapy for e.g. splinting and aids/adaptations)<br>Disease remission: e.g. through treatment with Disease Modifying Antirheumatic Drugs (DMARDs) (corticosteroids may be given to control symptoms until DMARDs work)<br>Surgical joint stabilisation or replacement | Discussion of pain management and monitoring its success<br>Pre- and post-operative care if joint replacement surgery<br>Working closely with the multi-disciplinary team<br>Discussion of activities of daily living and usefulness of modifications |

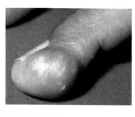

Gouty tophi with uric acid crystals exuding from the fingertip

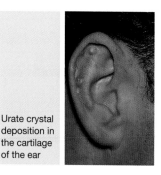

Urate crystal deposition in the cartilage of the ear

Source: Davey P (ed), 2014. Reproduced with permission of Wiley.

### Dietary advice for gout should include discussion of:

- Their usual diet: consider how this may be modified to reduce foods high in purines (e.g. liver, game, offal, sardines, anchovies, crab, herring, mackerel, yeast products, some vegetables e.g. asparagus, spinach and peas) and alcohol particularly spirits, beer and red wines. There is some evidence to suggest increased vitamin C is useful so discuss increasing vitamin C intake in diet. Low fat dairy products are also suggested as beneficial
- Weight loss may also be required (but not rapid) so advice should be given about slow reduction of weight and moderate exercise

Likely points of access to the healthcare system are general practice, walk-in-clinic, out-of-hours (OOH) service, emergency department, and ambulance service

# Key facts

- Nurses frequently provide care in primary care or in hospital for people with dislocations of joints or joint disease (arthropathy). There are several types of joint disease (above).
- Osteoarthritis is a progressive degenerative joint disease. It is the most common joint disease found in older people.
- Osteoarthritis is characterised by progressive cartilage damage and loss together with changes in the nearby bones due to the formation of osteophytes (bony projections/spurs).
- Gout and pseudogout are crystal-related joint disorders. In gout crystals of monosodium urate accumulate in joints: in pseudogout the crystals are calcium pyrophosphate dihydrate. Both result in synovitis (inflammation of the synovial membrane).
- Gout is more common in men than women.
- Pseudogout is a common age-related problem mostly found in people over 60 years of age.
- Rheumatoid arthritis (RA) is a systemic auto-immune disorder. The effects range from mild to severe. Although RA commonly centres on joints, extra-articular signs including splinter haemorrhages in nails and skin ulceration due to vasculitis may be present; there may also be kidney, lung and heart involvement.
- Rheumatoid arthritis is more common in younger women than younger men but by 65 years of age there is no difference between the sexes.
- Arthritis is also linked to infections. This may be as a direct result of infection in the joint (septic arthritis), as a symptom of a systemic infection e.g. hepatitis, mumps or as a reactive arthritis (aseptic inflammation of the joint) triggered from an infection at a distant site usually in the gastro-intestinal or urinary tract.
- Nurses will care for people having joint replacements (e.g. hip and knee).

# Essentials of best practice: arthropathies

The nursing care required by someone with an inflammation of their joints depends on the particular arthropathy (above) as well as its severity and location. Attention should also be paid to any systemic signs and symptoms and infections. Care is most likely to be provided in primary care via the GP or as an out-patient. Nurses will also routinely meet people with arthropathies who are admitted to hospital for other reasons – in these situations care will need to focus on the limitations presented by the arthropathy, for example dietary restrictions, modifications to daily living activities (e.g. the use of aids such as specially adapted cutlery) and the use of mobility aids.

Some people will be hospitalised for joint stabilisation or replacement and so the principles of pre- and post-operative care should be adhered to: some procedures will require special post-operative care and attention should always be paid to minimising the risks of immobility (e.g. VTE and pressure ulcers).

For many people the mainstay of treatment will be pain relief and rehabilitation and adaptation; so working closely with physiotherapists and occupational therapists is essential. Reinforcing exercise routines and the use of aids is a key nursing responsibility.

Nurses may also seek advice from specialist nurses for rheumatology and pain.

Care will largely focus on:

✓ Accurate assessment and regular monitoring (e.g. if surgery - pre- and post-operative care (see Section 1) including haemorrhage, shock, VTEs, infection, wound care and positioning)

✓ Communication with the healthcare team, patient and family

✓ Symptom control and management (e.g. pain relief, immobility, rehabilitation regimen)

✓ Health education and promotion (e.g. about levels of activity, pain relief and diet (e.g. gout opposite))

✓ Risk assessment and management (e.g. pressure ulcer risk, VTE risk)

✓ Discharge planning (post-discharge medication and advice about signs and symptoms of complications following joint replacement, e.g. infections: advice about mobilisation and positioning)

## Patient information

There are several useful charities and support groups focusing on joint disorders:
Arthritis Care www.arthritiscare.org.uk.
National Rheumatoid Arthritis Society (NRAS) www.nras.org.uk.
The Arthritic Association www.arthriticassociation.org.uk.
The UK Gout Society www.ukgout.org.
You will find very helpful patient-centred fact sheets at www.patient.co.uk.

# Nursing people with muscle disorders

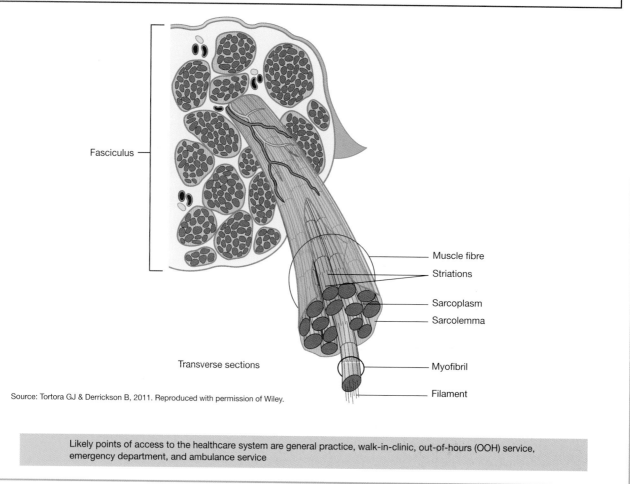

**Skeletal muscle fibre**

Fasciculus

Transverse sections

Muscle fibre

Striations

Sarcoplasm

Sarcolemma

Myofibril

Filament

Source: Tortora GJ & Derrickson B, 2011. Reproduced with permission of Wiley.

Likely points of access to the healthcare system are general practice, walk-in-clinic, out-of-hours (OOH) service, emergency department, and ambulance service

*Adult Nursing at a Glance*, First Edition. Andrée le May. © 2015 John Wiley & Sons, Ltd. Published 2015 by John Wiley & Sons, Ltd.
Companion website: www.ataglanceseries.com/nursing/adult

# Key facts

- Nurses infrequently provide care for people with disorders of their muscles without support from the multi-disciplinary team – especially physiotherapists and occupational therapists.
- Disorders of muscles can range from aches and strains to degenerative myopathies, which can result in extreme and debilitating muscle weakness.
- Strains result from torn or stretched muscle fibres. They may occur because of an accident or taking part in sports or other vigorous activities. The most common strains are to hamstrings and the calf, quadriceps and lumber muscles.
- Nurses may treat people with strains in primary care, walk-in-clinics or the ED. Care usually focuses on self-help treatments which include **P**rotecting and **R**esting the injured muscle, applying **I**ce and **C**ompression and **E**levating the affected limb (sometimes you may see this set of actions referred to as PRICE). Analgesics may also need to be recommended (or prescribed). Advice may also be given about anticipated recovery times and return to sport and about doing warming up and warming down exercises once fit. Referral to a specialist sports physiotherapist may be useful.
- There are several types of myopathy, many of which are inherited and described as primary myopathies (e.g. Duchenne muscular dystrophy).
- Muscular dystrophies lead to progressive muscle wasting and weakness.
- Nurses may routinely care for people with primary myopathies who need nursing care, not because of their muscle weakness and related limitations, but because they are ill from another cause. In these situations care must focus on both the presenting illness *and* any lasting problems linked to the myopathy.
- Other myopathies may be secondary to metabolic or endocrine diseases, for example associated with myxoedema, hyperthyroidism, Addison's disease or diabetes mellitus. Others may be linked to inflammation, for example dermatomyositis, or infection, for example HIV, or result from medications such as statins or steroids. Medical treatment and nursing care, in these instances, will depend on the underlying condition.
- For some conditions muscle biopsy and electromyography may be needed to reach a diagnosis; careful explanation of these procedures is a nursing responsibility.
- Myopathies can occur in any muscle not just skeletal muscles.
- Where muscle weakness is degenerative, the use of mobility aids and adaptive devices will be needed. Occupational therapists and physiotherapists will play a large part in this element of treatment. Ongoing support and encouragement from nurses is also a vital part of care.

- Musculo-skeletal complications from myopathies include the formation of contractures and chest and spinal deformities such as scoliosis.
- Nurses may be involved in genetic counselling and pre-natal diagnostic testing.
- Neuromuscular diseases such as myasthenia gravis cause significant muscle weakness of the limbs and fatigue. Myasthenia gravis is an auto-immune disease with relapsing/remitting symptoms. Other neuromuscular diseases result in problems related to mobility (Chapter 86).
- Older people experience age-related changes as their muscles age and lose elasticity and size. These changes can make movement harder because of reduced flexibility, strength and stamina and put an older person at risk of falls, isolation and loss of confidence in relation to their mobility. Recovery from muscle injury may also be prolonged.

# Essentials of best practice

Nursing care will depend on the presenting signs and symptoms.
Care will largely focus on:
✓ Accurate assessment and regular monitoring (e.g. in those recovering from injury)
✓ Communication with the healthcare team, patient and family
✓ Symptom control and management (e.g. pain relief, immobility, rehabilitation regimen and confidence building)
✓ Health education and promotion (e.g. about levels of activity and pain relief following injury: advice to older people about exercise to prevent muscle loss (this is important in earlier life too) and promote flexibility in order to prevent, for instance, falls)
✓ Risk assessment and management (e.g. falls and pressure ulcers due to immobility, VTE)
✓ Discharge planning (post-discharge rehabilitation regimens, outpatient appointments, advice about mobilisation and use of aids and adaptive devices)

## Patient information

There are several useful charities and support groups focusing on muscle disorders:
The Muscular Dystrophy Campaign provides information and support about muscular dystrophy and other related conditions. www.muscular-dystrophy.org.uk.
You will find very helpful patient-centred fact sheets at www.patient.co.uk.

# 80 Nursing people with nervous system disorders

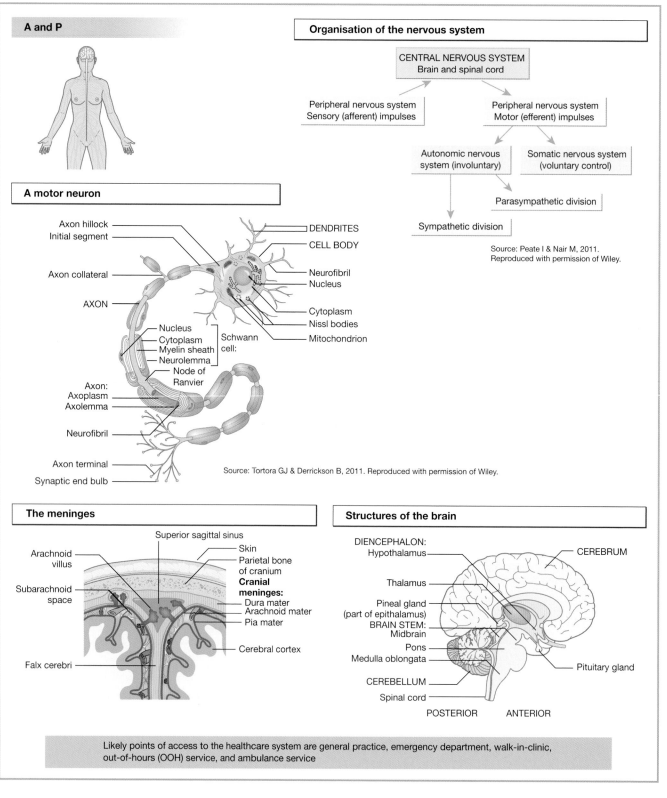

**A and P**

**A motor neuron**

- Axon hillock
- Initial segment
- Axon collateral
- AXON
  - Nucleus
  - Cytoplasm
  - Myelin sheath
  - Neurolemma
  - Node of Ranvier
  - Schwann cell:
- Axon:
  - Axoplasm
  - Axolemma
- Neurofibril
- Axon terminal
- Synaptic end bulb

- DENDRITES
- CELL BODY
- Neurofibril
- Nucleus
- Cytoplasm
- Nissl bodies
- Mitochondrion

Source: Tortora GJ & Derrickson B, 2011. Reproduced with permission of Wiley.

**Organisation of the nervous system**

CENTRAL NERVOUS SYSTEM
Brain and spinal cord

Peripheral nervous system
Sensory (afferent) impulses

Peripheral nervous system
Motor (efferent) impulses

Autonomic nervous system (involuntary)

Somatic nervous system (voluntary control)

Parasympathetic division

Sympathetic division

Source: Peate I & Nair M, 2011.
Reproduced with permission of Wiley.

**The meninges**

- Arachnoid villus
- Subarachnoid space
- Falx cerebri
- Superior sagittal sinus
- Skin
- Parietal bone of cranium
- **Cranial meninges:**
  - Dura mater
  - Arachnoid mater
  - Pia mater
- Cerebral cortex

**Structures of the brain**

DIENCEPHALON:
- Hypothalamus
- Thalamus
- Pineal gland (part of epithalamus)

BRAIN STEM:
- Midbrain
- Pons
- Medulla oblongata

CEREBELLUM
Spinal cord

CEREBRUM

Pituitary gland

POSTERIOR          ANTERIOR

Likely points of access to the healthcare system are general practice, emergency department, walk-in-clinic, out-of-hours (OOH) service, and ambulance service

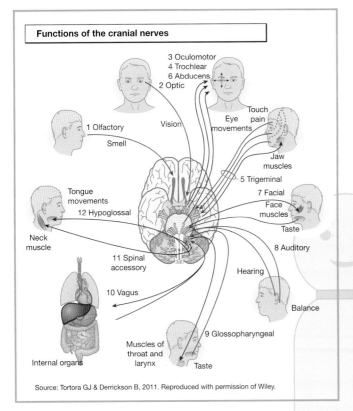

Functions of the cranial nerves

3 Oculomotor
4 Trochlear
6 Abducens
2 Optic

1 Olfactory

Smell

Vision

Eye movements

Touch pain

Jaw muscles

5 Trigeminal

7 Facial

Face muscles

Tongue movements

12 Hypoglossal

Taste

Neck muscle

8 Auditory

11 Spinal accessory

Hearing

10 Vagus

Balance

9 Glossopharyngeal

Internal organs

Muscles of throat and larynx

Taste

Source: Tortora GJ & Derrickson B, 2011. Reproduced with permission of Wiley.

## Key facts

- The nervous system is a highly organised, complex network. It influences many of the body's organs and functions as well as homeostasis.
- The nervous system can be divided into two interlinked parts – the central nervous system (CNS) (the brain and the spinal cord) and the peripheral nervous system (PNS). The PNS carries motor impulses *from* the CNS and sensory impulses *to* the CNS (above). The autonomic nervous system is part of the PNS.
- The nervous system works with other systems, particularly the endocrine system (see Chapter 66).
- Disorders of the nervous system can result in acute or chronic conditions.

## Common disorders of the nervous system

- Infections (e.g. meningitis and encephalitis)
- Epilepsy
- Space occupying lesions (benign or malignant)
- Vascular disorders
- Multiple sclerosis
- Parkinson's disease
- Dementias.

Each is covered in the following pages. See Chapter 81 for common signs, symptoms and emergencies.

## A and P

- The CNS comprises the brain and the spinal cord. Its role is to process and integrate information received from the sensory nerve fibres (afferent) of the peripheral nervous system and to respond to this information via the motor nerve fibres (efferent) of the PNS (above).
- The PNS includes the cranial and spinal nerves (above) and the autonomic nervous system (ANS).
- Sensory information comes from receptors/nerves found throughout the body (e.g. in the eyes, ears, tongue, nose, skin; baroreceptors and proprioceptors).

- Motor responses to sensory impulses occur through either the activation of the ANS (involuntary, e.g. vasoconstriction when cold) or the somatic nervous system (voluntary, e.g. putting on a jumper).
- There are two parts to the ANS: sympathetic and parasympathetic. The sympathetic part (thoracolumbar) is associated with 'fight or flight' responses to stressful situations: the parasympathetic (craniosacral) part is most active at rest and, for example, constricts bronchioles, decreases heart rate, increases peristalsis. The two systems work together.
- Neurons (nerve cells) receive, conduct and transmit impulses (messages).
- A neuron comprises a dendrite, a cell body and an axon (opposite). PNS axons are covered in a protective and insulating myelin sheath: these sheaths speed up the passage of electrical impulses.
- Impulses are generated and conducted by the movement of ions (mainly sodium and potassium) into and out of the neuron – this movement generates an electrical charge which travels along the axon. This involves the creation of action potentials (APs) and their movement along the axon: refractory periods when the neuron cannot receive another impulse occur between APs. Watch APs on YouTube www.youtube.com/watch?v=ifD1YG07fB8.
- The impulse then passes from one neuron to another (axon to dendrite) or to a muscle or gland using a chemical neurotransmitter. Neurotransmitters either stimulate or inhibit the impulse's passage across the gaps between, for example, two nerve cells (synaptic junction).
- Different neurotransmitters work in different parts of the nervous system, for example the sympathetic nervous system releases noradrenalin (called norepinephrine in the US) and the parasympathetic nervous system releases acetylcholine.
- The brain can be divided into four regions (cerebrum, diencephalon, brain stem and cerebellum) (opposite). Different areas of the brain are responsible for different functions (e.g. the cerebellum coordinates balance, posture and voluntary muscle movement).
- The brain is surrounded by three layers of protective connective tissue: the meninges (pia mater, arachnoid mater and dura mater) (above).
- The spinal cord links the brain and the PNS. It runs from the medulla oblongata to the upper part of the second lumbar vertebra: it is enclosed in the spinal canal and protected by the spinal meninges (pia mater, arachnoid mater and dura mater) and cerebrospinal fluid (CSF).
- CSF, a thin fluid similar to plasma, is produced by the choroid plexus in the ventricles. CSF circulates around the brain, in the ventricles and the spinal canal. It protects the brain, helps to maintain a uniform pressure around the brain and spinal cord and enables nutrient and waste exchange.
- Spinal nerves are attached to the spinal cord. Each spinal nerve innervates a group of muscles (myotome) and an area of skin (dermatome) (Chapter 81).

## Essentials of best practice

Nursing someone with any disorder of the nervous system requires you to be aware of all of the essentials of best practice. These will be expanded for the disorders listed above in the subsequent pages.

See Chapter 81 for more details about assessment of this system.

### Patient information

There are several patient support groups and charities focusing on disorders of the nervous system. You can find most of them on the Self Help UK website www.self-help.org.uk.
You will also find very helpful patient-centred fact sheets at www.patient.co.uk/.

# 81 Signs, symptoms, assessment and emergencies

**Important assessments of the nervous system are made through neurological observations** (based on Dougherty and Lister, 2011)

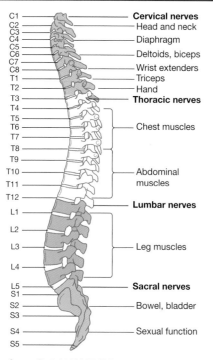

Assessment involves monitoring:
- Level of consciousness (the Glasgow Coma Scale should be used to give consistent findings)
  - o Arousability
  - o Awareness
- Pupillary activity (reactions to light, size, shape, equality). Do both eyes move together? Do either or both eyes deviate upwards/downwards?
- Motor function (muscle strength, tone, coordination, reflexes (blink, gag, swallow, oculocephalic and plantar) and abnormal movements, e.g. seizures, tics, tremors)
- Sensory function (central and peripheral vision, clarity of vision, hearing and ability to understand conversations, sensations, e.g. superficial (light touch) and deep sensations (muscle pain))
- Vital signs (respirations, temperature, pulse and blood pressure). Raised blood pressure, slowed pulse and slowed and irregular respirations may be indicative of increased intracranial pressure. Pyrexia may occur as a result of damage to the hypothalamus or infection

Record observations and report any deviations from the norm or the person's previous condition immediately

NB Changes in a person's neurological condition can occur rapidly or slowly over time – being alert to both is vital to ensuring a quick medical response

---

### The spinal nerves and their areas of innervation

| Segment | Area of innervation |
|---------|---------------------|
| C1 | **Cervical nerves** |
| C2 | Head and neck |
| C3 | |
| C4 | Diaphragm |
| C5 | |
| C6 | Deltoids, biceps |
| C7 | |
| C8 | Wrist extenders |
| T1 | Triceps |
| T2 | Hand |
| T3 | **Thoracic nerves** |
| T4 | |
| T5 | |
| T6 | Chest muscles |
| T7 | |
| T8 | |
| T9 | |
| T10 | Abdominal muscles |
| T11 | |
| T12 | |
| L1 | **Lumbar nerves** |
| L2 | |
| L3 | Leg muscles |
| L4 | |
| L5 | **Sacral nerves** |
| S1 | |
| S2 | Bowel, bladder |
| S3 | |
| S4 | Sexual function |
| S5 | |

Source: Peate I & Nair M, 2011.
Reproduced with permission of Wiley.

---

*Adult Nursing at a Glance*, First Edition. Andrée le May. © 2015 John Wiley & Sons, Ltd. Published 2015 by John Wiley & Sons, Ltd.
Companion website: www.ataglanceseries.com/nursing/adult

# Common signs and symptoms

There are a wide range of signs and symptoms related to neurological disorders. They include:

- Pain/discomfort: for example headache, eyes
- Photophobia
- Neck stiffness
- Nausea, vomiting
- Dizziness: loss of balance
- Altered vision: for example double vision, blurring, visual loss
- Altered movement: lack of coordination, pins and needles, paralysis, unsteadiness, clumsiness, falls, tremor
- Muscle weakness and wasting
- Difficulty speaking
- Difficulty swallowing
- Cramps and spasm of muscles
- Seizures
- Agitation
- Confusion and disorientation: loss of consciousness, loss of memory, cognitive impairment
- Skin rashes (petechiae, purpura)
- Altered heart rate, rhythm, BP, respiratory rate
- Pyrexia.

# Neurological emergencies

Recognising and responding to sudden deteriorations in a patient's neurological condition is vital. Three situations where rapid intervention can be life-saving are bacterial meningitis (see Chapter 82) spinal cord compression and raised intracranial pressure.

## Acute spinal cord compression is a medical emergency

Spinal cord compression may occur because of, for example:

- Secondary tumours from breast, prostate or lung cancers.
- Prolapsed intervertebral discs.
- Abscesses or other inflammatory lesions.

Acute spinal cord compression presents with rapidly deteriorating motor dysfunction largely of the lower limbs. If this happens to any of your patients call for immediate medical assistance or an emergency ambulance.

Diagnosis is usually made by MRI scanning and the treatment, if possible, is surgical decompression.

Initial nursing care is likely to focus on rapid preparation for surgery – be sure to remain calm and give clear explanations and information to the patient and their family/carers. Ongoing care will involve specialised post-operative care and support that will depend on the nature of any residual problems.

## Raised intracranial pressure is a medical emergency

Head injuries or other intracranial (e.g. cerebral abscess, haematomas or other space occupying lesions such as malignant or benign tumours) or extracranial (e.g. hepatic encephalopathy) pathologies may cause the pressure in the skull to rise, which in turn may result in coma, irreversible brain damage or death.

Common signs and symptoms of raised intracranial pressure which nurses need to be aware of and act on immediately are:

- Any alterations in consciousness.
- Focal neurological deficits such as limb weakness or speech deficits: pupil changes, double vision.

Alterations to vital signs, that is slowed and irregular respiratory rate, slowed heart rate and increased blood pressure, may follow but are not always the first signs to be present. Elevated temperature may occur due to compression of the hypothalamus.

Check observations and record assessment against Early Warning System/Glasgow Coma Scale. Call for immediate help, stay with the patient and monitor closely.

Ongoing nursing care will depend largely on medical treatment and the patient's condition but may include:

✓ Accurate, frequent monitoring of vital signs (+intracranial pressure, if measured – normal limits equal to or less than 15 mmHg). Be alert to changes in respiration, blood pressure and pulse. Changes to the cardiovascular system will mean less blood reaching the already compromised brain. Report alterations in BP (systolic <90 or >160 mmHg: diastolic <50 or >100 mmHg) and pulse (<50 or >100 beats/minute)

✓ Maintenance of their airway

✓ Accurate assessment and monitoring of level of consciousness: be alert to even the slightest change (e.g. agitation, restlessness, taking longer to respond than before)

✓ Care of infusions and urinary catheter and infection control

✓ Administration of prescribed medications

✓ Skilled, reassuring communication with the patient and their family and carers regardless of level of consciousness

✓ Rapid communication of deterioration to the medical team

✓ If surgery is needed post-operative observations should focus on continuous assessment of neurological state and immediate reporting of alterations: giving appropriate medications

# 82 Nursing people with CNS infections

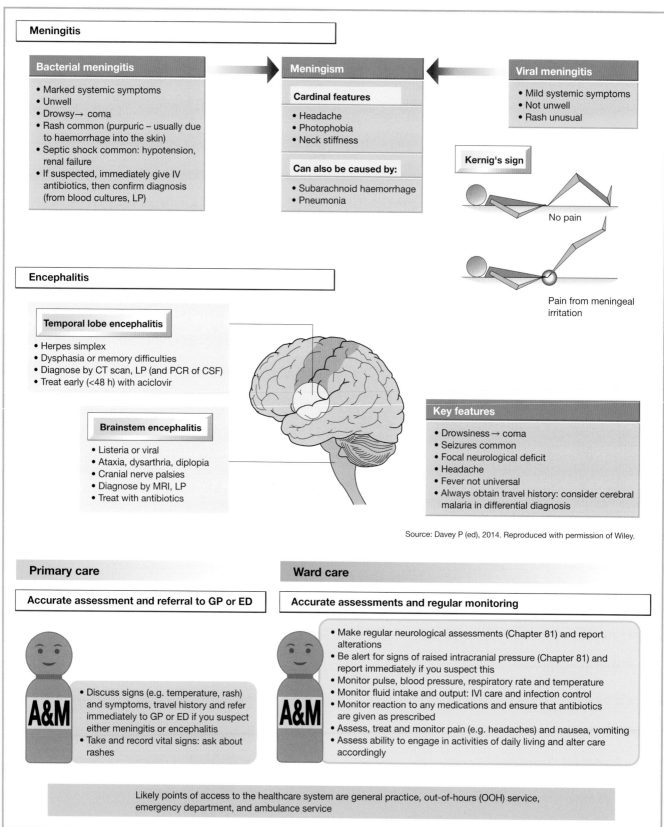

### Meningitis

#### Bacterial meningitis

- Marked systemic symptoms
- Unwell
- Drowsy→ coma
- Rash common (purpuric – usually due to haemorrhage into the skin)
- Septic shock common: hypotension, renal failure
- If suspected, immediately give IV antibiotics, then confirm diagnosis (from blood cultures, LP)

#### Meningism

**Cardinal features**

- Headache
- Photophobia
- Neck stiffness

**Can also be caused by:**

- Subarachnoid haemorrhage
- Pneumonia

#### Viral meningitis

- Mild systemic symptoms
- Not unwell
- Rash unusual

**Kernig's sign**

No pain

Pain from meningeal irritation

### Encephalitis

#### Temporal lobe encephalitis

- Herpes simplex
- Dysphasia or memory difficulties
- Diagnose by CT scan, LP (and PCR of CSF)
- Treat early (<48 h) with aciclovir

#### Brainstem encephalitis

- Listeria or viral
- Ataxia, dysarthria, diplopia
- Cranial nerve palsies
- Diagnose by MRI, LP
- Treat with antibiotics

#### Key features

- Drowsiness → coma
- Seizures common
- Focal neurological deficit
- Headache
- Fever not universal
- Always obtain travel history: consider cerebral malaria in differential diagnosis

Source: Davey P (ed), 2014. Reproduced with permission of Wiley.

### Primary care

#### Accurate assessment and referral to GP or ED

**A&M**

- Discuss signs (e.g. temperature, rash) and symptoms, travel history and refer immediately to GP or ED if you suspect either meningitis or encephalitis
- Take and record vital signs: ask about rashes

### Ward care

#### Accurate assessments and regular monitoring

**A&M**

- Make regular neurological assessments (Chapter 81) and report alterations
- Be alert for signs of raised intracranial pressure (Chapter 81) and report immediately if you suspect this
- Monitor pulse, blood pressure, respiratory rate and temperature
- Monitor fluid intake and output: IVI care and infection control
- Monitor reaction to any medications and ensure that antibiotics are given as prescribed
- Assess, treat and monitor pain (e.g. headaches) and nausea, vomiting
- Assess ability to engage in activities of daily living and alter care accordingly

Likely points of access to the healthcare system are general practice, out-of-hours (OOH) service, emergency department, and ambulance service

*Adult Nursing at a Glance*, First Edition. Andrée le May. © 2015 John Wiley & Sons, Ltd. Published 2015 by John Wiley & Sons, Ltd.
Companion website: www.ataglanceseries.com/nursing/adult

# Key facts

- Both bacterial meningitis and encephalitis are serious, potentially fatal infections requiring prompt diagnosis, treatment and hospitalisation.
- Viral meningitis is usually milder and self-limiting; however, some viruses can cause severe debilitation and functional and intellectual impairment.
- Some types of bacterial meningitis present with septicaemia induced disseminated intravascular coagulation (DIC). Anyone with this type of meningitis will be seriously ill and require intensive nursing and medical care. Recovery may be prolonged and functional (e.g. because of amputations) and intellectual impairment may remain.
- Encephalitis may also leave people functionally and intellectually impaired – sometimes to the extent that they require long-term ongoing care.
- Both bacterial meningitis and encephalitis can have a rapid onset (above).
- Immunisation is available against some types of meningitis and encephalitis.
- After discharge from hospital following bacterial or viral meningitis, some people continue to have minimal residual problems (e.g. headaches, poor concentration and fatigue), others may have functional deficits needing ongoing rehabilitation with physiotherapists and adaptations to be made to enable easier daily living by occupational therapists.

# Diagnosis

- Physical examination
- History taking
- Blood tests and culture
- Lumbar puncture
- CT scans and MRI
- Electroencephalography (EEG).

# Essentials of best practice

Any infection of the CNS is debilitating and frightening. Nursing largely focuses on monitoring the patient's condition and being alert to early signs of deterioration (and progress). Management of medications and addressing symptoms are also essential.

Nursing care will encompass:
- ✓ Accurate assessments and regular monitoring
- ✓ Communication with the healthcare team, patient and family
- ✓ Symptom control and management
- ✓ Discharge planning

## Patient information

Meningitis Now offers support and information to people who have had meningitis and their families www.meningitisnow.org.
The Encephalitis Society provides support and information about encephalitis: www.encephalitis.info/.
You will also find very helpful patient-centred fact sheets at www.patient.co.uk/.

# 83 Nursing people with epilepsy

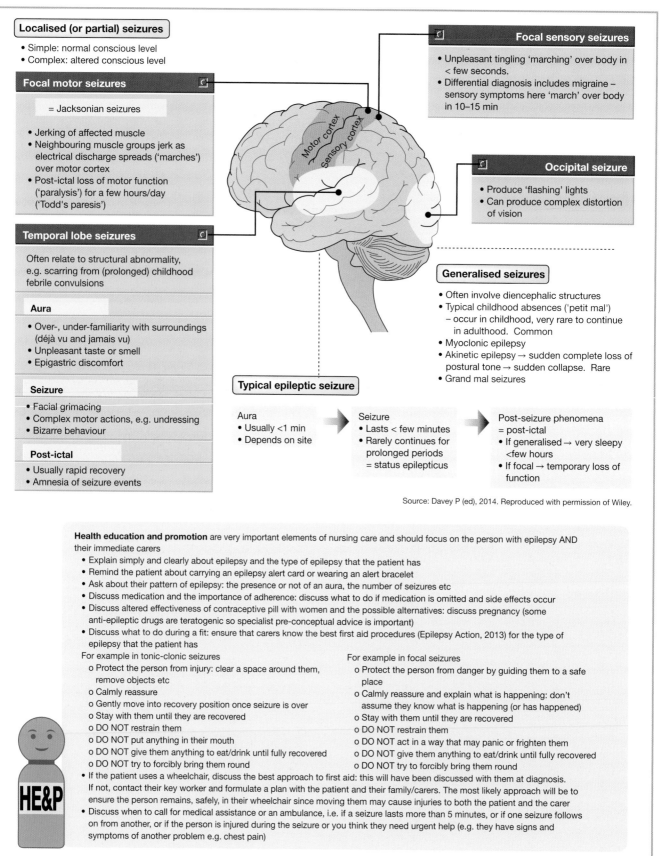

**Localised (or partial) seizures**

- Simple: normal conscious level
- Complex: altered conscious level

**Focal motor seizures**

= Jacksonian seizures

- Jerking of affected muscle
- Neighbouring muscle groups jerk as electrical discharge spreads ('marches') over motor cortex
- Post-ictal loss of motor function ('paralysis') for a few hours/day ('Todd's paresis')

**Temporal lobe seizures**

Often relate to structural abnormality, e.g. scarring from (prolonged) childhood febrile convulsions

**Aura**

- Over-, under-familiarity with surroundings (déjà vu and jamais vu)
- Unpleasant taste or smell
- Epigastric discomfort

**Seizure**

- Facial grimacing
- Complex motor actions, e.g. undressing
- Bizarre behaviour

**Post-ictal**

- Usually rapid recovery
- Amnesia of seizure events

**Focal sensory seizures**

- Unpleasant tingling 'marching' over body in < few seconds.
- Differential diagnosis includes migraine – sensory symptoms here 'march' over body in 10–15 min

**Occipital seizure**

- Produce 'flashing' lights
- Can produce complex distortion of vision

**Generalised seizures**

- Often involve diencephalic structures
- Typical childhood absences ('petit mal') – occur in childhood, very rare to continue in adulthood. Common
- Myoclonic epilepsy
- Akinetic epilepsy → sudden complete loss of postural tone → sudden collapse. Rare
- Grand mal seizures

**Typical epileptic seizure**

Aura
- Usually <1 min
- Depends on site

Seizure
- Lasts < few minutes
- Rarely continues for prolonged periods = status epilepticus

Post-seizure phenomena = post-ictal
- If generalised → very sleepy <few hours
- If focal → temporary loss of function

Source: Davey P (ed), 2014. Reproduced with permission of Wiley.

**Health education and promotion** are very important elements of nursing care and should focus on the person with epilepsy AND their immediate carers

- Explain simply and clearly about epilepsy and the type of epilepsy that the patient has
- Remind the patient about carrying an epilepsy alert card or wearing an alert bracelet
- Ask about their pattern of epilepsy: the presence or not of an aura, the number of seizures etc
- Discuss medication and the importance of adherence: discuss what to do if medication is omitted and side effects occur
- Discuss altered effectiveness of contraceptive pill with women and the possible alternatives: discuss pregnancy (some anti-epileptic drugs are teratogenic so specialist pre-conceptual advice is important)
- Discuss what to do during a fit: ensure that carers know the best first aid procedures (Epilepsy Action, 2013) for the type of epilepsy that the patient has

For example in tonic-clonic seizures
- o Protect the person from injury: clear a space around them, remove objects etc
- o Calmly reassure
- o Gently move into recovery position once seizure is over
- o Stay with them until they are recovered
- o DO NOT restrain them
- o DO NOT put anything in their mouth
- o DO NOT give them anything to eat/drink until fully recovered
- o DO NOT try to forcibly bring them round

For example in focal seizures
- o Protect the person from danger by guiding them to a safe place
- o Calmly reassure and explain what is happening: don't assume they know what is happening (or has happened)
- o Stay with them until they are recovered
- o DO NOT restrain them
- o DO NOT act in a way that may panic or frighten them
- o DO NOT give them anything to eat/drink until fully recovered
- o DO NOT try to forcibly bring them round

- If the patient uses a wheelchair, discuss the best approach to first aid: this will have been discussed with them at diagnosis. If not, contact their key worker and formulate a plan with the patient and their family/carers. The most likely approach will be to ensure the person remains, safely, in their wheelchair since moving them may cause injuries to both the patient and the carer
- Discuss when to call for medical assistance or an ambulance, i.e. if a seizure lasts more than 5 minutes, or if one seizure follows on from another, or if the person is injured during the seizure or you think they need urgent help (e.g. they have signs and symptoms of another problem e.g. chest pain)

*Adult Nursing at a Glance*, First Edition. Andrée le May. © 2015 John Wiley & Sons, Ltd. Published 2015 by John Wiley & Sons, Ltd.
Companion website: www.ataglanceseries.com/nursing/adult

## Primary care

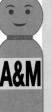

**A&M**
- Discuss epilepsy control and satisfaction with it: discuss any new pattern to seizures – a symptom diary may be useful
- Discuss (and monitor) medication regimen, side-effects and adherence: consider problems if any. If compliance is difficult discuss a system of reminders that would be feasible e.g. reminders from relatives/friends/mobile phone/computer alerts
- To monitor effectiveness of any nursing care plan, arrange a re-visit or telephone or email
- Refer to specialist epilepsy nurse/team if needed
- If you suspect depression (a possible accompaniment to epilepsy) discuss this and make a referral to the GP

**C**
- Accurate, clear and simple communication that is also reassuring is important. Epilepsy can be frightening for everyone
- Supplement verbal communication with written information
- Make sure that the patient/family knows how to get in touch with you
- If you suspect depression (a possible accompaniment to epilepsy) discuss this and make a referral to the GP
- Try to put patients and their families in touch with support groups to provide psychological, practical and social support (e.g. Epilepsy Action)

Likely points of access to the healthcare system are general practice, out-of-hours (OOH) service, emergency department, and ambulance service

## Key facts

- Epilepsy is an intense burst of electrical activity in the brain which causes a temporary disruption to the way the brain normally works: this means that the brain's messages get 'mixed up' (Epilepsy Action, 2013) and alterations occur to motor, sensory or psychological functions. The disordered electrical discharge can happen in different parts of the brain so epilepsy manifests in different ways (above).
- Sudden onset epilepsy can also be the first indication of another CNS disorder such as a space occupying lesion. New seizures should always be investigated thoroughly.
- Regardless of the way epilepsy manifests itself, it will be seen at first as a frightening condition by the patient and their family/friends/carers. Epilepsy is a condition surrounded by stigma, myths and old wives' tales so appropriate health education and promotion is an essential element of skilled nursing care (below).
- Epilepsy is an ongoing condition that is controlled by medication. Successful management of epilepsy rather than cure is the objective of care.
- Some people experience side-effects due to their medication and so for this reason (and sometimes others) compliance with medication can be poor.
- Medication for epilepsy can also interact with other medications (e.g. oral contraceptives) and so discussion of the range of medications taken is important.
- Women with epilepsy who are considering pregnancy will need to discuss medication and epilepsy control with their medical specialists before conception. Some drugs used to treat epilepsy are teratogenic.
- People living with epilepsy and their family/carers will require support from practice nurses, occupational health nurses and nurses working in the ED or acute wards if their epilepsy is not well controlled by medication (see below). Family planning nurses may also be involved in discussions about contraceptive effectiveness and pre-conceptual care with women of child-bearing age (above).
- When epilepsy is poorly controlled either through poor drug compliance or for example hypoglycaemia or alcohol withdrawal, seizures can happen continuously (status epilepticus). They may occur one after another or a seizure may appear to last longer than normal.
- Status epilepticus is a very serious condition requiring immediate medical intervention. Untreated status epilepticus has high morbidity and mortality due to cerebral oedema and cardiorespiratory arrest.

## Diagnosis

History taking from the patient and reliable observers is probably the most important element of diagnosis and will be used in conjunction with electroencephalographs (EEGs) and brain imaging.

## Essentials of best practice

Nursing care will largely focus on health education and promotion and accurate assessments and regular monitoring and will mostly occur in primary care (above). Occupational health nurses may also advise about maintaining a person's safety at work.

People with epilepsy may be admitted to hospital after their first seizure for diagnosis and treatment. They may subsequently be admitted if their seizures become poorly controlled, more frequent or they have continuous seizures (status epilepticus). Status epilepticus is a medical emergency requiring immediate attention. Medical care largely focuses on terminating the seizures, for example IV diazepam or anti-epileptics and maintaining the airway and cardiac output.

Nursing care in this situation should focus on:

✓ Accurate assessments and regular monitoring (immediate attention to ABCDE and blood glucose monitoring: ongoing monitoring of neurological status, vital signs and seizures)

✓ Symptom control and management (IVI and medications)

✓ Communication with the healthcare team, patient and family

✓ Risk assessment and management (safety, e.g. padded bed rails; maintenance of secure IVI if continual seizures)

## Patient information

Epilepsy Action provides support and information about different types of epilepsy www.epilepsy.org.uk.
You will also find very helpful patient-centred fact sheets at www.patient.co.uk/.

# 84 Nursing people with vascular disorders of the brain

## Types of vascular disorders

| Vascular disorder | Symptoms and signs | Pathology | Treatment |
|---|---|---|---|
| Stroke<br><br>(NB Transient Ischaemic Attacks (TIA) suggest a risk of strokes and require urgent investigation and possible surgical carotid endarterectomy. Nurses need to be alert to this and advise prompt medical consultation) | Sudden onset<br>Symptoms and signs will depend on the location of the stroke: they may include hemiplegia, language dysfunction, dyspraxia, denial of existence of affected body side, diplopia, visual loss, unsteadiness, dysphagia, unilateral weakness including facial weakness, amnesia, pyrexia, severe headache*, coma, death | Either vaso-occlusive infarct – emboli from another part of the body leading to major vessel blockage or an in situ vascular blockage of small vessel<br>Or haemorrhage (due to e.g. hypertension + anticoagulant therapy: thrombolysis)*<br>Location of damaged brain tissue determines presentation, prognosis and effects | Depends on type:<br>Infarct: thrombolysis within 3 hours of symptom onset<br>Haemorrhage: lower BP: surgical evacuation of blood may be needed<br>Prevention of VTE e.g. use of TED stockings<br>Symptom management<br>Long-term reduction of risk of further stroke |
| Subarachnoid haemorrhage (SAH) | Sudden onset<br>Severe headache as if being 'hit by cricket bat'<br>Loss of consciousness for some people | Arterial bleed from a ruptured Berry aneurysm or arteriovenous malformation | Surgical or endovascular repair<br>Symptom management<br>Long-term control of blood pressure if necessary |
| Subdural haemorrhage (SDH) | Slow onset<br>Focal neurological deficit<br>Decreased mobility in older people<br>Decreased mental agility in older people | Venous bleed with blood slowly oozing into subdural space and sucking in fluid from extracellular space – this acts like a space occupying lesion. Trauma, brain atrophy (chronic alcoholism) and old age are linked to SDHs | Surgical drainage |
| Venous sinus thrombosis | Rare (more common in women)<br>Various symptoms and signs: headache, seizures, disorders of consciousness, papilloedema | Cerebral venous sinus thrombosis can be associated with many things (e.g. pregnancy, oral contraception, inherited thrombophilia) | Anticoagulation<br>Surgical evacuation<br>Raised intracranial pressure management<br>Symptom management |

## Hospital care immediately following a stroke

- **If unilateral body weaknesses** ensure that you (and others) talk to the patient from the affected side: place drinks, call bells etc. on that side so they can reach over to them with unaffected limb. Position the patient on their affected side if lying in bed so they can use their unaffected side. Support affected side using e.g. pillows when they are sitting up in bed or chairs
- **If swallowing difficulties** do not give anything by mouth until an assessment has been made by a speech and language therapist. Insertion of a naso-gastric (NG) tube may be needed until swallowing is reinstated to ensure nourishment, hydration and administration of oral medication. If swallowing becomes a persistent problem nutrients may be given via a percutaneous endoscopic gastrostomy (PEG) or intravenously using total parenteral nutrition (TPN) (see Chapter 5)
- **Restricted range of movement** may predispose the person to contractures, pressure ulcer formation and VTE so regular changes in position, appropriate postural positioning, passive movement and the use of pressure relieving equipment are essential. TED stockings should be used. Working closely with the physiotherapist is essential to ensure correct care. Encourage the patient to participate in movement ensuring safety at all times (e.g. be aware of unexpected spasm, altered ability due to fatigue at the end of the day or after a poor night's sleep, altered sensations)
- **Balance difficulties** should be considered when mobilising
- **Unclear speech and difficulty understanding** require attentive and patient listening and observation and clear, simple communication
- **Difficulties with other activities of daily living** will need individualised assessment and care (e.g. continence – requiring catheter care or the use of continence aids; help may be needed with washing, mouth care, clothes changing)
- **Be alert to deteriorations in level of consciousness and vital signs or extensions of original signs and symptoms** – report immediately. Remember **ABCDE**

Likely points of access to the healthcare system are general practice, out-of-hours (OOH) service, ambulance service, and emergency department

*Adult Nursing at a Glance*, First Edition. Andrée le May. © 2015 John Wiley & Sons, Ltd. Published 2015 by John Wiley & Sons, Ltd.
Companion website: www.ataglanceseries.com/nursing/adult

# Key facts

- There are several vascular disorders of the brain (above). Each has its own associated treatment and management (above). Nursing care will link to each of these and each person's developing condition and may include for example pre- and post-operative care (Section 1), medicines management, neurological assessment and monitoring (Chapter 81), monitoring of vital signs, looking for signs of raised intracranial pressure (Chapter 81) and symptom control and management (above).
- The most common vascular disorder of the brain is stroke.
- Stroke – damage to the brain tissue due to either thrombosis or bleeding in the brain – can occur at any age although it is most prevalent after the age of 65 years. Stroke is the largest cause of disability in the UK and the third largest cause of death after heart disease and cancer.
- Stroke prevention is important – with raised blood pressure being one of the most easily modifiable risk factors (see Chapter 28): practice nurses, particularly, have a central role to play in prevention.
- Early recognition of stroke (or TIA) can be lifesaving. The Act FAST campaign (www.nhs.uk/actfast) is an example of public health education and promotion related to early recognition and action. FAST is an abbreviation for:
  - Face (face fallen to one side, inability to smile);
  - Arms (inability to raise arms and keep them raised);
  - Speech (slurring or inability to speak or understand);
  - Time (call 999 immediately if you see any of the above).
- Nursing care in both hospitals and the community (in people's homes, residential homes and nursing homes) will focus on the immediate management of stroke and rehabilitation.
- Providing the best stroke care involves every member of the healthcare multi-disciplinary team as well as colleagues working in social services and housing departments.
- Immediate acute stroke care will focus on minimising brain damage and resultant physical, cognitive and communication disabilities, providing appropriate and accurate information and reassurance to the patient and their family/carers, ensuring the patient is nursed in a safe and comfortable environment (e.g. careful positioning in bed, chairs ensuring appropriate support of e.g. weakened limbs) and dealing with symptoms as they present (e.g. swallowing, speech and cognition difficulties as well as alterations to mobility and the ability to undertake usual activities of daily living).
- Following stabilisation of a person's condition nursing attention should re-focus to observations for deterioration due to, for example, a second stroke, infection (pneumonia) or VTE and rehabilitation. Rehabilitation will involve working closely with physiotherapists, occupational therapists, speech and language therapists and the patient's family/carers.
- People who have had strokes recover in different ways – some make a complete recovery, some have minimal residual disabilities, some have severe disabilities and require ongoing complete care.

Everyone recovers at a different pace so individualised care is especially important.
- After a stroke, people may have ongoing problems that require skilled advice and help from practice nurses, community nurses and specialist stroke nurses. These problems could include:
  - one-sided weakness of their body affecting, for example, mobility and day-to-day functioning;
  - balance and coordination resulting in, for example, falls, unsteadiness, loss of confidence and isolation;
  - swallowing resulting in, for example, drooling, choking, aspiration pneumonia and malnutrition;
  - speech, communication and cognition (e.g. finding the correct words, not being able to speak, not being able to understand);
  - visual difficulties (e.g. double vision or loss of visual field);
  - inappropriate emotions (e.g. crying or laughing for no particular reason);
  - tiredness.
- Depression is a common sequel to stroke and nurses should be aware of this and make a referral to the GP or consultant if they suspect it.

# Diagnosis

- History taking
- Examination
- Brain imaging (CT and MRI)
- Scan of carotid arteries
- Blood tests.

# Essentials of best practice

Nursing care needs to focus skilfully and sensitively on the individual's presenting and residual signs and symptoms. Stroke is a sudden, frightening and, for many, devastating, illness with long-term physical, emotional, psychological and social implications affecting many aspects of life.

Nursing care is likely to focus on:
✓ Accurate assessments and regular monitoring
✓ Symptom control and management
✓ Communication with the healthcare team, patient and family
✓ Health education and promotion
✓ Risk assessment and management
✓ Discharge planning

---

**Patient information**

The Stroke Association offers information, a helpline and funds research into stroke: www.stroke.org.uk.
Age UK www.ageuk.org.uk.
You will also find very helpful patient-centred fact sheets www.patient.co.uk/.

# 85 Nursing people with multiple sclerosis

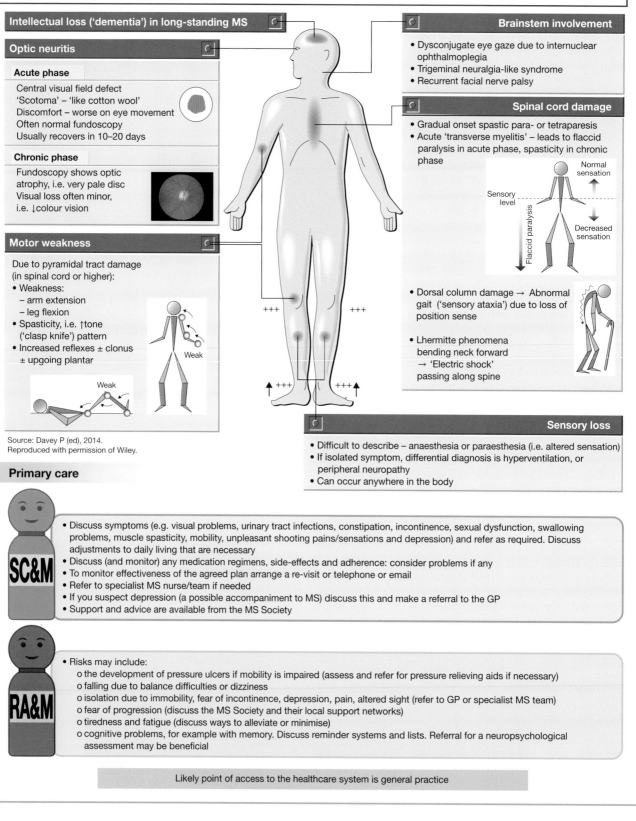

**Multiple sclerosis**

**Intellectual loss ('dementia') in long-standing MS**

**Optic neuritis**

**Acute phase**

Central visual field defect
'Scotoma' – 'like cotton wool'
Discomfort – worse on eye movement
Often normal fundoscopy
Usually recovers in 10–20 days

**Chronic phase**

Fundoscopy shows optic atrophy, i.e. very pale disc
Visual loss often minor, i.e. ↓colour vision

**Motor weakness**

Due to pyramidal tract damage (in spinal cord or higher):
• Weakness:
 – arm extension
 – leg flexion
• Spasticity, i.e. ↑tone ('clasp knife') pattern
• Increased reflexes ± clonus ± upgoing plantar

Weak

Weak

+++ +++

+++ +++

Source: Davey P (ed), 2014.
Reproduced with permission of Wiley.

**Brainstem involvement**

• Dysconjugate eye gaze due to internuclear ophthalmoplegia
• Trigeminal neuralgia-like syndrome
• Recurrent facial nerve palsy

**Spinal cord damage**

• Gradual onset spastic para- or tetraparesis
• Acute 'transverse myelitis' – leads to flaccid paralysis in acute phase, spasticity in chronic phase

Normal sensation

Sensory level

Flaccid paralysis

Decreased sensation

• Dorsal column damage → Abnormal gait ('sensory ataxia') due to loss of position sense

• Lhermitte phenomena bending neck forward → 'Electric shock' passing along spine

**Sensory loss**

• Difficult to describe – anaesthesia or paraesthesia (i.e. altered sensation)
• If isolated symptom, differential diagnosis is hyperventilation, or peripheral neuropathy
• Can occur anywhere in the body

**Primary care**

**SC&M**

• Discuss symptoms (e.g. visual problems, urinary tract infections, constipation, incontinence, sexual dysfunction, swallowing problems, muscle spasticity, mobility, unpleasant shooting pains/sensations and depression) and refer as required. Discuss adjustments to daily living that are necessary
• Discuss (and monitor) any medication regimens, side-effects and adherence: consider problems if any
• To monitor effectiveness of the agreed plan arrange a re-visit or telephone or email
• Refer to specialist MS nurse/team if needed
• If you suspect depression (a possible accompaniment to MS) discuss this and make a referral to the GP
• Support and advice are available from the MS Society

**RA&M**

• Risks may include:
 o the development of pressure ulcers if mobility is impaired (assess and refer for pressure relieving aids if necessary)
 o falling due to balance difficulties or dizziness
 o isolation due to immobility, fear of incontinence, depression, pain, altered sight (refer to GP or specialist MS team)
 o fear of progression (discuss the MS Society and their local support networks)
 o tiredness and fatigue (discuss ways to alleviate or minimise)
 o cognitive problems, for example with memory. Discuss reminder systems and lists. Referral for a neuropsychological assessment may be beneficial

Likely point of access to the healthcare system is general practice

*Adult Nursing at a Glance*, First Edition. Andrée le May. © 2015 John Wiley & Sons, Ltd. Published 2015 by John Wiley & Sons, Ltd.
Companion website: www.ataglanceseries.com/nursing/adult

## Key facts

• Multiple sclerosis (MS) is caused by a loss of myelin in the brain and spinal cord. This compromises the passage of the nerve impulse. As myelin loss increases more axons fail to function and permanent disabilities arise. MS is an ongoing, progressive condition that cannot be cured.

• MS is a relatively common disease (lifetime risk = 2–5/1000 in the UK) diagnosed in people usually between the ages of 20–40. More women than men have MS.

• MS is thought to be an altered immune response to parts of the CNS. It may have genetic and/or environmental (e.g. viral or toxins) triggers.

• MS presents with a variety of signs and symptoms (above).

• MS is generally, initially, characterised by periods of relapse and remission. This remitting/relapsing pattern is unpredictable and so can be disquieting for both the patient and their family.

• As MS progresses in different ways and at different speeds in different people it is important to care for each person as an individual and address each of their difficulties as they occur. Nursing (and multi-disciplinary) care should focus on physical, environmental, social and psychological aspects of care.

• Medical treatments may focus on reducing the severity and length of acute relapses (corticosteroids may be used, although over time they may become less effective) and symptom management. Some drugs (e.g. β-interferon, copaxone) can reduce the number of relapses but nothing is yet available to cure MS or stop its progression.

• In the longer term, as MS progresses and remissions cease or become infrequent, care may focus on symptom management and the adaptations needed to manage the disease alongside daily living. In this instance the importance of physiotherapy and occupational therapy is immense.

• People with MS may experience problems such as urinary tract infections, constipation, incontinence, sexual dysfunction, muscle spasticity, immobility, unpleasant shooting pains/sensations and depression. Each will need to be addressed in a way to suit the patient and their family/carers. People with MS may also be at risk of pressure ulcers if their mobility is compromised.

• Nurses in primary care and those working in the community, occupational health nurses and acute hospital nurses may all provide care to people with MS. As MS is a progressive disease, nurses providing palliative and end of life care may also work with people with MS and their families and carers (although MS may not significantly shorten life-span).

## Diagnosis

• History taking
• Examination
• Brain imaging.

## Essentials of best practice

Nursing care will largely focus on risk assessment and management and symptom control and management and will mostly occur in primary care (above). Specialist nurses for MS are available for advice both within the NHS and through the MS Society.

Nursing care is likely to focus on:

✓ Accurate assessments and regular monitoring
✓ Symptom control and management
✓ Communication with the healthcare team, patient and family
✓ Risk assessment and management

### Patient information

Multiple Sclerosis Society provides support and information about MS: www.mssociety.org.uk/.
You will also find very helpful patient-centred fact sheets at www.patient.co.uk/.

# 86 Nursing people with Parkinson's disease

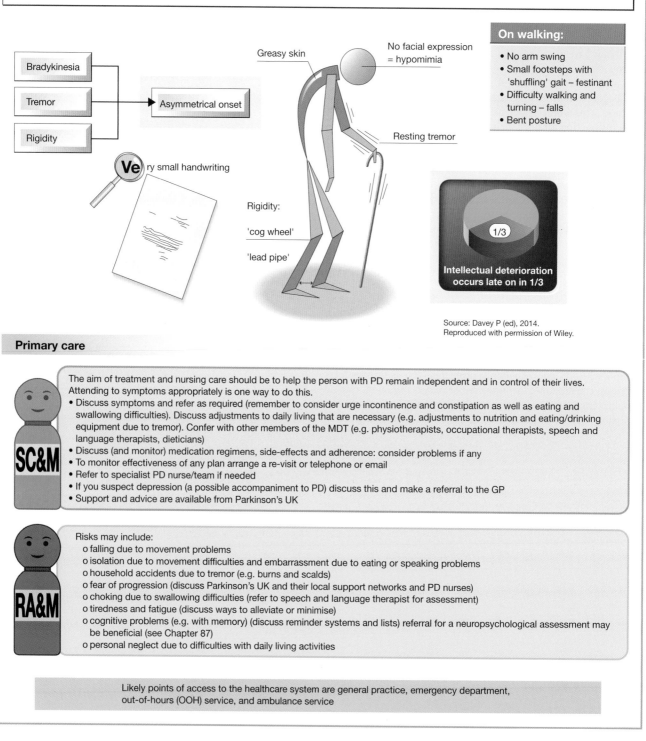

**Parkinson's disease**

Bradykinesia

Tremor

Rigidity

Asymmetrical onset

Greasy skin

No facial expression = hypomimia

**On walking:**
- No arm swing
- Small footsteps with 'shuffling' gait – festinant
- Difficulty walking and turning – falls
- Bent posture

Resting tremor

**Ve**ry small handwriting

Rigidity:

'cog wheel'

'lead pipe'

1/3

Intellectual deterioration occurs late on in 1/3

Source: Davey P (ed), 2014.
Reproduced with permission of Wiley.

## Primary care

**SC&M**

The aim of treatment and nursing care should be to help the person with PD remain independent and in control of their lives. Attending to symptoms appropriately is one way to do this.
- Discuss symptoms and refer as required (remember to consider urge incontinence and constipation as well as eating and swallowing difficulties). Discuss adjustments to daily living that are necessary (e.g. adjustments to nutrition and eating/drinking equipment due to tremor). Confer with other members of the MDT (e.g. physiotherapists, occupational therapists, speech and language therapists, dieticians)
- Discuss (and monitor) medication regimens, side-effects and adherence: consider problems if any
- To monitor effectiveness of any plan arrange a re-visit or telephone or email
- Refer to specialist PD nurse/team if needed
- If you suspect depression (a possible accompaniment to PD) discuss this and make a referral to the GP
- Support and advice are available from Parkinson's UK

**RA&M**

Risks may include:
- o falling due to movement problems
- o isolation due to movement difficulties and embarrassment due to eating or speaking problems
- o household accidents due to tremor (e.g. burns and scalds)
- o fear of progression (discuss Parkinson's UK and their local support networks and PD nurses)
- o choking due to swallowing difficulties (refer to speech and language therapist for assessment)
- o tiredness and fatigue (discuss ways to alleviate or minimise)
- o cognitive problems (e.g. with memory) (discuss reminder systems and lists) referral for a neuropsychological assessment may be beneficial (see Chapter 87)
- o personal neglect due to difficulties with daily living activities

Likely points of access to the healthcare system are general practice, emergency department, out-of-hours (OOH) service, and ambulance service

*Adult Nursing at a Glance*, First Edition. Andrée le May. © 2015 John Wiley & Sons, Ltd. Published 2015 by John Wiley & Sons, Ltd.
Companion website: www.ataglanceseries.com/nursing/adult

# Key facts

- Parkinson's disease (PD) is characterised by slow movements, resting tremor, rigidity and postural instability (above). All of these may result in falls. For some people intellectual deterioration, incontinence and constipation can also occur.
- PD is caused by a loss, in the brain, of dopamine-producing cells in the substantia nigra and the presence of Lewy bodies. Lewy bodies are small proteins that alter the action of dopamine and acetylcholine. Dopamine is essential for the control of movement, posture and coordination.
- PD cannot be cured and is a progressive disease. Symptoms can usually be controlled by treatments that increase dopamine levels in the CNS. L-dopa may be one treatment; others may focus on stimulating CNS dopamine receptors (e.g. dopamine agonists – pramipexole or apomorphine).
- Drug side-effects such as involuntary movement disorders (dyskinesia) can occur. In some people dopamine agonists may induce bizarre side-effects such as excessive gambling and hyper-sexuality and so their effects should be monitored carefully.
- PD is usually associated with increased age; however this is not always the case.
- Some types of PD may be linked to particular gene mutations. Some PD types are hereditary.
- PD will progress differently in different people so it is important to care for each person as an individual and address each of their difficulties as they occur. Nursing (and multi-disciplinary) care should focus on physical, environmental, social and psychological aspects of care.
- PD-like symptoms may also be a side-effect of some drugs such as anti-emetics, neuroleptics and lithium. Stopping the drug should stop the symptoms.

- Nurses in primary care and those working in the community, occupational health nurses and acute hospital nurses may all provide care to people with PD. As PD is a progressive disease, nurses providing palliative and end of life care may also become involved in care.

# Diagnosis

- History taking: falls may be the reason for consultation
- Examination (opposite for signs and symptoms)
- Brain imaging is likely to be normal.

# Essentials of best practice

Nursing care will mostly occur in primary care (above). Specialist nurses for PD are available for advice both within the NHS and from Parkinson's UK.
Nursing care is likely to focus on:
✓ Accurate assessments and regular monitoring
✓ Symptom control and management
✓ Communication with the healthcare team, patient and family
✓ Risk assessment and management

## Patient information

Parkinson's UK provides support and information about PD: www. parkinsons.org.uk/.
You will also find very helpful patient-centred fact sheets at www. patient.co.uk/.

# 87 Nursing people with dementia

## Types of dementia

| Dementia | Symptoms and signs | Pathology | Treatment |
|---|---|---|---|
| Alzheimer's disease | Episodic memory loss with gradual worsening. Initially new memory cannot be laid down but long-term memory may be intact – later no memory recalled<br>Confusion<br>Altered reasoning/thinking abilities<br>Mood changes<br>Difficulty communicating<br>Relentless deterioration | Cortical neuron loss (loss of cholinergic neurons)<br>Some familial inheritance seen | e.g. Aricept maintains existing levels of acetylcholine so may be beneficial for a short period of time<br>Symptom management |
| Vascular dementia | Progressive cognitive impairment (loss of memory and reasoning/thinking abilities) due to multiple small infarcts<br>Episodic deterioration<br>Difficulty with visuoperceptual tasks<br>Small stepping gait | Vascular lesions in brain | e.g. reducing vascular diseases risk factors (treating hypertension) and low dose aspirin may slow progress<br>Symptom management |
| Dementia with Lewy bodies (DLB) | Fluctuating cognitive abilities<br>Nocturnal visual hallucinations<br>Disordered REM sleep<br>Slow movements, stiffness, tremor, loss of facial expression (similar to PD) | The presence of Lewy bodies disrupts normal brain function by altering the action of the neurotransmitters dopamine and acetylcholine. (DLB shares some of the characteristics of PD and Alzheimer's disease) | Symptom management |
| Frontotemporal dementia (FTD) | Personality change<br>Disinhibited behaviours<br>Loss of interest in people and activities<br>Memory may be preserved<br>Language may be affected (slow hesitant speech: poor understanding of sentences) | Atrophy of the frontal and temporal lobes | Symptom management |

## Primary and hospital care

**SC&M**

The aim of treatment and nursing care should be to help the person with dementia remain independent and in control of their lives for as long as possible: attending to symptoms appropriately and supporting family/carers in doing this is one way to achieve this
- Discuss symptoms and review regularly with the person with dementia and their family/carers (remember to consider incontinence, behaviour changes and risks related to worsening or new symptoms)
- Discuss adjustments to daily living that are necessary with the person with dementia and their family/carers. Confer with other members of the MDT (e.g. physiotherapists, occupational therapists, speech and language therapists, psychologists, specialist dementia nurses and CMHNs)
- Discuss (and monitor) any medication regimens, side-effects and adherence: consider problems if any
- To monitor effectiveness of new care plans, arrange a re-visit or telephone or email
- Refer to specialist dementia nurse/team if needed
- If you suspect depression (a possible accompaniment to dementia for both the person with dementia and their carers) discuss this and make a referral to the GP/mental health team
- Support and advice is available from many charities and support groups (below), encourage carers to access this

**RA&M**

Risks may include:
  o wandering and falls
  o isolation due to cognitive impairment or behavioural change
  o disorientation due to memory loss (the need for constant reminders is important but may be frustrating/wearing for carers)
  o household accidents (e.g. forgetting about food left cooking, irons etc. left on, front doors open)
  o tiredness and fatigue of carers (discuss ways to alleviate or minimise)
  o inability to undertake daily living activities

Likely points of access to the healthcare system are general practice, emergency department, out-of-hours (OOH) service, and ambulance service

*Adult Nursing at a Glance*, First Edition. Andrée le May. © 2015 John Wiley & Sons, Ltd. Published 2015 by John Wiley & Sons, Ltd.
Companion website: www.ataglanceseries.com/nursing/adult

# Key facts

- Dementia is a global impairment of cognition with normal levels of consciousness (NB: by contrast in acute confusional states consciousness is impaired).
- Dementia is generally a disease of old age. The more common types are detailed opposite. However, younger people may have dementia due to HIV, vasculitis, new variant CJD (Creutzfeldt-Jakob disease) or end-stage multiple sclerosis.
- The early stages of dementia can be hard to detect reliably so referral to the GP or memory clinic is important.
- It is sometimes hard to determine the specific type of dementia that affects people, so it is wise to focus on the impact of the dementia and how nursing care can be best used to improve the quality of life of not only the person with dementia but also their family and carers.
- Having dementia will result in increased dependence on others to maintain activities of daily living.
- Dementia cannot be cured and is a progressive disease: progress can be slowed in some people by early treatments (below).
- For the majority of people with dementia, deterioration in memory and thinking abilities will also eventually be accompanied by physical decline (e.g. incontinence of urine and faeces).
- Providing the best care for someone with dementia will require the efforts of the entire multi-disciplinary team since attention will need to be given to the physical, environmental, social, emotional and psychological aspects of care. Family and carers will also need high levels of support and advice. Balancing the needs of the family/carer with the needs of the person with dementia is sometimes complex and challenging.
- Dementia will progress differently in different people so it is important to care for each person as an individual and address each of their difficulties as they occur. The goal of nursing is to achieve person-centred care delivered in a safe environment.
- All nurses will provide care to people with dementia either focusing specifically on dementia care or on other acute illnesses or disorders experienced by a person with dementia. As dementia is a progressive disease, and naturally associated with the later stages of life, nurses providing palliative and end of life care will also become involved.
- Some nurses specialise in dementia care (e.g. those working in community mental health teams and Admiral Nurses working alongside Dementia UK). Many wards in acute hospitals will have a nurse identified as a dementia champion too: these nurses have specialist knowledge of the needs of people with dementia.

# Diagnosis

- History taking from the patient and family
- Examination (including mental tests focusing on orientation, long- and short-term memory and concentration)
- Blood tests largely to assess general health
- Brain imaging (CT and MRI)

# Essentials of best practice

Nursing care will mostly occur in the community either through community nurses visiting older people for other reasons or practice nurses monitoring dementia progression. Much of the care needed around activities of daily living will be given by healthcare support workers and close liaison between them and the nursing team is required to ensure high quality seamless care.

In hospital, particularly, people with dementia may feel isolated and disorientated: they will easily forget why they are there, what they have been asked to do and who you are. Providing the best nursing care may feel challenging but can be achieved through ensuring that a consistent approach to care is given by all nurses involved. Repeated gentle reminders about the reason for their stay in hospital, your name and who you are and the treatments/care you are proposing are all important ways through which nurses can increase a person's compliance with care and also their feelings of safety and security. Creating a 'dementia friendly' environment is another way of doing this and can be achieved through the use of easily readable signs, colour coding different areas in the wards (e.g. toilets and bathroom floors/doors painted a different colour to others) and the reduction of distracting noises such as TVs, radios. Ensuring privacy and time to talk about what is happening is also an important facet of care.

Understanding and integrating the person's individual dementia focused needs with the specifics of care required by their hospitalisation (e.g. infection, fracture, exacerbation of underlying chronic illness) is the goal of care during hospital admissions. This will require nurses to work creatively with the multi-disciplinary team and the patient's family and carers.

Nursing care is likely to focus on:

✓ Accurate assessments and regular monitoring
✓ Symptom control and management
✓ Communication with the healthcare team, patient and family
✓ Risk assessment and management

## Patient information

Dementia UK provides support and information about various types of dementia and advice about Admiral Nurses www.dementiauk.org.uk/.
Advice and information may also be obtained from:
The Alzheimer's Society www.alzheimers.org.uk.
Alzheimer Scotland www.alzscot.org.
Age UK www.ageuk.org.uk.
Frontotemporal Dementia Support Group www.ftdsg.org/.
Lewy Body Society www.lewybody.org.
You will also find very helpful patient-centred fact sheets at www.patient.co.uk/.

# Nursing people with disorders of the eye or ear

## A and P

### The eye

Superior view of transverse section of right eyeball

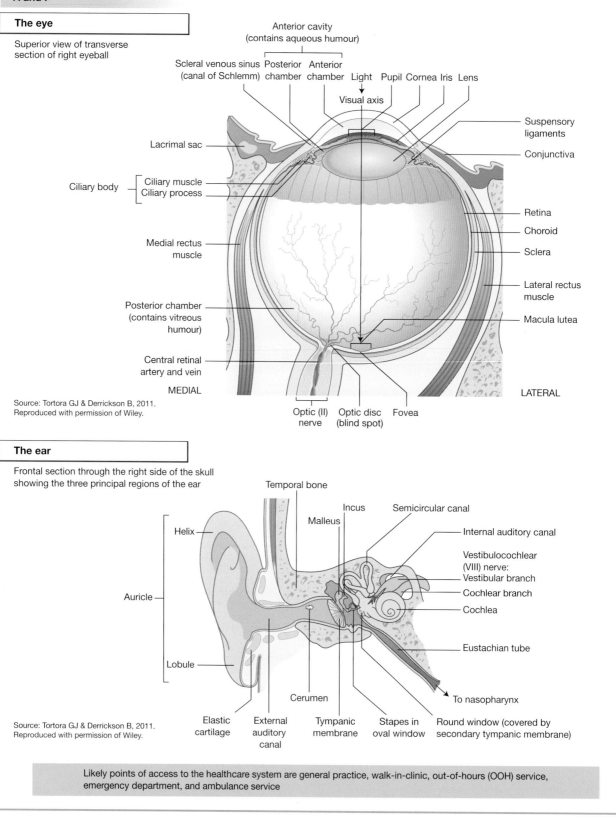

Source: Tortora GJ & Derrickson B, 2011.
Reproduced with permission of Wiley.

### The ear

Frontal section through the right side of the skull showing the three principal regions of the ear

Source: Tortora GJ & Derrickson B, 2011.
Reproduced with permission of Wiley.

Likely points of access to the healthcare system are general practice, walk-in-clinic, out-of-hours (OOH) service, emergency department, and ambulance service

*Adult Nursing at a Glance*, First Edition. Andrée le May. © 2015 John Wiley & Sons, Ltd. Published 2015 by John Wiley & Sons, Ltd.
Companion website: www.ataglanceseries.com/nursing/adult

# Key facts

• Seeing and hearing are central to understanding what is going on around us and communication. Alterations in our ability to do either (or both) can be disorientating and isolating.

• Assessing the eye can tell healthcare professionals a lot about a person's general health and specific illnesses (e.g. the sclera may be yellowed in jaundice: pupil size and reactivity can reveal neurological problems).

# Common eye disorders

• Red eye
• Glaucoma
• Cataract
• Macular degeneration.

# Common ear disorders

• Hearing loss
• Vertigo
• Tinnitus.

Each of the above is covered in the following pages together with associated signs and symptoms.

# A and P

## The eyes

• The eye's structure (opposite) comprises a three layered wall surrounding two main cavities (the anterior cavity and the posterior chamber – sometimes called the vitreous chamber): the anterior cavity is also divided into an anterior and posterior portion. The anterior cavity is filled with aqueous humour which brings nutrients to and takes waste from the eye. The posterior chamber is filled with shape-stabilising vitreous humour.

• The three-layered wall of the eye is made up of a fibrous tunic, vascular tunic and neural tunic. The fibrous outer tunic contains the tough, protective sclera (the white of the eye) and the cornea (transparent). The middle layer, the vascular tunic (also called the uvea), contains blood and lymph vessels as well as smooth muscles. It is made up of:

  • the iris (central coloured part of the eye) which regulates light entry. The pupil is the opening at the centre of the iris and is controlled by pupillary constrictor and dilator muscles; these in turn are controlled by the nervous system. The iris is attached to the muscular ciliary body, which contracts and relaxes to change the shape of the lens when focusing on objects at varying distances;

  • the choroid is a vascular, dark brown layer between the fibrous tunic and the neural tunic. This layer's capillaries take oxygen and nutrients to the retina.

• The neural tunic (retina) is associated with light absorption. Two types of photosensitive nerves, rods (which enable seeing in low levels of light) and cones (which enable seeing in bright light, colour vision and seeing detail) are found in the retina. The eye's lens focuses light onto the retina. Information is then sent from the retina, via the optic nerve (cranial nerve II) for deciphering by the brain. The macula is the central area of the retina where the main focus of the light falls and because of the density of the cones in this area it allows detailed vision.

• The retina is a delicate web of millions of specialised nerve cells and can become detached from the choroid, spontaneously or after injury, causing blindness.

• Accessory structures around the eye prevent damage (e.g. the eyelids blink continuously to keep each eye free from dust and the surface of the eye lubricated: eye lashes keep foreign matter from falling into the eye: tears wash the eyes and keep the conjunctiva clean (they are bactericidal) and lubricated).

## The ears

• The ear comprises the outer ear, the middle ear and the inner ear (opposite). The external auditory canal (meatus) is a narrow, s-shaped passage that extends from the auricle to the tympanic membrane (ear drum). It can become blocked with wax or foreign bodies. Sound travels along the meatus to the bones of the middle ear.

• The middle ear (tympanic cavity) is a small, air-filled cavity closed at one end by the ear drum and at the other by bone with two openings – the oval and the round windows. The eustachian tube (linked so it can equalise pressures on both sides of the ear drum) connects the middle ear and the nasopharynx. The malleus (hammer), incus (anvil) and stapes (stirrup) bones conduct sound vibrations between the ear drum and the receptors in the inner ear.

• The inner ear is associated with hearing and balance. It comprises a series of canals which form what is known as a labyrinth (the bony labyrinth and the membranous labyrinth).

• The bony labyrinth contains the semi-circular canals and the vestibule (balance) and the cochlea (hearing): it also contains the fluid filled sacs of the membranous labyrinth.

• The hair cell cilia in the organ of Corti in the cochlear duct are critical to hearing, distorting as sound passes through them and releasing neurotransmitters.

• Information about these sounds is then transferred to the brain by the cochlear branch of the vestibulocochlear nerve (cranial nerve VIII) for processing.

# Essentials of best practice

Disorders of the eyes and ears can range from mild to severe. Nursing someone with any of these disorders may take place in the GP surgery, the person's home, the ED or OOH service or in a specialist hospital ward or out-patient's clinic. All nurses will at some time in their careers provide care to people who have either (or both) visual or auditory problems, since diminishing sight and hearing are a natural consequence of growing older. The essentials of best practice required to care for people with common disorders of the eye and ear are covered in the subsequent pages.

## Patient information

There are several patient support groups and charities focusing on disorders of the eye/ear. You can find most of them on the Self Help UK website www.self-help.org.uk.
You will also find very helpful patient-centred fact sheets at www.patient.co.uk/.

# 89 Nursing people with disorders of the eye

## Red Eye

| Diagnosis | How common 1 = very common 6 = very rare | Symptoms especially | | Signs | Treatment |
|-----------|------------|---------------------|--|-------|-----------|
| **Conjunctivitis** Infective Dry eye Allergic | 1 1 2 | Sticky Gritty Itchy Stringy discharge | | Redness entire surface, eye and two lid linings | Topical chloramphenicol Topical lubricants Topical mast stabiliser |
| **Episcleritis** | 2 | Irritation | | Sectorial redness, eye only | None? |
| **Iritis** (anterior uveitis) | 3 | Pain, moderate Photophobia | | Redness, eye only around cornea ± small pupil | Topical corticosteroid and dilate |
| **Corneal** (keratitis) | 4 | Pain, sharp Photophobia Watering | | Local redness and corneal stain | Topical antiviral |
| **Scleritis** | 5 | Pain, may be severe, may increase on eye movement | | Intense redness, eye only | Systemic with corticosteroid and cytotoxic? |
| **Acute glaucoma** | 6 | Pain, aching Vomit | | Intense redness, eye only ± large fixed pupil | Topical after diagnosis Acetazolamide also? |

Source: Davey P (ed), 2014. Reproduced with permission of Wiley.

## Assessment of the eye includes:

**A&M**

- Asking about symptoms (above), their history and precipitating factors: check about pain and photophobia (NB: photophobia may be indicative of some infections, e.g. meningitis)
- Looking in both eyes (comparing one with the other) (you may need to use a pen torch and gloves). Looking at both eyes (e.g. for one-sided eyelid drooping or uneven pupils)
- Asking about sight and alterations to normal habits (e.g. reading, TV watching) or activities (NB: poor sight may be linked to falls, isolation and loss of confidence): remember to ask about glasses/lens, when optician was last visited
- Asking about distortions of vision (blurred, tunnel, double vision, flashing lights, difficulty in seeing in the dark) and headaches
- Advising about actions – referral to a GP or optician

## Some useful pointers for good eye health include:

**HE&P**

- Having regular eye tests and contacting an optician/GP if changes to vision occur
- Wearing sunglasses with a UV filter (strong sunlight can be damaging, e.g. cataracts)
- Eating a balanced diet rich in vitamin A
- Smoking has been linked to cataract formation and macular degeneration so stopping smoking should be advised
- Keeping within a healthy weight is also important in preventing age related diabetes which in turn may impact on sight (diabetic retinopathy)
- Wearing eye protection when doing tasks that might cause eye injury
- Seeking advice if eyes become infected/red from the GP
- Keeping a check on underlying health problems that might affect the eyes (e.g. diabetes, hypertension)

*Adult Nursing at a Glance*, First Edition. Andrée le May. © 2015 John Wiley & Sons, Ltd. Published 2015 by John Wiley & Sons, Ltd.
Companion website: www.ataglanceseries.com/nursing/adult

# Key facts

- Disorders of the eye are usually associated with infection, allergy and/or ageing.
- Red eye (above) is caused by inflammation of the eye's surface (either the conjunctiva or the episclera). Treatment is usually topical directly applied to the eye either as ointments/drops: some problems may require oral corticosteroids.
- Being diagnosed with a long-term eye condition is likely to cause anxiety because of fear of sight loss. Sensitive and appropriate education, reassurance and monitoring should form the basis of skilled nursing care in these instances.
- Some eye disorders such as glaucoma can be inherited so regular monitoring by an ophthalmologist will be needed.
- Glaucoma causes damage to the optic nerve because of increased intra-ocular pressure. Glaucoma may occur at any age but more commonly after the age of 40. Glaucoma may be acute (above) or chronic. In chronic glaucoma symptoms are usually noticed when peripheral vision lessens (tunnel-like). The aim of treatment in both acute and chronic glaucoma is to reduce damage (repair of already acquired loss of vision is not possible in chronic glaucoma): options include eye drops to lower intraocular pressure by reducing the amount of aqueous fluid produced and increasing the opening of the drainage channels in the eye. Laser surgery, performed under local anaesthetic as a day case/out-patient, may also be used to improve drainage. Nursing care for people with glaucoma will focus on teaching eye drop use and monitoring compliance (in some instances, if e.g. manual dexterity is compromised, drops will need administering). If surgery is performed, care will focus also on information giving and reassurance.
- Many people, as they grow older, experience age-related changes to their eyes such as macular degeneration and the formation of cataracts.
- It is particularly important that older people are screened for macular degeneration (and are aware of what to look out for). Age-related macular degeneration (AMD) affects a small area of the retina called the macula causing distortion (e.g. wavy rather than straight lines) and blurring of central vision which may eventually progress to seeing just a blank patch. AMD won't lead to total loss of sight and is not painful but is very distressing as it impacts on daily living and recreational activities (e.g. reading, watching television, films, looking at photographs etc.). Regular review by an ophthalmologist is important if a person is diagnosed with AMD.
- There are two types of age-related macular degeneration – wet and dry. Wet AMD is the more serious but less common (~10–15% of people with AMD). In wet AMD new blood vessels replace defective ones; however, they grow in the wrong place causing bleeding and swelling below the macula, resulting in macular scarring. If untreated wet AMD can progress rapidly causing severe damage to central vision. Rapid treatment to stop blood vessel growth is needed.
- Dry AMD progresses more slowly. There is no treatment and so attention focuses on environmental changes (e.g. better lighting, magnifiers) to make the most of remaining central vision. Referral to a low vision service linked to the local hospital/local authority may be helpful.
- Cataracts form when the lens of the eye becomes opaque as a result of ageing/trauma/disease (e.g. diabetes). Cataracts are common so nurses will frequently care for a person with cataracts – being aware of their effects is therefore important.
- Seeing through a cataract is often described as looking through a frosted window (e.g. a gradual dimming, reduced distance vision and alterations to colour and depth perception). These alterations will impact on a person's usual activities making some routines difficult (e.g. reading small print, seeing the edge of stairs, feeling confident walking in unfamiliar places). Replacing the opaque lens with an artificial lens (intraocular lens implantation) under a local anaesthetic is the preferred treatment. Lens replacement usually requires a short stay in hospital as a day patient, preceded by pre-operative assessment of eye and general health; after the operation ongoing care at home is focused on the instillation of eye drops (usually by the person although for some people extra help will be required to do this effectively).

# Essentials of best practice

Nursing someone with an eye disorder will mainly occur in the community (within a person's home/nursing home/residential home), GP practices, specialist out-patients' departments, walk-in-clinics or in a specialist eye unit (usually as a day case). Care will largely focus on:

✓ Accurate assessment and regular monitoring (e.g. cataracts)
✓ Communication with the healthcare team, patient and family
✓ Symptom control and management (e.g. advise about low vision equipment and referral to support services)
✓ Health education and promotion (e.g. about diet, medication and maintaining good eye health (above))
✓ Risk assessment and management (e.g. extra attention to prevent trips or falls)
✓ Discharge planning (post-discharge medication and signs and symptoms of complications e.g. infections)

Help may be needed, in or out of hospital, with activities of daily living if a patient has vision problems.

Some people may also need advice about supplementary benefits to enable them to make significant changes to their lives and referral to a social worker, specialist occupational therapist/sensory team or Citizen's Advice Bureau may be helpful.

---

**Patient information**

There are several useful charities and support groups:
The RNIB supports blind and partially sighted people and provides easily accessible information about sight www.rnib.org.uk.
The International Glaucoma Association: www.glaucoma-association.com.
The Macular Society: www.macularsociety.org.
You will also find very helpful patient-centred fact sheets at www.patient.co.uk.

# 90 Nursing people with disorders of the ear

### Assessment of the ear includes:

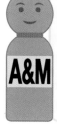

**A&M**

- Asking about hearing (e.g. muffled, tinnitus) and balance and any alterations over a given period of time to either or both of these. Ask how dizziness (vertigo) manifests so it can be distinguished from faintness/light headedness. (NB: dizziness may be linked to falls, poor hearing to isolation and loss of confidence). Ask how hearing/balance alteration affects usual routines
- Asking about symptoms related to hearing problems/vertigo, their history, effects and if any precipitating factors. For instance, people with ears blocked by wax may complain of a feeling of fullness, muffled hearing, squeaking and discomfort. Check for ear discharge and pain
- Observing for hearing difficulties (e.g. understanding conversations, loudness of speech, attentiveness to others): hearing aids (check batteries: and if appropriate connecting tubes for blockages)
- Observing for balance difficulties (holding onto chairs/furniture)
- Looking in both ears (comparing one with the other) e.g. for wax (cerumen) or other foreign objects in the external auditory canal
- Advising about actions – referral to a GP (if discharge for example) or audiologist

### Communicating with an older person who has a hearing loss should include:

**C**

- Finding out what helps the person to hear better: making sure hearing aids work and are correctly inserted (having a piece of paper and pen may also be useful: some people may prefer to use iPads/mobile phones to record information)
- Using charts, pictures etc. to help explain important points
- Facing the person when you're talking to them (many people lip read): ensuring that if they wear glasses they have them on to see you better
- Keeping your hands away from your face when speaking so you don't hide your mouth or facial expressions (which help to get your points across)
- Gaining the person's attention before beginning to speak (touch may be useful)
- Making sure you don't talk when you are moving around or when you have your back to them
- Reducing background noise prior to a conversation
- Checking understanding: restating information using different words if need be
- Leaving the call bell within reach if a person is in hospital or a nursing/residential home
- Considering other techniques that might help the person to hear you (ask relatives if there are particular things that help)

### Some useful pointers for good ear health include:

**HE&P**

- Having regular hearing tests may be just as important as regular eye tests for older people, especially if hearing is impaired. Finding out about hearing loss (and monitoring alterations) means that hearing aids and other resources may be used/updated quickly
- Contacting the practice nurse/GP for advice/information is always a good starting point. Practice nurses and health visitors should ask about hearing in routine health checks for older people
- Wearing hearing aids if fitted (sometimes people keep these for 'best' and then find it hard to fit or tolerate them). Maintaining hearing aids as advised by manufacturers and having them regularly serviced
- Removing wax if necessary. This involves a visit to (or from) the practice nurse or community nurse for ear irrigation (this process should adhere to the relevant local policy and guideline)

*Adult Nursing at a Glance*, First Edition. Andrée le May. © 2015 John Wiley & Sons, Ltd. Published 2015 by John Wiley & Sons, Ltd.
Companion website: www.ataglanceseries.com/nursing/adult

# Key facts

- The ear is responsible for hearing and balance.
- Disorders of the ear are usually associated with infection, trauma and/or ageing.
- Disorders associated with balance (vestibular problems) can occur for several reasons ranging from acute (or chronic) labyrinthitis (viral or inflammatory) to Ménière's disease (recurrent attacks of vertigo, tinnitus and hearing loss) to benign paroxysmal positional vertigo (associated with changing head positions). People with any of these will largely be cared for by GPs or at out-patients' appointments, thereby requiring minimal input from nurses.
- People affected by hearing loss, on the other hand, are often encountered by nurses working in many settings and need care tailored to their individual needs.
- Hearing loss in adults may be congenital or acquired, for example as a result of trauma (e.g. excess noise, head injury), illness (e.g. Ménière's disease) or ageing.
- There are two categories of hearing loss – conductive and sensorineural.
- Acute hearing loss may be caused by foreign bodies or an accumulation of wax in the external auditory canal or infection (e.g. otitis media). These sorts of problems prevent sound waves passing through to the cochlear (conduction deafness). Conductive hearing loss may be alleviated by removal of wax or foreign bodies or the treatment of infection with, if appropriate, antibiotics.
- Sensorineural deafness (e.g. age-related hearing loss, congenital malformations, Ménière's disease) is likely to be a result of a defect in the cochlea or its connecting nerve.
- Age-related hearing loss (presbycusis) is characterised by an inability to hear both high and low frequencies.
- Having a long-term hearing loss is likely to cause anxiety because of fear of social alienation.
- Hearing loss can result in exclusion from conversations, the usual hubbub of life, information, leisure activities and family and friends. All of these things can lead to isolation, frustration and depression.
- Sensitive and appropriate education, reassurance, referral for aids (e.g. hearing aids, amplified, vibrating and flashing phones/alarms) and monitoring of the use and effectiveness of any hearing aids should form the foundation of skilled nursing care for people with a hearing loss.
- Many people, as they grow older, experience natural age-related changes to their hearing so it is particularly important that older people, if they (or their family/friends) notice a hearing loss, are assessed and treated quickly. If hearing loss is confirmed, regular review by an audiologist is important to ensure the best hearing possible is achieved using aids and other hearing technologies.

# Essentials of best practice

Nursing someone with hearing loss can occur anywhere in the health and social care system.

Care will largely focus on:

✓ Communication with the healthcare team, patient and family (above)

✓ Symptom control and management (e.g. advise about hearing equipment and referral to support services)

✓ Health education and promotion (e.g. about hearing equipment and its use *and* maintenance: advice should be written and spoken)

✓ Risk assessment and management (e.g. extra attention to traffic and identifying alternative warning systems e.g. flashing, vibrating, and amplified fire alarms)

✓ Discharge planning (from any ward or unit in a hospital)

Hearing loss is isolating – some people will benefit from advice about clubs or societies which will cater for their needs as well as provide means through which they can join in activities they might have enjoyed in the past (e.g. going to specially signed theatre/cinema productions) and wish to continue enjoying. It is important for nurses to meet the social and psychological needs of people with sensory deficits and capitalise on their remaining abilities as well as meeting any physical/treatment needs they may have.

Some people may need advice about supplementary benefits to enable them to make significant changes to their lives, and referral to a social worker, specialist occupational therapist/sensory team or Citizen's Advice Bureau may be helpful.

## Patient information

There are several useful charities and support groups:

Action on Hearing Loss supports people with hearing disorders and provides easily accessible information and advice about hearing enhancing technologies: www.actiononhearingloss.org.uk.

The Ménière's Society: www.meniers.org.uk.

British Sign Language: www.britishsignlanguage.com.

You will also find very helpful patient-centred fact sheets at www.patient.co.uk.

# 91 Nursing people with disorders of the reproductive system and breast

## A and P

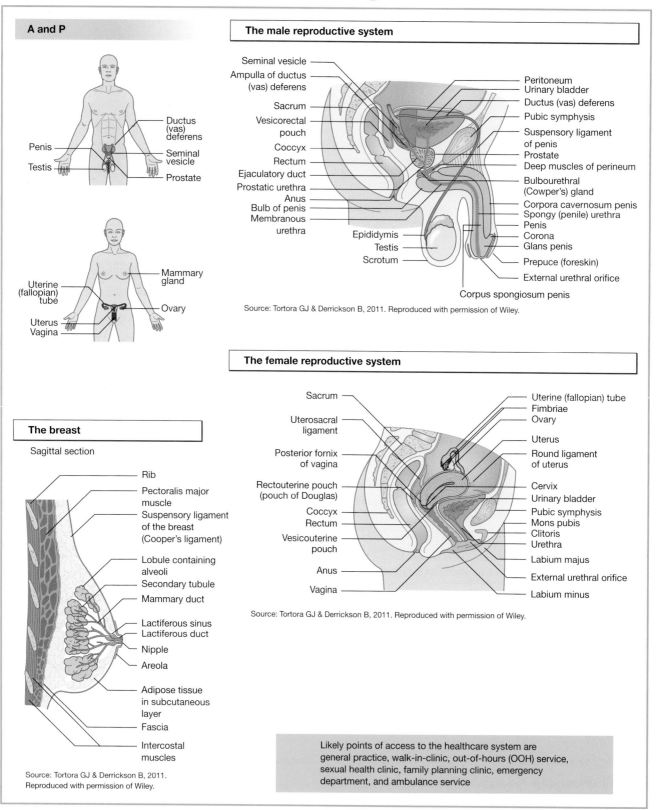

- Penis
- Testis
- Ductus (vas) deferens
- Seminal vesicle
- Prostate

- Uterine (fallopian) tube
- Uterus
- Vagina
- Mammary gland
- Ovary

## The male reproductive system

- Seminal vesicle
- Ampulla of ductus (vas) deferens
- Sacrum
- Vesicorectal pouch
- Coccyx
- Rectum
- Ejaculatory duct
- Prostatic urethra
- Anus
- Bulb of penis
- Membranous urethra
- Epididymis
- Testis
- Scrotum
- Peritoneum
- Urinary bladder
- Ductus (vas) deferens
- Pubic symphysis
- Suspensory ligament of penis
- Prostate
- Deep muscles of perineum
- Bulbourethral (Cowper's) gland
- Corpora cavernosum penis
- Spongy (penile) urethra
- Penis
- Corona
- Glans penis
- Prepuce (foreskin)
- External urethral orifice
- Corpus spongiosum penis

Source: Tortora GJ & Derrickson B, 2011. Reproduced with permission of Wiley.

## The female reproductive system

- Sacrum
- Uterosacral ligament
- Posterior fornix of vagina
- Rectouterine pouch (pouch of Douglas)
- Coccyx
- Rectum
- Vesicouterine pouch
- Anus
- Vagina
- Uterine (fallopian) tube
- Fimbriae
- Ovary
- Uterus
- Round ligament of uterus
- Cervix
- Urinary bladder
- Pubic symphysis
- Mons pubis
- Clitoris
- Urethra
- Labium majus
- External urethral orifice
- Labium minus

Source: Tortora GJ & Derrickson B, 2011. Reproduced with permission of Wiley.

## The breast

Sagittal section

- Rib
- Pectoralis major muscle
- Suspensory ligament of the breast (Cooper's ligament)
- Lobule containing alveoli
- Secondary tubule
- Mammary duct
- Lactiferous sinus
- Lactiferous duct
- Nipple
- Areola
- Adipose tissue in subcutaneous layer
- Fascia
- Intercostal muscles

Source: Tortora GJ & Derrickson B, 2011. Reproduced with permission of Wiley.

Likely points of access to the healthcare system are general practice, walk-in-clinic, out-of-hours (OOH) service, sexual health clinic, family planning clinic, emergency department, and ambulance service

*Adult Nursing at a Glance*, First Edition. Andrée le May. © 2015 John Wiley & Sons, Ltd. Published 2015 by John Wiley & Sons, Ltd.
Companion website: www.ataglanceseries.com/nursing/adult

# Key facts

• The reproductive system is the only system that is significantly different in men and women. Its ultimate purpose is to produce children however sexual reproduction is far more complex than just procreation because of its close ties to emotions and sexual desires.

• The breast is often seen as an integral part of the reproductive system in women because of its links, in many cultures, to sexuality and also the nurturing of babies.

• Whilst this section focuses mainly on anatomical and physiological aspects of the reproductive system and breasts, it is important to remember the importance of social, cultural and psychological norms and influences on sexual behaviour, sexuality and body image.

• The reproductive systems and breasts are influenced by (or influence) other systems particularly the endocrine system (see Chapter 66).

• Disorders of the reproductive systems and breasts can result in acute or chronic conditions.

# Common disorders

• Urethritis
• Vaginal discharge
• Prostatic hypertrophy
• Prostate cancer
• Uterine and ovarian disorders
• Breast lumps.

Each is covered in the following pages. Signs and symptoms associated with disorders of these systems are discussed in the following pages rather than collectively in one section.

# A and P

• The male reproductive system (above) comprises a penis, two testes held in a scrotum; the testes are made up of many sections containing 1–4 seminiferous tubules within which sperm are made. The Leydig cells situated between these tubules secrete testosterone and other male sex hormones. Once formed, sperm are transported to the epididymis to complete their maturation before moving to a vas deferens (there are two) and seminal vesicles. Each vas deferens and the duct of the seminal vesicles merge forming the paired ejaculatory ducts. Sperm are bathed in a fluid produced by the vas deferens, the seminal vesicles and the prostate gland ready for ejaculation from the ejaculatory ducts. This mix of sperm and fluid (semen) then passes through the prostate gland past the bulbourethral glands (which produce clear salty secretions lubricating the urethra) into the urethra of the penis and is expelled. Around 300 million sperm mature every day.

• Male sex hormones (androgens) (Chapter 67) control the functioning of the testes and also the development of the reproductive system during adolescence. Androgens include testosterone (androgens are also found, to a lesser extent, in women).

• The female reproductive system (opposite) comprises the vagina, clitoris, labia majora and minora, cervix, uterus, two fallopian tubes and two ovaries.

• The ovaries and uterus undergo cyclical changes during a woman's reproductive years under the control of many different hormones (above). These cycles can be altered by emotional and psychological factors, excessive exercise and malnutrition. They can also be artificially controlled with hormones or drugs, for example oral contraception pills/implants or infertility treatments.

• Breasts (also called mammary glands) are made of adipose (fat) tissue, fibrous connective tissue and glandular tissue (above). Breasts have several functions in women linked to sexual attractiveness and sexual arousal as well as milk production under the influence of prolactin (Chapter 67). Men's breasts are not as developed as women's and do not normally lactate.

# Essentials of best practice

Nursing someone with any disorder of the reproductive system or breasts requires you to be aware of all of the essentials of best practice. These will be expanded for the disorders listed above in the subsequent pages.

It is also important that nurses talk about sexuality, body image and sexual function in their overall assessments of people with, for example, long-term conditions which can affect sexual functioning (e.g. cardiac or respiratory conditions which might limit exercise and therefore be thought to impact on sexual activity too) or conditions which could alter perceptions of body image and attractiveness (e.g. skin conditions, disfiguring surgery of any kind).

## Patient information

There are several patient support groups and charities focusing on disorders of the reproductive systems and breasts. You can find most of them on the Self Help UK website http://www.self-help.org.uk.

You will also find very helpful patient-centred fact sheets at www.patient.co.uk/.

# 92 Nursing people with vaginal discharge or urethritis

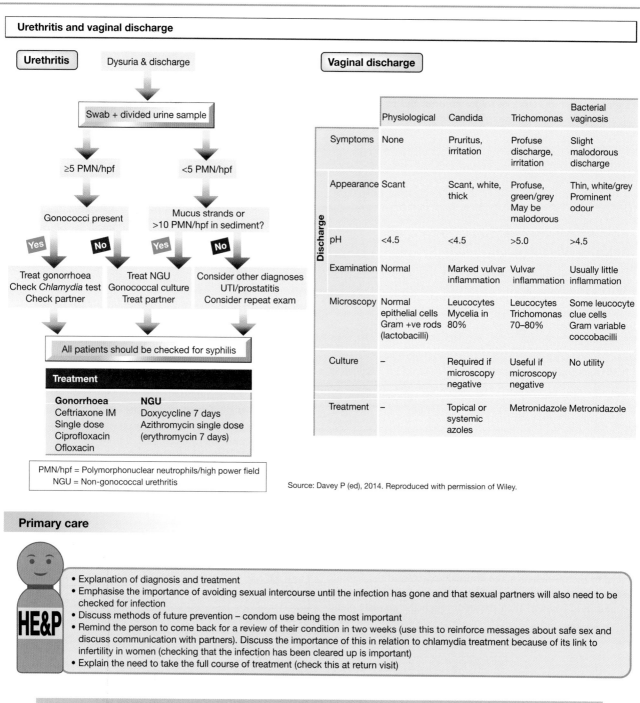

**Urethritis and vaginal discharge**

### Urethritis

Dysuria & discharge

↓

Swab + divided urine sample

↓                    ↓

≥5 PMN/hpf          <5 PMN/hpf

↓                    ↓

Gonococci present    Mucus strands or >10 PMN/hpf in sediment?

**Yes** / **No**        **Yes** / **No**

↓          ↓          ↓          ↓

Treat gonorrhoea / Check *Chlamydia* test / Check partner

Treat NGU / Gonococcal culture / Treat partner

Consider other diagnoses / UTI/prostatitis / Consider repeat exam

↓          ↓          ↓

All patients should be checked for syphilis

**Treatment**

| Gonorrhoea | NGU |
|---|---|
| Ceftriaxone IM | Doxycycline 7 days |
| Single dose | Azithromycin single dose |
| Ciprofloxacin | (erythromycin 7 days) |
| Ofloxacin | |

PMN/hpf = Polymorphonuclear neutrophils/high power field
NGU = Non-gonococcal urethritis

### Vaginal discharge

| Discharge | | Physiological | Candida | Trichomonas | Bacterial vaginosis |
|---|---|---|---|---|---|
| | Symptoms | None | Pruritus, irritation | Profuse discharge, irritation | Slight malodorous discharge |
| | Appearance | Scant | Scant, white, thick | Profuse, green/grey May be malodorous | Thin, white/grey Prominent odour |
| | pH | <4.5 | <4.5 | >5.0 | >4.5 |
| | Examination | Normal | Marked vulvar inflammation | Vulvar inflammation | Usually little inflammation |
| | Microscopy | Normal epithelial cells Gram +ve rods (lactobacilli) | Leucocytes Mycelia in 80% | Leucocytes Trichomonas 70–80% | Some leucocyte clue cells Gram variable coccobacilli |
| | Culture | – | Required if microscopy negative | Useful if microscopy negative | No utility |
| | Treatment | – | Topical or systemic azoles | Metronidazole | Metronidazole |

Source: Davey P (ed), 2014. Reproduced with permission of Wiley.

## Primary care

**HE&P**

- Explanation of diagnosis and treatment
- Emphasise the importance of avoiding sexual intercourse until the infection has gone and that sexual partners will also need to be checked for infection
- Discuss methods of future prevention – condom use being the most important
- Remind the person to come back for a review of their condition in two weeks (use this to reinforce messages about safe sex and discuss communication with partners). Discuss the importance of this in relation to chlamydia treatment because of its link to infertility in women (checking that the infection has been cleared up is important)
- Explain the need to take the full course of treatment (check this at return visit)

Likely points of access to the healthcare system are general practice, walk-in-clinic, family planning clinic, and sexual health clinic

*Adult Nursing at a Glance*, First Edition. Andrée le May. © 2015 John Wiley & Sons, Ltd. Published 2015 by John Wiley & Sons, Ltd.
Companion website: www.ataglanceseries.com/nursing/adult

# Key facts

• Vaginal discharge is one of the most common symptoms that women seek advice about either through their GP or practice nurses or from nurses working in family planning or sexual health clinics. There are several causes (not always related to sexually transmitted infections) for example allergy or contact dermatitis, irritants such as a soap or bath oils, panty-liners, spermicides and there is a range of treatments (above).

• There can also be a link between systemic disorders and vaginal discharge/urethritis (e.g. diabetes predisposes a person to candida).

• Urethritis is the most common presentation of sexually transmitted infections in men (opposite) although irritants, inflammation and foreign bodies can also cause similar symptoms.

• Nursing care is primarily associated with sample taking for diagnostic testing and with health education and promotion (below).

# Diagnosis

• Physical examination
• History taking
• Sample testing and urinalysis.

# Essentials of best practice

An infection of the reproductive system can be debilitating and to some extent embarrassing. Nurses need to be sensitive to the possibility of embarrassment and communicate in a straightforward, non-judgemental and informative way.

Nursing care will encompass:

✓ Communication with the healthcare team, patient and family
✓ Health education and promotion (above)
✓ Symptom control and management

## Patient information

Sexual health clinics that offer testing services and advice may be found through local GP practices or at the following websites:

Marie Stopes International www.mariestopes.org.uk.

Brook www.brook.org.uk/.

You will also find very helpful patient-centred fact sheets at www.patient.co.uk/.

# 93 Nursing men with disorders of the prostate gland

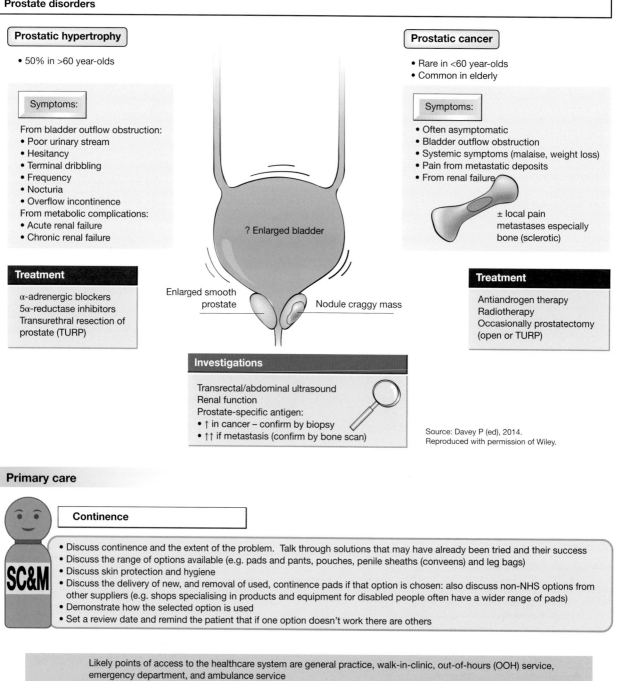

## Prostate disorders

### Prostatic hypertrophy

• 50% in >60 year-olds

**Symptoms:**

From bladder outflow obstruction:
• Poor urinary stream
• Hesitancy
• Terminal dribbling
• Frequency
• Nocturia
• Overflow incontinence
From metabolic complications:
• Acute renal failure
• Chronic renal failure

**Treatment**

α-adrenergic blockers
5α-reductase inhibitors
Transurethral resection of prostate (TURP)

? Enlarged bladder

Enlarged smooth prostate

Nodule craggy mass

### Prostatic cancer

• Rare in <60 year-olds
• Common in elderly

**Symptoms:**

• Often asymptomatic
• Bladder outflow obstruction
• Systemic symptoms (malaise, weight loss)
• Pain from metastatic deposits
• From renal failure

± local pain metastases especially bone (sclerotic)

**Treatment**

Antiandrogen therapy
Radiotherapy
Occasionally prostatectomy (open or TURP)

**Investigations**

Transrectal/abdominal ultrasound
Renal function
Prostate-specific antigen:
• ↑ in cancer – confirm by biopsy
• ↑↑ if metastasis (confirm by bone scan)

Source: Davey P (ed), 2014.
Reproduced with permission of Wiley.

## Primary care

**SC&M**

### Continence

• Discuss continence and the extent of the problem. Talk through solutions that may have already been tried and their success
• Discuss the range of options available (e.g. pads and pants, pouches, penile sheaths (conveens) and leg bags)
• Discuss skin protection and hygiene
• Discuss the delivery of new, and removal of used, continence pads if that option is chosen: also discuss non-NHS options from other suppliers (e.g. shops specialising in products and equipment for disabled people often have a wider range of pads)
• Demonstrate how the selected option is used
• Set a review date and remind the patient that if one option doesn't work there are others

Likely points of access to the healthcare system are general practice, walk-in-clinic, out-of-hours (OOH) service, emergency department, and ambulance service

# Key facts

- Prostate disorders are a common problem for men over the age of 60. They largely fall into two groups – benign prostatic hypertrophy and prostatic cancer (above).
- Benign prostatic hypertrophy often presents with problems associated with urination (e.g. hesitancy, dribbling, frequency, incontinence or more acutely retention of urine). Nursing care is therefore predominantly associated with the management of these symptoms (opposite). Some people may present with chronic renal failure (Chapter 56).
- Prostate cancer is common in older men and is often slow growing. Prostate cancer may also present with bladder problems (above).
- Surgery may be a treatment option for both benign prostatic hypertrophy and prostate cancer.
- In cancer, either a resection of the prostate (Transurethral Resection of the Prostate – TURP) or prostatectomy may be performed depending on the disease's progression. Nursing care may therefore focus on pre- and post-operative care (Section 1) or the management of related hormonal therapy or radiotherapy and any related side-effects.
- Whilst TURP may improve symptoms, quality of life and life expectancy for men with cancer, it can also cause retrograde ejaculation (semen is ejaculated into the bladder) resulting in a dry orgasm. There is also a low risk of impotence and temporary incontinence. All of these risks should be discussed with the person (and their partner) beforehand.
- Prostatectomy has a larger risk of impotence.

# Essentials of best practice

Apart from the obvious fear of cancer, prostatic disorders can be distressing because of their interference with usual activities of daily living. Nurses need to be sensitive to this and the possibility of embarrassment around the discussion of urinary and sexual difficulties: communication should be straightforward and informative.

Catheter care is important if inserted following acute retention of urine to avoid introducing infection (Chapter 58).

If a patient requires surgery, nursing care will focus on the principles of pre- and post-operative care described in Section 1. Post-operative complications may include bleeding (haematuria), clot retention in the bladder and urethra, VTE and infection. Nursing care will encompass:

✓ Accurate assessment and regular monitoring (e.g. following surgery, fluid balance whilst catheterised and observations for bleeding until catheter removed)

✓ Communication with the healthcare team, patient and family

✓ Health education and promotion (e.g. around skin care if using incontinence pads and medication regimens. After surgery remind the patient to drink plenty and avoid constipation)

✓ Symptom control and management (e.g. around urinary difficulties. Immediate post-surgical bladder irrigation, for up to 24 hours, may be used to prevent clot retention. For men with cancer, nurses will also need to consider the management of side-effects related to hormonal therapy or radiotherapy)

✓ Risk assessment and management (e.g. infection control following catheter insertion, management of IVI post-surgery, VTE)

✓ Discharge planning (remember to reinforce that the prostatic bed needs to heal before presenting symptoms will disappear: ensure the patient and their family/carers know to contact the GP if bleeding or blood in urine. Follow-up visits need to be arranged for men with cancer)

## Patient information

Prostate specific information may be obtained from:
Prostate Cancer UK www.prostatecanceruk.org.uk.
Macmillan for information about prostate cancer and support services and local networks www.macmillan.org.uk.
You will also find very helpful patient-centred fact sheets at www.patient.co.uk/.

# 94 Nursing women having hysterectomies

## The uterus, ovaries, fallopian tubes and cervix

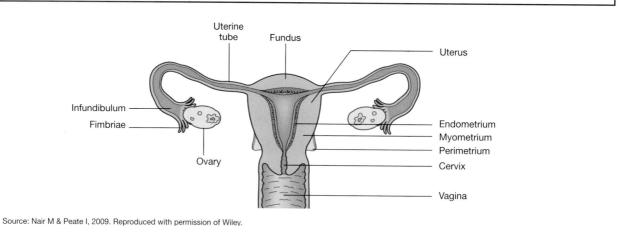

Source: Nair M & Peate I, 2009. Reproduced with permission of Wiley.

## Hospital care

### Post-hysterectomy

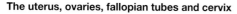

- Discuss what to expect (e.g. light vaginal bleeding post-operatively for around 6 weeks (if this becomes heavier or smelly contact the GP immediately: women may feel more tired than usual so advise them to rest as often as they can)
- Discuss taking light exercise and slowly building this up: full recovery will take between 6 to 8 weeks but some women take longer to feel that they are back to normal
- Discuss the emotional and psychological impact of having a hysterectomy (some women will be delighted – others distressed)
- Driving must be avoided until an emergency stop can be performed safely. Talking to the insurance company should clarify this
- Remind the women not to lift heavy things and avoid strenuous activity
- Discuss resuming sexual intercourse around 4–6 weeks after the operation and reinforce that having a hysterectomy does not physiologically affect sex drive but some women will feel it will (others may look forward to it improving it because of e.g. pre-hysterectomy pain or heavy bleeding). Talking these things through may be helpful, as will reminders about seeking advice early from the GP, consultant or specialist gynaecological nurse if needed
- If the cervix has not been removed, cervical smears should be done as usual
- Remember to supplement your discussions with written information. Useful websites are listed below

Likely points of access to the healthcare system are general practice, walk-in-clinic, and out-of-hours (OOH) service

# Key facts

• Hysterectomy is the surgical removal of the uterus. This may or may not be accompanied by removal of the cervix and ovaries (removal of the ovaries alone is called oophorectomy).

• Hysterectomy is a relatively common operation undergone by women before or after the menopause. It is usually the last resort (except when there is cancer) in a series of treatment options.

• Hysterectomy may be performed for the following reasons:
  • heavy or painful periods (menorrhagia);
  • fibroids;
  • prolapse;
  • endometriosis;
  • cancer of the uterus, cervix, fallopian tubes or ovaries.

• There are various types of hysterectomy
  • total hysterectomy (removal of the uterus and cervix but not the ovaries);
  • subtotal hysterectomy (removal of the uterus);
  • radical hysterectomy (removal of the uterus, cervix, fallopian tubes, ovaries, part of the vagina and lymph nodes – usually because of cancer).

• The uterus can be removed either through the vagina, through an abdominal incision or by key hole surgery.

• Recovery from surgery will depend on the type of surgery performed and the reason for it.

• Chemotherapy or radiotherapy will follow surgery for cancer and nursing care will need to focus on these treatments and their associated side-effects as well as supporting the woman (and her family/carers) emotionally and psychologically.

• If the ovaries are removed prior to menopause, hormone replacement therapy may be prescribed.

• Even if the ovaries are not removed menopause may be accelerated.

• Nursing care will largely focus on pre- and post-operative care (Section 1) although women may wish to discuss the possibility of hysterectomy with practice nurses, family planning nurses and specialist gynaecology nurses before they come to a final decision.

# Essentials of best practice

Nursing a woman following a hysterectomy should focus on the principles of pre- and post-operative care described in Section 1 and the signs and symptoms exhibited by the person at the time. Post-operative complications may include bleeding, VTE and infection.

Nursing care will encompass:

✓ Accurate assessment and regular monitoring (e.g. following surgery, fluid balance whilst catheterised and observations for bleeding from incision site)

✓ Communication with the healthcare team, patient and family

✓ Health education and promotion (above)

✓ Symptom control and management (e.g. pain management, preventing urinary retention)

✓ Risk assessment and management (e.g. infection control, VTE)

✓ Discharge planning (remember to reinforce information regarding activities during recovery and ensure the patient and their family/carers know to contact the GP if the wound site bleeds or pyrexia develops)

## Patient information

Information about hysterectomies and disorders of the uterus and other reproductive organs may be obtained from:

Women's Health Concern (WHC) provides general information for women about health www.womens-health-concern.org

The Hysterectomy Association provides information, a telephone helpline and peer support for women having hysterectomies www.hysterectomy-association.org.uk.

Macmillan provides information about reproductive system cancers and support services and local networks www.macmillan.org.uk.

You will also find very helpful patient-centred fact sheets at www.patient.co.uk/.

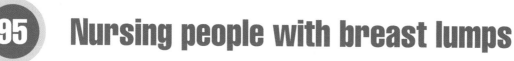

# 95 Nursing people with breast lumps

### Breast disease: likely causes with age

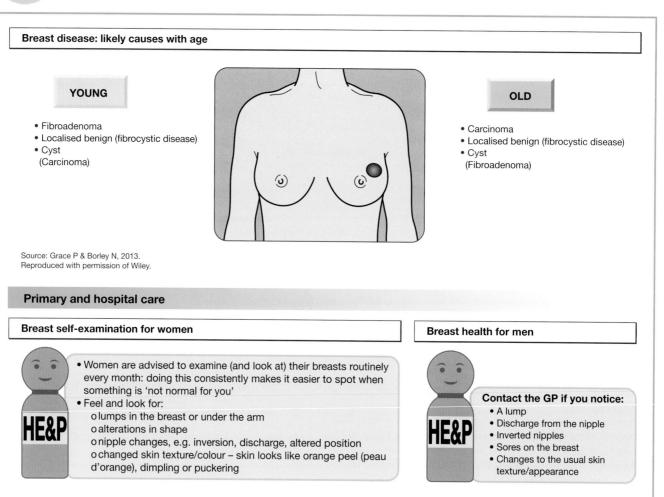

**YOUNG**

- Fibroadenoma
- Localised benign (fibrocystic disease)
- Cyst
  (Carcinoma)

**OLD**

- Carcinoma
- Localised benign (fibrocystic disease)
- Cyst
  (Fibroadenoma)

Source: Grace P & Borley N, 2013.
Reproduced with permission of Wiley.

### Primary and hospital care

#### Breast self-examination for women

**HE&P**

- Women are advised to examine (and look at) their breasts routinely every month: doing this consistently makes it easier to spot when something is 'not normal for you'
- Feel and look for:
  o lumps in the breast or under the arm
  o alterations in shape
  o nipple changes, e.g. inversion, discharge, altered position
  o changed skin texture/colour – skin looks like orange peel (peau d'orange), dimpling or puckering

#### Breast health for men

**HE&P**

**Contact the GP if you notice:**
- A lump
- Discharge from the nipple
- Inverted nipples
- Sores on the breast
- Changes to the usual skin texture/appearance

Likely points of access to the healthcare system are general practice, women's health clinic or mammography service

# Key facts

- A breast lump is a palpable mass in the breast.
- Breast lumps are a common and much feared occurrence in women. They are uncommon in men.
- Breast pain (mastalgia) is most commonly associated with inflammation, infection or menstrual cycles (cyclical mastalgia).
- Breast lumps are due to a number of causes in women (below).
- In men, enlargement of the breast may cause concern but may not in itself have serious health consequences. Breast enlargement is largely due to, for example, hyperplasia of glandular tissue caused by, for example, obesity, hyperprolactinaemia (high level of prolactin), systemic disease such as liver cirrhosis, chronic renal failure or an underlying hormone-secreting tumour.
- Men can however, although rarely, get breast cancer so any enlargement of breasts and the presence of lumps, alterations to nipples or skin texture (above) should be investigated.
- Investigations undertaken to determine the cause of the lump will include:
  - clinical examination and history;
  - imaging (ultrasound, mammography);
  - fine needle aspiration cytology/biopsy.
- The treatment of benign breast lumps depends on their cause, for example cysts may need draining.
- The treatment of breast cancer will depend on the results of disease staging, type of cancer and discussions with the patient and her/his family/carers about their preferred treatment. The options will include mastectomy and restoration of the breast, lumpectomy and breast conserving surgery followed by chemotherapy/radiotherapy. Sometimes ovaries are also removed (oophorectomy).
- If breast cancer is diagnosed, the person and their family will benefit from reassuring, honest communication to enable them to deal with not only the diagnosis of cancer but also an inevitable change in body image. Some women's cancer will be hereditary and so add the extra concern of passing the faulty gene on to their daughters. Genetic counselling may be recommended.
- After surgery, recovery will depend on the type of surgery performed and the subsequent outcome with regard to the need for chemotherapy and/or radiotherapy. Nursing care will then need to focus on these treatments and their associated side-effects as well as supporting the woman (and her family/carers) emotionally and psychologically.
- Women/men may wish to discuss all treatment possibilities with practice nurses, specialist breast care nurses, GPs and consultant oncologists/breast surgeons before coming to a final decision about treatment.
- Initial hospital nursing care for a patient with breast cancer will largely focus on pre- and post-operative care (Section 1).

# Essentials of best practice

Nursing someone following surgery for breast cancer should focus on the principles of pre- and post-operative care described in Section 1 and the signs and symptoms exhibited by the person at the time. Post-operative complications may include VTE and infection.

Specialist nursing advice will be available from breast care specialist nurses and consultant nurses.

Nursing care following surgery will encompass:

✓ Accurate assessment and regular monitoring (e.g. following surgery, fluid balance if catheterised and observations for bleeding from incision site and wound care)

✓ Communication with the healthcare team, patient and family

✓ Health education and promotion (e.g. levels of activity, dealing with fatigue, altered body image, discussion about further treatments, prostheses)

✓ Symptom control and management (e.g. pain management, psychological support)

✓ Risk assessment and management (e.g. infection control, VTE)

✓ Discharge planning (remember to reinforce information regarding activities during recovery and ensure the patient and their family/carers know to contact the GP if the wound site bleeds or pyrexia develops)

Following discharge from hospital, nurses in primary care and those working in the community may provide care to people with breast cancer. Despite excellent survival rates breast cancer can, for some, be a progressive disease so care from nurses providing palliative and end of life care may also be needed.

---

## Patient information

Information about disorders of the breast may be obtained from:
Women's Health Concern (WHC) provides general information for women about health www.womens-health-concern.org.
Breast Cancer Care is a charity providing information and peer support for people with benign breast conditions and cancer www.breastcancercare.org.uk.
Macmillan provides information about breast and other cancers, support services and local networks www.macmillan.org.uk.
You will also find very helpful patient-centred fact sheets at www.patient.co.uk/.

# 96 Nursing people with cancer

Early signs and symptoms of cancer depend on which of the many types of cancer it is, but may include unusual bleeding, altered routines (e.g. bowel habits), nausea, loss of appetite, lumps, pain, fatigue, breathlessness, or unintended weight loss.

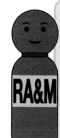

**Nurses play an important role in providing the right care to a person with neutropenia. This may be crucial to a person's survival and should include the following:** (see Dougherty and Lister, 2011) (see also Chapter 62)
- Protective isolation during hospitalisation may be required
- Education about food hygiene whilst in hospital and when discharged (include patient's family and carers)
  o some foods should be avoided because of infection risk e.g. soft cheeses, paté, take-away meals
  o fruit, salads should be washed and drained before eating
- Emphasise the importance of good hand hygiene at all times
- Remind the patient, once discharged, to avoid crowded areas and people with infections, gardening and cleaning
- Pets should not be allowed to lick the person's face and new pets should not be bought whilst the person is at risk of neutropenia
- **Any** signs and symptoms of infection should be reported to the GP or the patient's hospital

*Adult Nursing at a Glance*, First Edition. Andrée le May. © 2015 John Wiley & Sons, Ltd. Published 2015 by John Wiley & Sons, Ltd.
Companion website: www.ataglanceseries.com/nursing/adult

# Key facts

• Cancer can affect any of the body's systems; there are over 200 different types of cancer. Covering each of these is beyond the remit of this book.

• Cancer is when normal cells grow uncontrollably (e.g. as a tumour) damaging or destroying its tissue of origin and infiltrating and destroying neighbouring organs and tissues. Unlike other cells, cancer uses the blood and lymph systems to spread and grow also in other parts of the body (metastasise).

• The most common cancers in the UK are found in the lungs, bowel, breasts and prostate gland.

• Cells may become cancerous (malignant) as a result of exposure to various factors, for example chemicals, radiation, viruses or other organisms, and heredity.

• As cancer manifests itself in different ways depending on its location, stage of development and the person's overall health, signs and symptoms associated with cancer will vary and so in turn will nursing care. Many of these consequences and their management will be similar to those already dealt with in the earlier chapters of this section.

• There are many different ways to treat and manage cancer (e.g. surgery, chemotherapy, radiotherapy, immunotherapy, monoclonal antibodies or a combination of treatments).

• Cancer treatments may cause a number of unpleasant (e.g. nausea, vomiting, hair loss, fatigue, lymphodema) and dangerous (e.g. neutropenia) side-effects.

• The consequences of cancer are wide-ranging and will vary from complete cure to long-term management to rapid death. Nurses will care for people with cancer and their families/carers in many situations and in any setting where healthcare is delivered.

• Around 25% of all deaths are caused by cancer. However, many people live with cancer for years and do not die from it.

• The treatment and management of cancer has improved significantly so now more people than before survive cancer. Increased survival means that nurses' attention needs to focus on treatment management *and* on supporting people to live with (or with having had) cancer so they are able to make necessary readjustments to their life and retain confidence and control of their health and quality of life.

• Some cancers can be prevented such as lung cancer (smoking cessation), malignant melanoma (protection from sunshine), cervical cancer and some mouth cancers. Nurses have an important role in reducing the risk of cancer through developing and delivering health promotion and education campaigns as well as giving individually targeted education and advice. Health education and promotion is designed to alter people's risks of developing cancer through raising awareness of causative factors and changing behaviours. For example, the risk of cervical cancer may be reduced by altering sexual behaviour to incorporate the use of condoms, reducing human papilloma virus (HPV) infection; or the risk of mouth cancer may be reduced by altering the diet and social practices of Asian communities where betel nuts are chewed.

• The early diagnosis of cancer is an important aspect of successful treatment and so symptom recognition is central to many cancer awareness campaigns. Nurses need to refer patients to their GP, practice nurses or specialist cancer nurses if they experience unusual signs and symptoms (above). Some people find it hard to know when to seek advice, either being unduly worried about minor ailments ('the worried well') or seeking advice late when their cancer has developed beyond the early stages. Always refer someone for an expert opinion.

• Screening for cervical cancer, for example, through smear tests, colorectal cancer through testing for faecal occult blood, or breast cancer through mammography are also important ways to identify cancers early.

• Some people are genetically at greater risk of developing certain cancers than others. For example, some women have genes that predispose them to breast or ovarian cancer and because of this decide to have their breasts or ovaries removed to protect them from these cancers.

• Immunisations may also protect against cancer, for example immunisation against HPV in cervical cancer. This is now routinely offered to girls between the ages of 12 and 13.

• Having (or having had) cancer can leave a person with feelings of loss, altered body image, anxiety, uncertainty and fear of recurrence. Help with psychological adjustment to cancer as well as physical adjustment is an important facet of nursing care.

• For some people, cancer will cause their death and in these instances attention needs to seamlessly switch from treatment to palliation and when appropriate to end of life care (Chapter 13).

• Integrated, person-centred, multi-disciplinary, multi-agency care is essential regardless of the type, stage or location of the cancer.

# Essentials of best practice

The nursing care of people with cancer will vary from person to person and also for each person and their family/carers as their cancer progresses, remits or is cured. The principles of care for patients with cancer are likely to be similar to those mentioned in the systems earlier and in Section 1. Care will largely revolve around:

✓ Accurate assessments and regular monitoring
✓ Symptom control and management (see Section 1)
✓ Communication with the healthcare team, patient and family
✓ Risk assessment and management (e.g. for neutropenia see above and Chapter 62)
✓ Health education and promotion
✓ Discharge planning

## Patient information

There are several useful charities and support groups focusing on cancer including:
Macmillan Cancer Support www.macmillan.org.uk.
Cancer Research UK www.cancerresearchuk.org.
You will also find very helpful patient-centred fact sheets at www.patient.co.uk.

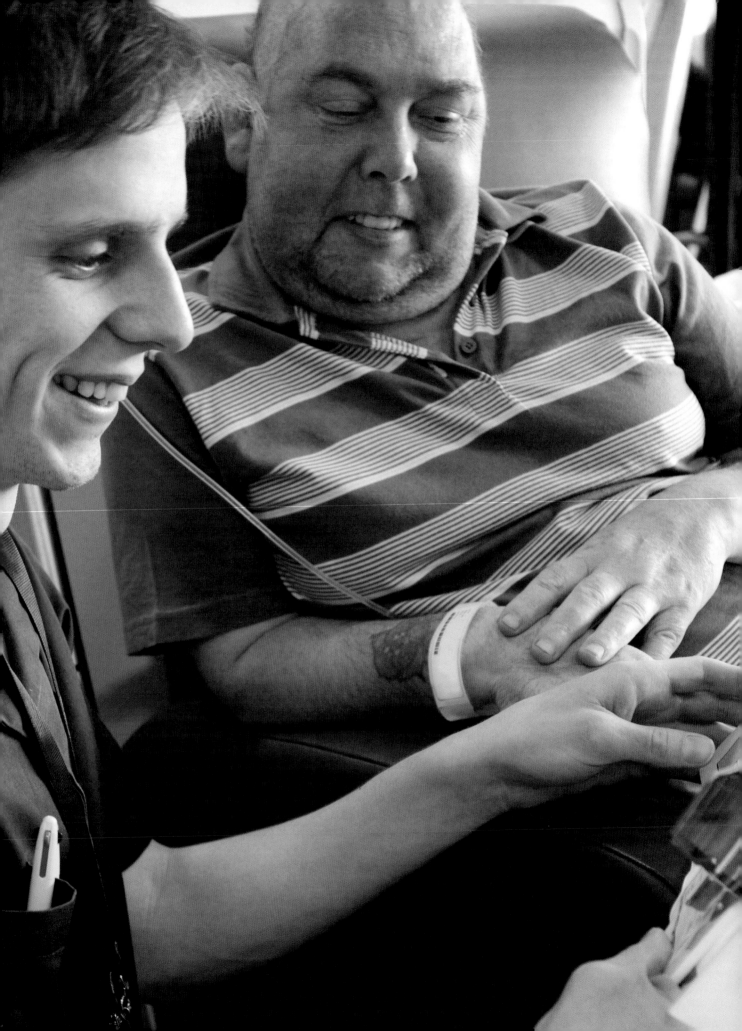

# Essential skills: leadership and organisational

## Chapters

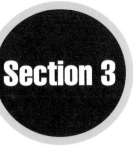

Don't forget to visit the companion website for this book at **www.ataglanceseries.com/nursing/adult** to do some practice MCQs on these topics.

# Organisational aspects of care

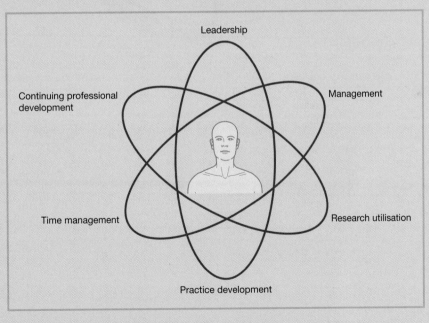

The previous two sections of this book have revealed the array of skilled practice that underpins high-quality individualised patient care. Section 3 explores other key skills essential to developing, organising and maintaining a supportive and efficient environment within which sensitive, effective nursing care can be delivered and advanced.

The following chapters focus on the interlinked skills of:
• Leadership
• Management

• Managing people and difficult situations
• Research utilisation
• Time management
• Continuing professional development
• Practice development.

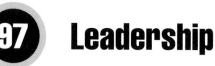

# 97 Leadership

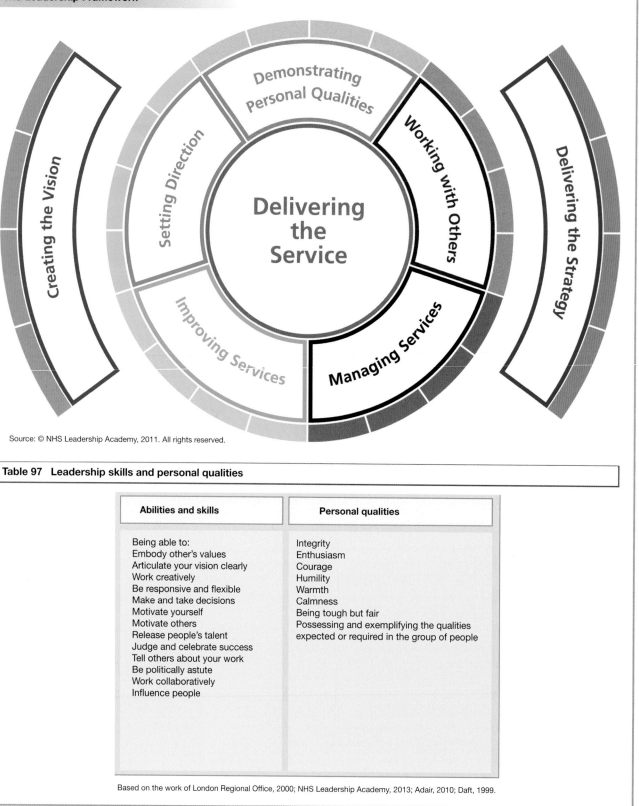

**The Leadership Framework**

Source: © NHS Leadership Academy, 2011. All rights reserved.

**Table 97  Leadership skills and personal qualities**

| Abilities and skills | Personal qualities |
|---|---|
| Being able to:<br>Embody other's values<br>Articulate your vision clearly<br>Work creatively<br>Be responsive and flexible<br>Make and take decisions<br>Motivate yourself<br>Motivate others<br>Release people's talent<br>Judge and celebrate success<br>Tell others about your work<br>Be politically astute<br>Work collaboratively<br>Influence people | Integrity<br>Enthusiasm<br>Courage<br>Humility<br>Warmth<br>Calmness<br>Being tough but fair<br>Possessing and exemplifying the qualities<br>expected or required in the group of people |

Based on the work of London Regional Office, 2000; NHS Leadership Academy, 2013; Adair, 2010; Daft, 1999.

*Adult Nursing at a Glance*, First Edition. Andrée le May. © 2015 John Wiley & Sons, Ltd. Published 2015 by John Wiley & Sons, Ltd.
Companion website: www.ataglanceseries.com/nursing/adult

# Nursing and leadership

Nurses are leaders in many situations – they lead episodes of care with patients and their friends and families; they lead teams of people providing care or those taking part in service development or improvement projects; they lead groups of students through mentorship and their peers through clinical supervision; and they lead health and social care organisations at various levels from team leader to chief executive. Whatever the situation that nurses are leading in, the core element in that leadership process/relationship is ensuring that the most appropriate and effective care possible is given and they often do that by influencing other people.

Leadership is a central feature of nursing emphasised by both the NMC and the RCN. Leadership, management and team working comprise the NMC's (2010) fourth domain of practice and are implicit in the RCN's eighth Principle of Nursing Practice (H). The RCN principle reminds us that the way nurses lead is also important 'Nurses and nursing staff lead by example, develop themselves and other staff, and influence the way care is given in a manner that is open and responds to individual needs' (see References and further reading).

# What is leadership?

Leadership is often described as being about our relationships with other people and the way we constructively influence them. If we think of it like this it is easy to identify three key interacting elements in this influencing relationship within nursing – the leader, the people/person being influenced (sometimes known as followers especially when we're thinking about teams of people) and the job/task being done. In nursing, particularly, the job/task often involves another group of people – either patients/service users and their families and carers or our other health and social care colleagues. Leadership then is largely about people and the way they communicate and behave.

Leading people successfully requires nurses to be creative and adapt their leadership style and approach to suit the range of different situations (and people) that they encounter every day. But whoever or whatever it is that nurses are leading, their leadership needs to be clear and strong in order to ensure that dignified care of a high quality is delivered within a positive working culture.

## Defining leadership

When you ask people to define leadership, they often start by saying that it's about influencing people and making things happen in teams, services and/or organisations. A commonly used definition is one by Daft (1995: 5) who says that 'Leadership involves influence, it occurs among people, those people intentionally desire significant changes, and the changes reflect purposes shared by leaders and followers. Influence means that the relationship between people is not passive; however, also inherent in this definition is the concept that influence is multidirectional and non-coercive' (Daft, 1999: 5).

The NHS Leadership Academy (2011) in their Leadership Framework (LF) (above) identifies five core domains essential for delivering good quality healthcare ('the service') and two domains relevant to more senior leaders (creating the vision and delivering the strategy. Each of these is made up of a number of elements – all of which are, to some extent, about influence. The component elements of the five core domains are:

- For Demonstrating Personal Qualities
  - developing self-awareness;
  - managing yourself;
  - continuing personal development;
  - acting with integrity.
- For Working with Others
  - developing networks;
  - building and maintaining relationships;
  - encouraging contribution;
  - working with teams.
- For Managing Services
  - planning;
  - managing resources;
  - managing people;
  - managing performance.
- For Improving Services
  - ensuring patient safety;
  - critically evaluating;
  - encouraging improvement and innovation;
  - facilitating transformation.
- Setting Direction
  - identifying the contexts for change;
  - applying knowledge and evidence;
  - making decisions;
  - evaluating impact.

You can read more about each of them on the NHS Leadership Academy website (www.leadershipacademy.nhs.uk). Some of these elements relate to the personal qualities, abilities and skills listed above.

Although the Leadership Framework incorporates a domain called managing services, it is important to remember that not all leaders are service managers and not all managers are leaders. It is possible to lead people without having management responsibility for them or organisational services and it is certainly possible to be a manager without having the skills and abilities of a leader (see Chapter 98 for more information on management).

You can learn how to lead more successfully, but before you start to do this you need to understand the importance of leadership to high-quality nursing care and organisational success, to recognise the difficulties and challenges of being a leader and to acquire and practice the skills and qualities detailed above and in the LF. You might find it helpful to start off by assessing yourself or finding out what others think about. You can find two useful tools for doing this (a self-assessment tool and the LF 360° feedback tool) at the NHS Leadership Academy website.

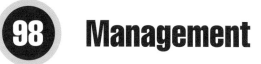

# 98 Management

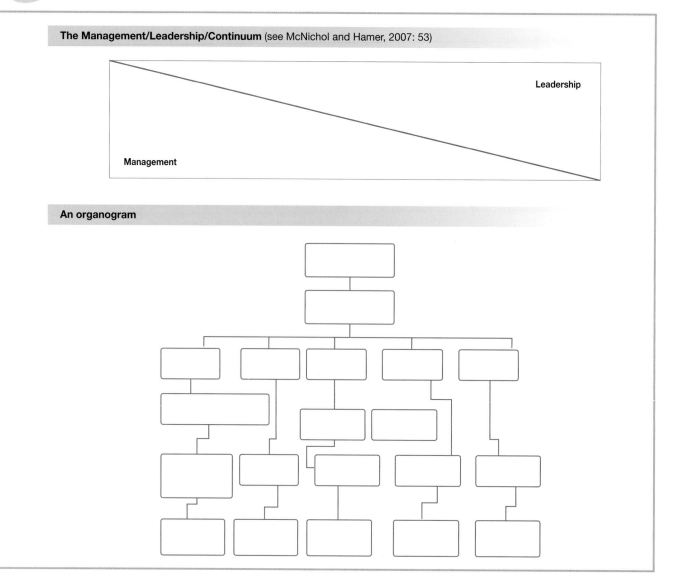

**The Management/Leadership/Continuum** (see McNichol and Hamer, 2007: 53)

Leadership

Management

**An organogram**

*Adult Nursing at a Glance*, First Edition. Andrée le May. © 2015 John Wiley & Sons, Ltd. Published 2015 by John Wiley & Sons, Ltd.
Companion website: www.ataglanceseries.com/nursing/adult

# What is management?

Management, just like leadership, is about working with and influencing people. Unlike leadership, the main purpose of management is to achieve the goals of the organisation. Management is therefore largely associated with specific, goal-orientated, functions. Leaders do not generally have to achieve the same goal-oriented work as managers do and so may be perceived as being more able to be creative in what they do.

However, there will be times when managers have to be leaders and leaders have to adopt some of the goal-oriented functions of management. McNichol and Hamer (2007) suggests that there is often a continuum between management and leadership (above).

Planning, organising, motivating and controlling are the common functions of management (la Monica Rigolosi, 2013). These functions are outlined below one by one – this makes it look as if they happen separately, but they are in fact interlinked.

# Management functions

**Planning** is about identifying problems, detailing long- and short-term goals, deciding on objectives and then working out how the goals and objectives are to be achieved. Goals and objectives need to be kept **s**imple, **m**eaningful, **a**chievable, and **r**ealistic: they also need to have a **t**imescale attached to them (this sometimes is referred to as setting SMART goals/objectives).

**Organising** is about getting all the resources needed to achieve your goals together – these resources include not only people with the right knowledge and skills but also finance and equipment.

**Motivating** other people to achieve the goals set is an important and sometimes challenging aspect of management. If people are not motivated they won't work effectively or efficiently and this will have a negative effect on the organisation's effectiveness. Goal setting must therefore not only reflect the abilities of the people involved and available resources but also the team and manager's motivation. (See Chapter 99)

**Controlling** doesn't mean controlling in terms of stopping people doing things or being manipulative: here controlling is about setting up ways to evaluate progress either at the end of a job/project (summative evaluation) or at points during the job in order to act on this feedback (formative evaluation) to make the job go better. This ongoing formative type of evaluation means that plans can be adjusted as jobs/projects progress if necessary. (Sometimes these evaluations are referred to as quality control checks or audits.)

# Management skills

Generally it is agreed that there are three critical sorts of skills that managers need. These are technical, human and conceptual. Sometimes technical skills are referred to as 'hard' skills and human skills as 'soft' skills. Technical skills are associated with using the appropriate knowledge, techniques and equipment to perform a task or achieve a goal (e.g. showing a junior member of the ward team how to set up an ECG or collating information using a particular software package). Human skills are about working with people and enabling them to contribute effectively to meeting goals. This involves understanding what motivates people and being able to communicate easily and clearly with them. Conceptual skills are about understanding the complexity of the organisation and recognising how what you and the various teams around you does fits with the overall goals of the organisation (e.g. how does managing trolley waits in the Emergency Department fit with the overall organisational goal of preventing people waiting longer than necessary anywhere in the hospital?).

In the main, managers combine all of these skills but sometimes people at different levels of management use some skills more than others. For instance, a ward sister/charge nurse is more likely to use more technical and human skills than conceptual ones, whereas a chief operating officer of a hospital would use more conceptual and human skills. The figure above shows an organogram – you might see these used to depict different levels of management in an organisation.

# Responsibility and accountability

In order to be effective, managers need to know what and who they are responsible and accountable for. They also need to know how much authority, or power, they have to make decisions about their area(s) of responsibility (McNichol and Hamer, 2007). Managers sometimes need to delegate responsibility to others. and in doing so they should make sure that they are confident that the other person can do the job they are delegating, explain clearly what is expected of them and how this delegated area of responsibility will be evaluated.

# Role models

Additionally, managers are important role models to others. Sometimes managers may encourage team members to shadow them so that they can begin to understand and learn the skills of management. If you get an opportunity to shadow a manager take it up!

# Managing care

Front-line nurses working on wards, in primary care and in the community might use all the functions (and skills) ascribed to management in their day-to-day care of patients. After all it is vital that nurses plan, organise and evaluate care and motivate their patients/clients and their families and friends to concur with care or more actively participate in it. It is also important that nurses motivate their colleagues to deliver and evaluate care as described in care plans and treatment regimes.

Additionally, every nurse needs to manage their time, appearance, level of knowledge and skills effectively in order to provide the best care possible to the patient.

Nursing is a very flexible career. Nurses who want to move away from managing day-to-day patient care have the opportunity to leave front-line practice and take on more management responsibilities through, for example, managing teams of nurses and nursing assistants who deliver care. Ultimately some nurses will reach the level of Chief Executive and run an organisation; in this sort of role they are likely to find a closer alignment of management and leadership.

# 99 Managing people and difficult situations

## Features of motivation

| | |
|---|---|
| Motivation is unique to the individual | What motivates one person may not motivate another |
| Motivation is usually intentional | The individual has a choice of whether to act or not |
| Motivation is multi-faceted | No single thing has been identified as being able to motivate every individual. The two most important aspects to consider are:<br>1. What gets a person in a 'ready state' to do something<br>2. What makes an individual engage in an activity |

Source: Cox & Le May, 2006. Reproduced with permission of Palgrave Macmillan.

*Adult Nursing at a Glance*, First Edition. Andrée le May. © 2015 John Wiley & Sons, Ltd. Published 2015 by John Wiley & Sons, Ltd.
Companion website: www.ataglanceseries.com/nursing/adult

# Managing people

There are many, many books written about managing people: this chapter just gives you some pointers about what works well and what doesn't. Almost without knowing it you will have been managing different people each day. You manage patients, their families and carers, your nursing colleagues and your colleagues from other disciplines. Managing people doesn't mean that you have to be their line manager and be responsible for how they do their jobs, it may simply mean that you interact with them and try to get the best from them. You will do this as a nurse regardless of your role in the organisation.

Managing people is primarily about:

- motivating them to get involved in something;
- communicating clearly and honestly;
- making sure they feel included and their views are respected;
- being sensitive to their needs.

## Motivating people

People are motivated by many things: not all people are motivated by the same things. The table above summarises the features of motivation.

In 1987, Herzberg suggested that working people's motivation might be affected by hygiene/maintenance factors (e.g. their working conditions or pay, level) and growth/motivational factors (e.g. a sense of achievement, recognition, responsibility). Hygiene factors are often associated with feelings of dissatisfaction and the motivational factors with satisfaction. A person's level of motivation and job satisfaction is about the interplay between these factors, that is which they value most. Successful people management is about finding out what is important to each person. Once you know this you will be better able to motivate them.

## Communicating clearly and honestly

Clear, honest and appropriately channelled communication is critical to the successful management of people. The key features of good communication are:

- Be clear about the purpose of the communication.
- Make sure the information is accurate.
- Use simple language.
- Make sure you give enough information.
- Make sure you don't give too much information.
- Use the right channel of communication (e.g. face-to-face, telephone, email, text, letter). Think about what you are trying to communicate, how urgent it is, how controversial it is, how confidential it is.

- Check that the other person has understood you.
- Always be considerate and polite.

## Making sure people feel included

People like to discuss things and feel included in decision making. Try to make opportunities for this either by talking to people individually or in small groups. When people are in a group, try to make sure that you encourage less vocal people to talk too. Talking informally over coffee about ideas is also a good way of hearing people's views and making them feel included. Remember that sometimes people need privacy to discuss what's happening, so allow them the space to do that and, if need be, without you.

## Being sensitive to their needs

It is very easy to unintentionally upset people, particularly if they are already feeling vulnerable. Try not to be judgemental or biased. Give people space to tell you their needs and once you know them be empathic. One useful tip is to think what you might do in their circumstances and tailor the way you interact with them accordingly.

# Managing difficult situations

As a nurse you are likely to find yourself in a variety of difficult situations. These may range from breaking bad news to people, to caring for people who are upset and emotionally drained, to working with people who are angry and frustrated. You might also find yourself dealing with differences of opinion between colleagues.

Every situation is different but here are some general pointers that you might find useful.

- Get as much information as you can about the situation. Find out what is really happening and don't act just on what other people have told you.
- Actively listen to what the people involved are saying.
- Clarify things. Ask lots of questions.
- Check out your understanding, don't just assume you have understood.
- Try to articulate the problem so everyone involved is talking about the same thing.
- Watch people's non-verbal cues – sometimes these can be more informative than what is being said.
- Don't be confrontational.
- Keep calm and act professionally.
- Use negotiation to try to reach a conclusion or solution that everyone can live with. This is sometimes called a win–win situation.
- If you don't think you are going to be able to reach a satisfactory conclusion, ask someone else to mediate for you.

# 100 Research utilisation

**Box 100  The process of evidence based practice** (Source: Sackett et al., 2004)

Asking clear questions about practice – usually about an individual patient.

Looking for answers to those questions – firstly searching for research findings.

Judging (critically appraising) the evidence for its rigour, validity (truthfulness) and usefulness to practice.

Integrating these findings with clinical expertise, patient's needs, and patients' preferences.

If appropriate, applying these findings to the patient's care.

Evaluating the outcome of our decisions/practice.

## Frameworks for guiding the implementation of research

| **Promoting Action on Research Implementation in Health Services (PARiHS) framework** (Rycroft-Malone, 2010) | **Ottawa Model of Research Use (OMRU)** (Logan and Graham, 2010) | **Knowledge-to-Action (KTA) framework** (Graham and Tetroe, 2010) | **Joanna Briggs Institute (JBI) framework for implementing evidence** (Pearson, 2010) |
|---|---|---|---|
| This framework emphasises that the success of implementation depends on the relationship between key factors: <br> - the nature of the evidence (research, clinical experience or patient experience) <br> - the context within which it is implemented (e.g. the culture of the organisation, leadership and the potential for evaluation) <br> - facilitation (this depends on the role of the facilitator and their attributes and skills). <br> Successful implementation occurs 'when evidence is scientifically robust and matches professional consensus and patients' preferences … the context receptive to change with sympathetic cultures, strong leadership, and appropriate monitoring and feedback systems … and, when there is appropriate facilitation of change with input from skilled external and internal facilitators' (112–3). This framework may be used to diagnose the receptiveness of each context to change and thereby tailor any facilitation to meet the needs of that specific context. | This model specifically focuses on getting valid research findings implemented. <br> There are six key structural elements <br> 1. the research-informed innovation <br> 2. the potential adopters <br> 3. the practice environment <br> 4. implementation interventions for transferring the research findings into practice <br> 5. the adoption of the innovation <br> 6. the outcomes – health related and others. <br> In addition there are three process elements (AME) that need to be considered – Assessment of barriers and supports (these are associated with the structural elements 1–3 above), Monitoring how the research-informed innovation is implemented, and Evaluation of the impact of the innovation (monitoring and evaluation are linked closely to structural elements 4–6). <br> This model can be applied to evidence-based practice projects and also quality improvement projects. | This framework is conceptually robust being derived from an analysis of 31 planned action/ change theories in health and social sciences, education and management. <br> The framework emphasises the importance of social interaction and of tailoring evidence to meet contextual and cultural needs. <br> The framework comprises a number of phases: <br> - identify problem/select knowledge <br> - adapt knowledge to the local context <br> - assess barriers to knowledge use <br> - implement tailored intervention <br> - monitor knowledge use <br> - evaluate outcomes (both those associated with the process of change and the outcomes in relation to healthcare) <br> - sustain knowledge use. | This framework is particularly focussed on the use of research evidence. <br> At its core there are four key components: <br> - healthcare evidence generation <br> - evidence synthesis <br> - evidence/knowledge transfer <br> - evidence utilisation. <br> Our primary concern is the use of evidence – this part of the framework focuses on practice change, embedding evidence through system/organisation-wide change and evaluating its impact. <br> The framework emphasises that the process of evidence utilisation is influenced by: <br> - resources <br> - education/expertise <br> - patient preference <br> - the availability of research <br> - staffing levels, skill mix <br> - policies. |

Source: Barton & le May, 2012. Reproduced with permission of Taylor and Francis.

*Adult Nursing at a Glance*, First Edition. Andrée le May. © 2015 John Wiley & Sons, Ltd. Published 2015 by John Wiley & Sons, Ltd.
Companion website: www.ataglanceseries.com/nursing/adult

# Why is using research important?

All nurses are expected to be aware of and able to utilise research findings and evaluate their usefulness in their everyday practice. Using the most up-to-date and appropriate research and tailoring it to meet the needs of each patient is a fundamental component of skilled, high-quality nursing care.

The term research utilisation is often used synonymously with evidence-based practice (EBP) (see above). EBP has been an important element of nursing's vocabulary since the mid 1990s but nurses started to think seriously about underpinning practice with research much earlier, in the mid-1970s, with the publication of the Briggs' Report. This report emphasised the need for nurses and midwives to become more familiar with and use research to enhance care. It also encouraged nurses to think more critically about what they were doing and why and not just follow instructions from others. Since then all nurses regardless of specialty and grade have been expected to use research findings, alongside factual and experiential knowledge, in their clinical practice.
Using research is important because it means:

**1** We can give the most up-to-date and appropriate research based care to patients and their families/carers.

**2** We can use research findings into working practices (e.g. how to communicate effectively in multi-disciplinary teams) to create environments within which we can deliver the best care possible.

**3** We can use research findings to justify our decisions.

**4** We can use research findings to argue for better resources or different ways of doing things rather than relying on hunches or doing what we have always done.

**5** We can use research findings to improve our working environment (e.g. through using the findings from RN4CAST) since this environment impacts not only on the health and wellbeing of staff but also of patients.

**6** We can use research findings to help us to think differently and be more creative in our practice.

In addition to using research findings to improve practice, nurses can also do research to develop nursing's specific knowledge base. Nursing research can focus on many different things, for example working out why one nursing intervention (e.g. a specific dressing) works better than another or how a group of patients feel about a particular service (e.g. specialist epilepsy nursing services) or experience an illness like Chronic Obstructive Pulmonary Disease (COPD). Try using Google to find some research on any of these.

# Utilising research in practice

However, using research in practice is not always as easy as it should be; there are barriers that will need to be overcome just as there are enablers to be exploited. The barriers might include:

- Lack of motivation to change practice.
- Fear of changing practice.
- Lack of opportunity to find the latest research.
- Pressure of workload.
- Active resistance from colleagues or patients.
- Acceptance of traditional practice.
- Not being able to understand the language (jargon) used by researchers in their papers or reports.

Add some of your own as you come across them and think about how you might solve them.
The enablers might include:
- Good role models who can help you.
- Having a research centre in your hospital or community setting.
- Being able to easily access information on the internet or at the library.
- Going on a specific course to help you to change practice.

Sometimes nurses have found it useful to use a framework to help them implement research when they want to change practice in a team or unit (see examples above). However, if you as a practitioner want to implement research findings in your own practice you don't always need to follow a step-by-step framework, it is perfectly possible for you use research without one. But before you do so make sure that you have assessed the quality of the research findings (e.g. their validity and reliability) and their clinical relevance and benefits to your patient(s). If you then think there is potential to use the research discuss how you are going to do this with your colleagues and then, once the nursing team has agreed, with your patients and their families.

If you do decide to use a framework to guide you, make sure that you pick one that you think will work in your practice environment. Getting a good match between the context you work in and want to change and the framework that you plan to use is often the key to the sustained use of research.

Whether you use a framework or not – remember to discuss any changes in care before you make them with your colleagues, patients and their relatives. It is important to remember that convincing other people to use the research findings or to comply with them is very important, so it's a good idea to make sure they feel part of the change process. It's also important to document the changes you have made and how successful (or not) they have been. One of the big mistakes nurses make is not to evaluate the effects of using research findings in their day-to-day practice: failing to do this evaluation means that we don't know how useful research actually is when it's put into practice. So once you have successfully implemented research findings tell other people how well they worked, what problems you had implementing them (if any) and how you got over them. When you're doing this think of yourself as a role model to others no matter how simple the change to practice seems to have been. And remember to record all of this in your Continuing Professional Development portfolio (see Chapter 102).

# Time management

---

### Box 101a    Things that stop you managing your time well

**Here are some examples:**

a) Other people's demands which do not relate to your priorities

b) Answering telephone calls and finding the person wanted on the phone

c) Not having prioritised your workload so that you are trying to do everything at once

**Now jot down some of your own and write some solutions against them**

---

### Box 101b    Reviewing your time management

Make a note of some examples of when your time management went well and why. Identify some other examples of where things could have gone better. Think about how you could improve the ones that didn't go so well and write down how you might do things differently next time.

| What went well and why? | What could be done better and how? |
|---|---|
|  |  |

---

*Adult Nursing at a Glance*, First Edition. Andrée le May. © 2015 John Wiley & Sons, Ltd. Published 2015 by John Wiley & Sons, Ltd.
Companion website: www.ataglanceseries.com/nursing/adult

# What is time management?

Although there are many definitions of time management, it is generally agreed that time management is simply about using time to your best advantage. This sounds easy – but in fact it is a very hard skill to accomplish. The difficulty lies in being able to stay in control of how you spend your time – be that at work, play or in learning!

If time management was just about you working out what to do with your time then everything would probably go smoothly, but in reality this is not the case because other people and their deadlines impact on your time. Sometimes these deadlines or demands can be negotiated so you can retain some control over them, but sometimes this is not possible and you have to prioritise them in relation to the amount of time available or delegate to someone else.

In nursing we usually work pre-determined shifts meaning that the time over which certain work 'tasks' have to be done is finite but luckily we have colleagues taking over from us at the end of each shift so we can pass unfinished work on to them. But within those shifts we have to work out what 'tasks' need to take priority and which, if any, could be delegated to someone else or handed on to colleagues on the next shift. We have to juggle (and prioritise) the demands and needs of many people, for example patients, their families and friends; colleagues within the nursing team and from across the multi-disciplinary team and our managers, especially when we are asked to add in extra 'tasks' because of staff shortages or because patients suddenly require a different level of care to be provided (see above). (Also, those of you undertaking courses have to fit in your teachers' deadlines for assessments.) Not all of these people will know your workload, your available time or your ability to use that time effectively. You are the only person who can see the whole picture and so you must become adept at managing your time. Here are some tips for helping you to do this in the workplace. (Of course you can also use them in other aspects of your life!)

# Time management tips

In order to manage your time well at work you need to make some decisions. There are three main things to decide:
1 What you need to spend your time on and how much time you need to spend on it.
2 What the competing demands on your time are.
3 How well (or poorly) you have managed your time in particular situations and what you need to learn from this.

## Deciding what you need to spend your time on and how much time you need to spend on it

Nursing is a varied, exciting and dynamic job. The variety means that rarely are two shifts the same and this, whilst being an advantage, presents an immediate problem in terms of time management because you cannot easily plan ahead. Starting every new shift means having to work out what you have to do. This requires assessing the situation that you find yourself in – how many patients are you caring for, how ill or dependent are they, what work is left over for you to do from the previous shift, what, if anything, is planned by others for you to do during this shift e.g. ward rounds you have to attend, patients who need to be transferred, discharged or admitted or meetings that need you to be there. Try to find out close to the start of the shift your work for the day. Naturally, there will be things you can't take into account at the start of the shift, but if you have identified the likely tasks and events that you are responsible for, or need to be involved in, then you will be more in control of your time than if you haphazardly went from task to task not knowing the complete picture or anticipating what might come up next.

So here the important tip is to find out as much as you can about what you need to do before doing anything. And to try to work out how long each 'task' will take you. If you think you cannot manage them all, say so, then some can either be delegated to others or rescheduled.

## Identifying what the competing demands on your time are

Sometimes it will seem as if you have to do everything at once and you'll want to prioritise what you need to do. Prioritisation might result in you:
• Having to prioritise the care of the most ill patient over that of others.
• Prioritising a number of routine tasks that can be done quickly so that they are completed before you need to spend an uninterrupted period of time with a patient or their relatives.
• Realising that many things need to be done at once – if this happens ask others if they can help you out.
• Negotiating with patients the best time for them to have. for example, certain procedures carried out or to go to sleep.
• Telling patients that you cannot attend to them at the moment but will be back in a given amount of time. It is important to tell them when you will be back – for example saying in 10 minutes rather that 'in a short while' which of course could mean anything.
• Having to re-plan your time when something unforeseen happens.
So here an important tip is to work out what needs to be done, in what order and confer with your colleagues and patients about how this fits with their plans and expectations. Another tip is to remember to ask for help and to remember to tell people when you haven't been able to complete all the jobs that you were required to do.

## Thinking about how well (or poorly) you have managed your time in particular situations and what you need to learn from this

Thinking about how you could have done things differently is always important but so too is recognising that you have done well! (above).

So here the important tip is to reflect on your shift and think first of all about what went well and why, and then if there were things that could have worked out better. When you reconsider the things you could improve, think about their timing and if doing them at a different time could have made a difference or whether if you had done something in a different way it would have worked better or taken less time.

Always remember to take breaks in the day to restore your energy – working through meal breaks won't help you manage your time any better!

# 102 Continuing professional development

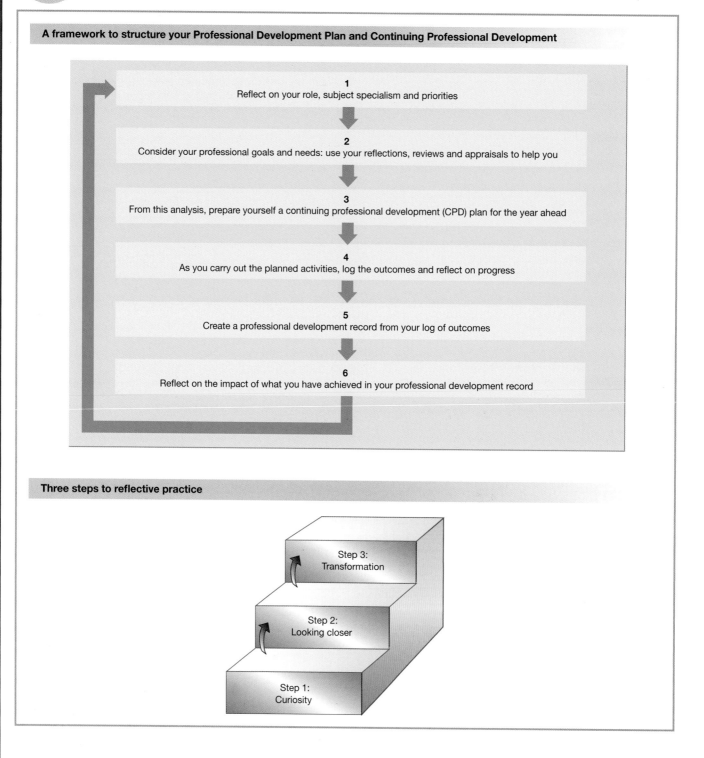

**A framework to structure your Professional Development Plan and Continuing Professional Development**

**1**
Reflect on your role, subject specialism and priorities

**2**
Consider your professional goals and needs: use your reflections, reviews and appraisals to help you

**3**
From this analysis, prepare yourself a continuing professional development (CPD) plan for the year ahead

**4**
As you carry out the planned activities, log the outcomes and reflect on progress

**5**
Create a professional development record from your log of outcomes

**6**
Reflect on the impact of what you have achieved in your professional development record

**Three steps to reflective practice**

Step 3:
Transformation

Step 2:
Looking closer

Step 1:
Curiosity

*Adult Nursing at a Glance*, First Edition. Andrée le May. © 2015 John Wiley & Sons, Ltd. Published 2015 by John Wiley & Sons, Ltd.
Companion website: www.ataglanceseries.com/nursing/adult

# Continuing professional development (CPD)

Continuing professional development (CPD) is about ensuring that your knowledge and skills are up-to-date and that you remain competent to practice throughout your career. CPD is something that every healthcare professional has to do.

CPD is sometimes described as continuing personal and professional development (CPPD) and this reflects the breadth of opportunities that can count as CPD.

The Nursing and Midwifery Council (NMC) requirements for CPD must be met every time you renew your registration. For nurses working in the UK, CPD may include regularly updating skills and knowledge, reflecting on practice and their day-to-day work and teaching/mentoring others. All of these involve continuous learning and development. Taking part in and implementing the learning gained from these activities enables nurses to give safe, up-to-date, highly skilled care.

CPD is not, for instance, just about going on courses and collecting certificates; it involves thinking about how you will use your learning to develop yourself as well as care. This self-development can be structured by writing a Personal Development Plan (PDP) and shared with your manager or mentor. A PDP helps you to plan what you intend to learn or improve in the future. You might use the steps outlined above to develop your PDP.

All CPD you do should be recorded in a portfolio. This will provide you with a useful record of what you have achieved which will be helpful for constructing your Curriculum Vitae or for presentation to the NMC if they check your CPD activities when you re-register. Your portfolio should document what you have done, what you have learnt from it and how it has influenced your practice: it should make reference to your PDP.

CPD doesn't just have to be about developing clinical knowledge and skills, it is important to develop other skills as well in order to enhance the care that you provide. For example, you might choose to develop some managerial skills, delegation skills or leadership skills – all of them will make you a more competent practitioner.

All-in-all CPD is about making you a more accomplished nurse.

## CPD and life-long learning

CPD is also closely linked with life-long learning. Many people think that once you graduate and become a nurse you stop learning – this is not the case, you will continue to learn new knowledge and develop new skills throughout the lifetime of your career. Once you have graduated and are working in your first job you will start with a period of preceptorship. During this time others will be helping you to settle into your new role and profession so that you become a competent member of the nursing team. After that, your learning and development will continue, although probably not in such a directed way, it will undoubtedly include clinical supervision, mentoring and teaching others and attending courses, conferences and seminars.

## Preceptorship

Preceptorship is 'a period of structured transition for newly registered practitioners during which [time] he or she will be supported by a preceptor, to develop their confidence as an autonomous professional, refine skills, values and behaviours and to continue on their journey to life-long learning' (DH, 2010:11).

## Clinical supervision

'Clinical supervision is a support mechanism for practising professionals within which they can share clinical, organizational, developmental and emotional experiences with another professional in a secure, confidential environment in order to enhance knowledge and skills. This process will lead to an increased awareness of other concepts including accountability and reflective practice.' (Lyth (2000:729).

## Mentoring

Being a mentor is about being a guiding teacher. In nursing, mentorship is traditionally linked to helping students to learn in practice. but you can be a mentor at any time in your life – to anybody. And you can also have a mentor whenever you need one. In nursing being a mentor helps you to continuously improve your own practice because you are working as a knowledgeable role model to others constantly seeking out and using the latest research and actively discussing your practice. In order to mentor nursing students you have to follow a set of responsibilities laid down by the NMC and have successfully completed a preparatory course.

# Reflective practice

Oelofsen's (2012) contemporary definition of reflective practice describes it as the process of making sense of events, situations and actions that occur in the workplace. He emphasises its importance to providing high quality care and advocates reflecting in a structured way using a simple three step model. The steps are shown above. They comprise:

1 **Curiosity** which involves noticing things, asking questions and questioning assumptions.

2 **Looking closer** which is about actively engaging with the questions generated from Step 1 and finding out more. Oelofsen calls this 'zooming in'.

3 **Transformation** which is about working out how to act on the findings from Step 2 and then making things happen to improve practices and care.

The important thing about reflective practice is not just to sit and think about care, but to willingly try to change your practice as a result of this reflective process. Oelofsen's third step emphasises this.

You might combine the frameworks in the figures above to develop your PDP and plan your CPD.

**Practice development**

A framework to structure your Professional Development Plan and Continuing Professional Development

Source: Reproduced with permission of Healthcare Improvement Scotland and NHS Education for Scotland.

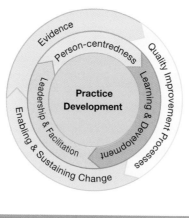

### Box 103    PDSA cycles

PDSA cycles were popularised by the Institute for Healthcare Improvement (IHI) (www.ihi.org/IHI/) in North America, and have been used across the world to make improvements to healthcare.  In this model there are three key questions that underpin improvement –

1.  What are we trying to accomplish?
2.  What change can we make that will result in an improvement?
3.  How will we know that a change is an improvement?

The PDSA cycle is used to 'test a change by developing a plan to test the change (Plan), carrying out the test (Do), observing and learning from the consequences (Study), and determining what modifications should be made to the test before applying it more widely (Act)'. (www.ihi.org/IHI/Topics/Improvement/ImprovementMethods/Tools/ Plan-Do-Study-Act%20(PDSA)%20Worksheet).

# What is practice development?

Practice development is about changing nursing practice to make care better and to improve the environment in which nurses and other members of the multi-disciplinary team work – and of course within which care is delivered. Practice development is not a new idea – it emerged from the first Nursing Development Units (NDUs) which started developing nursing practice in England in the 1980s. Since then many designated development units have grown up, but you don't need to work in one of these to make improvements to practice – all of you can do this either as part of your daily individual practice or more collectively as part of the nursing team.

Practice development has been defined as 'a continuous process of improvement towards increased effectiveness in patient-centred care. This is brought about by helping health care teams to develop their knowledge and skills and to transform the culture and context of care. It is enabled and supported by facilitators committed to systematic rigorous continuous processes of emancipatory change that reflect the perspectives of service users and service providers.' (McCormack, 2009:45; see also Garbett and McCormack, 2002).

One of the important features of practice development is that it is the people who actually deliver care who are involved in developing it – it is not a top-down managerial exercise: the essence of sound practice development is ownership and involvement which in turn may lead to feelings of empowerment and emancipation. Clark and Wilcockson (2002) stressed this in their writings: 'developing practice and developing care should be in the hands of the people who are doing it, because those people are the ones who are with the patients and public on a daily basis. These are the people who should understand the job and should understand how the job grows' (2002: 402).

# Developing practice

Practice development is a way of thinking *and* working which requires nurses to be innovative and entrepreneurial. NHS Scotland has designed a simple diagram (above) to help nurses remember the key elements of any successful practice development activity.

Their framework starts to be useful once you've identified an area for development and your colleagues want to support this development. When you have done this begin to look for **evidence** to base your development on (this could be research findings, guidelines, audit data, information from patient's experiences, professional opinion or policy). When you've got the evidence, think about how using that evidence would improve your current practice. You might want to structure this part of the development by using **improvement processes** such as PDSA (Plan: Do: Study: Act) (above). PDSA enables you to plan a change to improve care, make the change in, for example, a small group of patients, and then evaluate that small change before extending it to a whole unit. Once you've decided how to begin to implement your change get people involved so that they own the change (**enabling**), that way you are more likely to create **sustaining change** rather than a short-lived change which no-one wanted. Practice development should always promote **person-centredness.** Developing practice is not always easy and requires skilled **leadership and facilitation** but one thing that is certain is that everyone involved **learns** a lot and **develops** their skills and knowledge as the project unfolds. One thing missing from this is the need to explicitly evaluate the project and the importance of telling others about it (whether it was a success or not). (Remember that you can learn as much from something that went wrong as you can from something that has worked.)

You can use this framework in conjunction with the key principles of practice development outlined below. As you can see there is considerable overlap. Practice development projects need to:
- Be person-centred.
- Work from a clear set of values (e.g. respect, trust, dignity).
- Promote collaboration, participation and shared ownership.
- Use ways to facilitate critical reflection (e.g. action learning).
- Use the best evidence available (usually from research).
- Evaluate the way you did things (process) and the outcomes.
- Use a facilitative and inclusive style to enable change to occur.
- Tell other people what you've done and learnt.

(Based on work by McCormack et al., 2006:11)

When you are thinking about developing practice, you might also find it useful to structure your work using a change management model – there are a lot of them to choose from so make sure you pick one that fits with your approach to practice development (see Further reading).

It's always a good idea before you begin a practice development project to check out what other people have done. You can learn a lot by reading what others have achieved or finding out any problems that they have encountered so you can try to avoid them.

A good place to start is The Foundation of Nursing Studies' Innovation Centre and its series of 4-page easy to read project reports (fons.org/library/dissemination-series.aspx). Here you can read about many different types of project, ranging from developing nutritional care in an acute hospital ward to developing a nurse-led respite ward in a hospice. The reports also detail a variety of techniques that can be used to develop innovative practice.

# Appendix: summary of key features of arrhythmias

| Type of arrhythmia | Aetiology | Outcome | Treatment |
|---|---|---|---|
| Supraventricular tachycardia (SVT) or AV or AV node re-entrant tachycardias | Arises above ventricles<br>Extra electrical pathway | Tachyarrhythmia<br>Rapid palpitations<br>Regular, narrow QRS complex on ECG<br>Tachycardia >150 bpm<br>Intermittent problem<br>Rarely life threatening | Pharmacological<br>Cardioversion<br>Ablation |
| Atrial flutter | Arises above ventricles in atria<br>Usually underlying heart problem or thyroid problem | Tachyarrhythmia<br>May be asymptomatic or be associated with rapid palpitations or breathlessness<br>Regular rhythm around 150 bpm | Pharmacological<br>Cardioversion<br>Ablation |
| Atrial fibrillation (AF) | Arises above ventricles in atria<br>Uncoordinated firing of impulses in/around atria<br>May be caused by underlying heart problem, thyrotoxicosis, alcohol, pulmonary embolism, pneumonia, COPD | Tachyarrhythmia<br>Irregular heart rhythm<br>Pulse fast (>90–150 bpm) and irregular | Pharmacological<br>Cardioversion<br>Anticoagulation as thromboembolism is a risk in AF |
| Ventricular tachycardia (VT) | Arises from ventricles<br>Usually underlying heart problem associated often with myocardial damage | Tachyarrhythmia<br>*Regular* tachycardia (120–190 bpm) with broad QRS complexes = monomorphic VT<br>*Irregular* tachycardia = polymorphic and can degenerate to VF<br>Usually symptoms: palpitations, breathlessness, chest pain, sweating, nausea, collapse<br>Can cause cardiac arrest | Pharmacological<br>Cardioversion<br>Implantable defibrillators (ICDs)<br>Revascularisation |
| Ventricular fibrillation (VF) | Arises from ventricles<br>Usually linked to underlying heart problems | Tachyarrhythmia<br>Ventricles quiver but do not pump blood<br>Causes cardiac arrest | Resuscitation<br>Investigate cause and treat<br>Implantable defibrillators |
| Sinus bradycardia or sinus arrest | Sinoatrial node disease<br>Can be linked with AF (sick sinus syndrome/tachybrady syndrome) | Bradyarrhythmia<br>Symptoms may include dizziness or syncope<br>In sick sinus syndrome heart rate can sometimes be fast and sometimes slow | Pacemaker bradycardia + if sick sinus syndrome pharmacological control of fast beats |
| Atrioventricular block | Disease of AV node and/or conducting system<br>Failure to transmit P waves to ventricles<br>1st, 2nd, 3rd degree block depending on type of AV block. 3rd degree = complete heart block (CBH) | Bradyarrhythmia<br>Heart rate can be as low as <35 bpm in 3rd degree block<br>Symptoms of 2nd and 3rd degree heart block may include dizziness, syncope, tiredness, confusion, breathlessness or fluid retention | No treatment if minor – observe<br>Pacemaker if 2nd or 3rd degree block |
| Bundle branch block | Electrical impulses travel through ventricles more slowly than normal<br>Left and right bundle branch block (LBBB and RBBB)<br>RBBB can occur without heart disease<br>LBBB usually linked to underlying heart disease | | Bundle branch block doesn't need treatment but underlying problems might |

*Adult Nursing at a Glance*, First Edition. Andrée le May. © 2015 John Wiley & Sons, Ltd. Published 2015 by John Wiley & Sons, Ltd.
Companion website: www.ataglanceseries.com/nursing/adult

# References and further reading

Below you will find a combined list of references and further reading. Some suggestions for further reading are accompanied by a sentence or two to show why these texts are useful.

**NICE and SIGN guidelines, if they are available, should also be read in relation to each of the chapters in this book.**

## Fundamentals of nursing care
### Chapter 1
Francis R (2013) *Final Report of the Independent Inquiry into Care. Provided by Mid-Staffordshire NHS Foundation Trust*. London, Department of Health.

Matiti MR and Baillie L (2011) (Eds) *Dignity in Healthcare: A Practical Approach for Nurses and Midwives*. Oxford, Radcliffe Publishing Ltd.

RCN (2008) *RCN's definition of dignity*. www.rcn.org.uk/development/practice/dignity/rcns_definition_of_dignity

## Communication
### Chapters 2 & 3
Dougherty L & Lister S (Eds) (2011) *The Royal Marsden Hospital Manual of Clinical Nursing Procedures. Student Edition*, 8th edn. Oxford, Wiley Blackwell.

NMC (2009) *Record keeping: Guidance for nurses and midwives*. http://www.nmc-uk.org/Documents/NMC-Publications/NMC-Record-Keeping-Guidance.pdf

## Assessment and monitoring
### Chapters 4 & 5
Baillie L (2009) (Ed) *Developing Practice Adult Nursing Skills*. London, Hodder Arnold.

BAPEN (2003) *Malnutrition Universal Screening Tool*. http://www.bapen.org.uk/pdfs/must/must_full.pdf

Bond S (1997) (Ed) *Eating Matters*. University of Newcastle upon Tyne, Centre for Health Services Research and the Institute for Health of the Elderly.

Dougherty L and Lister S (2011) (Eds) *The Royal Marsden Hospital Manual of Clinical Nursing Procedures, Student Edition*, 8th edn.Oxford, Wiley-Blackwell.

O'Brien L (2012) (Ed) *District Nursing Manual of Clinical Procedures*. Oxford, Wiley-Blackwell.

## Symptom control and management
### Chapters 6, 7, 8, 9, 10, 11, 12 & 13
Davey P (Ed) (2014) *Medicine at a Glance*, 4th edn. Oxford, Wiley Blackwell.

Dougherty L & Lister S (Eds) (2011) *The Royal Marsden Hospital Manual of Clinical Nursing Procedures. Student Edition*, 8th edn. Oxford, Wiley Blackwell.

McCaffrey R (2002) *Nursing Management of the Patient with Pain*, 3rd edn. Philadelphia: Lippincott.

O'Brien L (2012) (Ed) *District Nursing Manual of Clinical Procedures*. Oxford, Wiley-Blackwell.

## Risk assessment and management
### Chapters 14, 15, 16, 17, 18, 19, 20 & 21
Dougherty L & Lister S (Eds) (2011) *The Royal Marsden Hospital Manual of Clinical Nursing Procedures. Student Edition*, 8th edn. Oxford, Wiley Blackwell.

Lapham R & Agar H (2009) *Drug Calculations for Nurses: A Step-by-step Approach*, 3rd edn. London: Hodder Arnold.

Nursing and Midwifery Council (2013 update) *Medicines Management Standards* www.nmc-uk.org/Documents/NMC-Publications/NMC-Standards-for-medicinesmanagement.pdf

## Health education and promotion
### Chapter 22
Dougherty L & Lister S (Eds) (2011) *The Royal Marsden Hospital Manual of Clinical Nursing Procedures. Student Edition*, 8th edn. Oxford, Wiley Blackwell.

## Research and service development
### Chapter 25
Petrie A & Sabin C (2009) *Medical Statistics at a Glance*. Oxford, Wiley Blackwell.

## Nursing people with cardiovascular disorders
### Chapters 26, 27, 28, 29, 30, 31, 32, 33, 34 & 35
Aaronson PI, Ward JPT & Connolly MJ (2012) *The Cardiovascular System at a Glance*, 4th edn. Oxford, Wiley Blackwell.

Davey P (Ed) (2014) *Medicine at a Glance*, 4th edn. Oxford, Wiley Blackwell.

Dougherty L & Lister S (Eds) (2011) *The Royal Marsden Hospital Manual of Clinical Nursing Procedures. Student Edition*, 8th edn. Oxford, Wiley Blackwell.

Grace P & Borley N (Eds) (2009) *Surgery at a Glance*. Oxford, Wiley Blackwell.

*Adult Nursing at a Glance*, First Edition. Andrée le May. © 2015 John Wiley & Sons, Ltd. Published 2015 by John Wiley & Sons, Ltd.
Companion website: www.ataglanceseries.com/nursing/adult

Peate I & Nair M (2011) *Fundamentals of Anatomy and Physiology*. Oxford, Wiley Blackwell.

Tortora GJ & Derrickson B (2011) *Essentials of Anatomy and Physiology*, 8th edn. Oxford, Wiley Blackwell.

## Nursing people with respiratory disorders
### Chapters 36, 37, 38, 39, 40 & 41

Davey P (Ed) (2014) *Medicine at a Glance*, 4th edn. Oxford, Wiley Blackwell.

Dougherty L & Lister S (Eds) (2011) *The Royal Marsden Hospital Manual of Clinical Nursing Procedures. Student Edition*, 8th edn. Oxford, Wiley Blackwell.

Nair M & Peate I (2009) Fundamentals of Applied Pathophysiology. Oxford, Wiley Blackwell.

Tortora GJ & Derrickson B (2011) Essentials of Anatomy and Physiology, 8th edn. Oxford, Wiley Blackwell.

## Nursing people with digestive disorders
### Chapters 42, 43, 44, 45, 46, 47, 48, 49, 50 &51

Davey P (Ed) (2014) *Medicine at a Glance*, 4th edn. Oxford, Wiley Blackwell.

Dougherty L & Lister S (Eds) (2011) *The Royal Marsden Hospital Manual of Clinical Nursing Procedures. Student Edition*, 8th edn. Oxford, Wiley Blackwell.

O'Brien L (Ed) (2012) *District Nursing Manual of Clinical Procedures*. Oxford, Wiley Blackwell.

Peate I & Nair M (Eds) (2011) *Fundamentals of Anatomy and Physiology for Student Nurses*. Oxford, Wiley Blackwell.

Tortora GJ & Derrickson B (2011) *Essentials of Anatomy and Physiology*, 8th edn. Oxford, Wiley Blackwell.

## Nursing people with urinary disorders
### Chapters 52, 53, 54, 55, 56, 57 & 58

Davey P (Ed) (2014) *Medicine at a Glance*, 4th edn. Oxford, Wiley Blackwell.

Dougherty L & Lister S (Eds) (2011) *The Royal Marsden Hospital Manual of Clinical Nursing Procedures. Student Edition*, 8th edn. Oxford, Wiley Blackwell.

O'Brien L (Ed) (2012) *District Nursing Manual of Clinical Procedures*. Oxford, Wiley Blackwell.

Peate I & Nair M (Eds) (2011) *Fundamentals of Anatomy and Physiology for Student Nurses*. Oxford, Wiley Blackwell.

Tortora GJ & Derrickson B (2011) *Essentials of Anatomy and Physiology*, 8th edn. Oxford, Wiley Blackwell.

## Nursing people with blood/lymph disorders
### Chapters 59, 60, 61, 62, 64, 64 & 65

Davey P (Ed) (2014) *Medicine at a Glance*, 4th edn. Oxford, Wiley Blackwell.

Dougherty L & Lister S (Eds) (2011) *The Royal Marsden Hospital Manual of Clinical Nursing Procedures. Student Edition*, 8th edn. Oxford, Wiley Blackwell.

Tortora GJ & Derrickson B (2011) *Essentials of Anatomy and Physiology*, 8th edn. Oxford, Wiley Blackwell.

Peate I & Nair M (Eds) (2011) *Fundamentals of Anatomy and Physiology for Student Nurses*. Oxford, Wiley Blackwell.

## Nursing people with endocrine disorders
### Chapters 66, 67 & 68

Davey P (Ed) (2014) *Medicine at a Glance*, 4th edn. Oxford, Wiley Blackwell.

## Nursing people with immune disorders
### Chapters 69, 70 & 71

Davey P (Ed) (2014) *Medicine at a Glance*, 4th edn. Oxford, Wiley Blackwell.

Nair M & Peate I (2009) *Fundamentals of Applied Pathophysiology*. Oxford, Wiley Blackwell.

Peate I & Nair M (Eds) (2011) *Fundamentals of Anatomy and Physiology for Student Nurses*. Oxford, Wiley Blackwell.

## Nursing people with skin disorders
### Chapters 72, 73 & 74

Davey P (Ed) (2014) *Medicine at a Glance*, 4th edn. Oxford, Wiley Blackwell.

Nair M & Peate I (2009) *Fundamentals of Applied Pathophysiology*. Oxford, Wiley Blackwell.

## Nursing people with musculoskeletal disorders
### Chapters 75, 76, 77, 78 & 79

Davey P (Ed) (2014) *Medicine at a Glance*, 4th edn. Oxford, Wiley Blackwell.

Peate I & Nair M (Eds) (2011) *Fundamentals of Anatomy and Physiology for Student Nurses*. Oxford, Wiley Blackwell.

Tortora GJ & Derrickson B (2011) *Essentials of Anatomy and Physiology*, 8th edn. Oxford, Wiley Blackwell.

## Nursing people with nervous system disorders
### Chapters 80, 81, 82, 83, 84, 85, 86 & 87

Davey P (Ed) (2014) *Medicine at a Glance*, 4th edn. Oxford, Wiley Blackwell.

Dougherty L & Lister S (Eds) (2011) *The Royal Marsden Hospital Manual of Clinical Nursing Procedures. Student Edition*, 8th edn. Oxford, Wiley Blackwell.

Peate I & Nair M (Eds) (2011) *Fundamentals of Anatomy and Physiology for Student Nurses*. Oxford, Wiley Blackwell.

Tortora GJ & Derrickson B (2011) *Essentials of Anatomy and Physiology*, 8th edn. Oxford, Wiley Blackwell.

## Nursing people with disorders of the eye or ear
### Chapters 88, 89 & 90

Davey P (Ed) (2014) *Medicine at a Glance*, 4th edn. Oxford, Wiley Blackwell.

Tortora GJ & Derrickson B (2011) *Essentials of Anatomy and Physiology*, 8th edn. Oxford, Wiley Blackwell.

## Nursing people with disorders of the reproductive system and breast
### Chapters 91, 92, 93, 94 & 95

Davey P (Ed) (2014) *Medicine at a Glance*, 4th edn. Oxford, Wiley Blackwell.

Grace P & Borley N (Eds) (2009) *Surgery at a Glance*. Oxford, Wiley Blackwell.

Nair M & Peate I (2009) *Fundamentals of Applied Pathophysiology*. Oxford, Wiley Blackwell.

Tortora GJ & Derrickson B (2011) *Essentials of Anatomy and Physiology*, 8th edn. Oxford, Wiley Blackwell.

## Nursing people with cancer
## Chapter 96

Dougherty L & Lister S (Eds) (2011) *The Royal Marsden Hospital Manual of Clinical Nursing Procedures. Student Edition*, 8th edn. Oxford, Wiley Blackwell.

## Essential skills: leadership and organisational
## Chapters 97, 98, 99, 100, 101, 102 & 103

Adair J (2010) *Not Bosses but Leaders,* 3rd edn. London, Kogan Page.

Aiken L et al. (2012) Patient safety, satisfaction, and quality of hospital care: cross sectional surveys of nurses and patient in 12 countries in Europe and the United States. *BMJ,* 344,e1717.

Barton D & le May A (2012) *Adult Nursing: Preparing for Practice.* London, Hodder Arnold.

Clarke C and Wilcockson J (2002) Seeing need and developing care: exploring knowledge for and from practice. *International Journal of Nursing Studies,* 39(4), 397–406.

Cox Y & le May A (2006) Leadership for Practice. In: Brown J & Libberton P (Eds) *Principles of Professional Studies in Nursing.* London, Palgrave Macmillan.

Daft R (1999) *Leadership Theory and Practice.* Fort Worth, Harcourt Brace.

DH (2010) *Preceptorship Framework for Newly Registered Nurses, Midwives and Allied Health Professionals.* London, Department of Health.

Gabbay J and le May A (2011) *Evidence Based Health Care: Clinical Knowledge in Practice.* London, Routledge. This book describes how doctors and nurses develop, share and implement knowledge in their practice.

Garbett R and McCormack B (2002) A concept analysis of practice development. *NT Research* 7(2), 87–100.

Iles V and Cranfield S (2004) *Developing Change Management Skills.* London, NCCSDO.

Le May A (2012) In: Barton D and le May A (Eds) *Adult Nursing Preparing for Practice.* London, Hodder Arnold.

Le May A & Holmes S (2012) *Introduction to Nursing Research: Developing Research Awareness.* London, Hodder Arnold. An easy to read introduction to research.

London Regional Office (2000) *Embodying Leadership.* London, Department of Health.

Lyth G (2000) Clinical supervision: a concept analysis. *Journal of Advanced Nursing* 31(3), 722–729.

McCormack B, Dewar B, Wright J et al. (2006) *A Realist Synthesis of Evidence Relating to Practice Development: Final Report To NHS Education For Scotland and NHS Quality Improvement Scotland.* http://www.healthcareimprovementscotland.org/previous_resources/archived/pd_-_evidence_synthisis.aspx

McCormack B (2009) Practitioner Research. In: Hardy S, Titchen A, McCormack B and Manley K (Eds) *Revealing Nursing Expertise Through Practitioner Inquiry.* Oxford, Wiley-Blackwell.

McKenzie C and Manley K (2011) Leadership and Responsive Care: Principle of Nursing Practice H. *Nursing Standard*, 25, 35, 35–37.

## A summary and case study about clinical leadership

McNichol E and Hamer S (2007) *Leadership and Management: A 3-Dimensional Approach.* Cheltenham, Nelson Thornes.

Oelofsen N (2012) Using reflective practice in frontline nursing. *Nursing Times,* 108(24), 22–24.

Rigolosi E (2013) *Management and Leadership in Nursing and Health Care*, 3rd edn. New York, Springer.

RN4CAST (2009) RN4CAST Articles http://www.rn4cast.eu/articles.php. Information from the RN4CAST nursing research project.

Sacket D, Strauss S, Richardson W et al. (2004) *Evidence Based Medicine: How to Practice and Teach EBM.* London, Churchill Livingstone.

Walsh D (2010) *The Nurse Mentor's Handbook: Supporting Students in Clinical Practice.* Maidenhead, Open University Press.

# Index

*Adult Nursing at a Glance*, First Edition. Andrée le May. © 2015 John Wiley & Sons, Ltd. Published 2015 by John Wiley & Sons, Ltd.
Companion website: www.ataglanceseries.com/nursing/adult